D1046978

Exercise and Sport Sciences Reviews

Volume 18, 1990

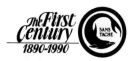

EXERCISE AND SPORT SCIENCES REVIEWS

Volume 18, 1990

Editors

KENT B. PANDOLF, Ph.D.

Director, Military Ergonomics Division
U.S. Army Research Institute of Environmental Medicine
Natick, Massachusetts

Adjunct Professor of Health Sciences
Sargent College of Allied Health Professions
Boston University
Boston, Massachusetts

Adjunct Clinical Professor of Sports Biology
Springfield College
Springfield, Massachusetts

JOHN O. HOLLOSZY, M.D.

Professor of Medicine
Department of Internal Medicine
Washington University School of Medicine
St. Louis, Missouri

American College of Sports Medicine Series

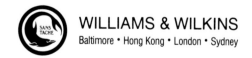

WILLIAMS & WILKINS
Baltimore • Hong Kong • London • Sydney

Editor: John P. Butler
Associate Editor: Marjorie Kidd Keating
Copy Editor: Klementyna L. Bryte
Designer: Norman Och
Illustration Planner: Lorraine Wrzosek
Production Coordinator: Raymond E. Reter

Printed in the United States of America

Library of Congress Catalog Card Number 72-12187

ISBN 0-683-00047-0

90 91 92 93
1 2 3 4 5 6 7 8 9 10

Preface

Exercise and Sport Sciences Reviews is an annual publication sponsored by the American College of Sports Medicine that reviews current research concerning behavioral, biochemical, biomechanical, clinical, physiological, and rehabilitational topics involving exercise science. The Editorial Board for this series currently consists of 12 recognized authorities who have assumed the responsibility for one of the following general topics: biochemistry, exercise physiology, psychology, motor control, athletic medicine, rehabilitation, sociology of sport, environmental physiology, biomechanics, growth and development, epidemiology, and physical fitness. The organization of the Editorial Board should help foster the commitment of the American College of Sports Medicine to publish timely reviews in broad areas of interest to clinicians, educators, exercise scientists, and students. The goal for this Editorial Board is to provide at least one review in each of these 12 areas for each volume of *Exercise and Sport Sciences Reviews*. Further, the Editor shall select three or four additional topics to be developed into chapters based on current interest, timeliness, and importance to the above audience. Volume 18 of this series features for the first time a research topic that is debated from two somewhat different points of view (Chapters 1 and 2).

The contributors for each volume are selected by the Editorial Board members and the Editor. Although the majority of these reviews are invited, unsolicited manuscripts of potential chapter topics will be received by the Editor and reviewed by him and/or various members of the Editorial Board for possible inclusion in future volumes. The completion of Volume 18 of this series signals the end of the tenure of Kent B. Pandolf, Ph.D., as Editor. Dr. Pandolf was the Editor of Volumes 14 through 18. Future correspondence should be directed to John O. Holloszy, M.D., Washington University School of Medicine, 2nd Floor, West Building, 4566 Scott Avenue, Campus Box 8113, St. Louis, MO 63110, who assumes the role of sole Editor of *Exercise and Sport Sciences Reviews* commencing with Volume 19.

Kent B. Pandolf, Ph.D.
John O. Holloszy, M.D.
Editors

Guest Referee Editors

The Editors of *Exercise and Sport Sciences Reviews* gratefully acknowledge the services of the following Guest Referee Editors who assisted the Editorial Board in the review of these chapters.

Elizabeth S. Bressan

Gary A. Dudley

Bo Fernhall

Richard E. Grindeland

Everett A. Harman

Brad D. Hatfield

Donald Hellison

Ira Jacobs

John B. Ryan

Michael L. Sachs

Contributors

Bruce E. Baker, M.D., F.A.C.S.M.
Department of Orthopedic Surgery
Madison Irving Medical Center
Syracuse, New York

Richard N. Baumgartner, Ph.D.
Division of Human Biology
Department of Pediatrics
Wright State University School of Medicine
Dayton, Ohio

Claude Bouchard, Ph.D., F.A.C.S.M.
Physical Activity Sciences Laboratory
Laval University
Sainte-Foy, Quebec, Canada

Brenda Jo Light Bredemeier, Ph.D.
Department of Physical Education
University of California, Berkeley
Berkeley, California

George A. Brooks, Ph.D., F.A.C.S.M.
Exercise Physiology Laboratory
Department of Physical Education
University of California, Berkeley
Berkeley, California

Wm. Cameron Chumlea, Ph.D.
Division of Human Biology
Department of Pediatrics
Wright State University School of Medicine
Dayton, Ohio

Victor A. Convertino, Ph.D., F.A.C.S.M.
Life Sciences Research Office
National Aeronautics and Space Administration
Kennedy Space Center, Florida

Marsha Cressler-Chaviz, M.S.
Lynn Maguire Physical Therapy Clinic
Las Vegas, Nevada

Jean-Pierre Després, Ph.D.
Physical Activity Sciences Laboratory
Laval University
Sainte-Foy, Quebec, Canada

Lawrence E. Hart, M.B., B.Ch., M.Sc., F.R.C.P.(C)
Departments of Clinical Epidemiology and Biostatistics, and Medicine
Health Science Centre
McMaster University
Hamilton, Ontario, Canada

Melbourne F. Hovell, Ph.D., M.P.H.
Graduate School of Public Health
San Diego State University
San Diego, California

Robert K. Jensen, Ph.D.
School of Human Movement and Centre for Research in Human
    Development
Laurentian University
Sudbury, Ontario, Canada

Abram Katz, Dr.Med.Sci.
Department of Kinesiology
University of Illinois
Urbana, Illinois

Barry Lavay, Ph.D.
Department of Physical Education
California State University, Long Beach
Long Beach, California

Robert M. Malina, Ph.D., F.A.C.S.M.
Department of Kinesiology and Health Education
University of Texas
Austin, Texas

Penny McCullagh, Ph.D.
Department of Kinesiology
University of Colorado at Boulder
Boulder, Colorado

T. Christian North, Ph.D.
North and Associates
Boulder, Colorado

Greg Reid, Ph.D.
Department of Physical Education
McGill University
Montreal, Quebec, Canada

J. Gavin Reid, Ph.D.
Department of Anatomy
School of Physical and Health Education
Queen's University
Kingston, Ontario, Canada

Alex F. Roche, M.D., Ph.D.
Division of Human Biology
Department of Pediatrics
Wright State University School of Medicine
Dayton, Ohio

Kent Sahlin, Dr.Sci.
Department of Clinical Physiology
Karolinska Institute
Huddinge University Hospital
Huddinge, Sweden

George J. Salem, M.S.
Department of Kinesiology
University of California, Los Angeles
Los Angeles, California

James F. Sallis, Ph.D.
Department of Psychology
San Diego State University
San Diego, California

Wendell N. Stainsby, Sc.D., F.A.C.S.M.
Department of Physiology
College of Medicine
University of Florida
Gainesville, Florida

Zung Vu Tran, Ph.D., F.A.C.S.M.
College of Human Performance and Leisure Studies
University of Northern Colorado
Greeley, Colorado

Arthur C. Vailas, Ph.D., F.A.C.S.M.
Biodynamics Laboratory
University of Wisconsin
Madison, Wisconsin

Stephen D. Walter, Ph.D.
Department of Clinical Epidemiology and Biostatistics
Health Science Centre
McMaster University
Hamilton, Ontario, Canada

Maureen R. Weiss, Ph.D.
Department of Physical Education and Human Movement Studies
University of Oregon
Eugene, Oregon

Andrew J. Young, Ph.D., F.A.C.S.M.
Physiology Branch, Military Ergonomics Division
U.S. Army Research Institute of Environmental Medicine
Natick, Massachusetts

Ronald F. Zernicke, Ph.D., F.A.C.S.M.
Department of Kinesiology
University of California, Los Angeles
Los Angeles, California

Contents

Exercise and Sport Sciences Reviews

Volume 18, 1990

1
Role of Oxygen in Regulation of Glycolysis and Lactate Production in Human Skeletal Muscle

ABRAM KATZ, Dr. Med. Sci.
KENT SAHLIN, Dr. Sci.

INTRODUCTION

In the past century, considerable effort has been put into investigating the regulation of carbohydrate metabolism in skeletal muscle. Specifically, the regulation of and the role of oxygen (O_2) availability in glycolysis and lactate production have been of interest. Part of this interest undoubtedly stems from the association between these processes and muscle fatigue under various but not all conditions [106].

Glycolysis is defined as the degradation of 6-carbon to 3-carbon sugars. This process occurs in the cytosol and is accomplished in the aldolase reaction (Fig. 1.1). It is, however, generally accepted to view glycolysis as the flux through phosphofructokinase (PFK), an enzyme that catalyzes an irreversible reaction in vivo [93]. The endpoint of glycolysis is pyruvate. Subsequent metabolism of pyruvate depends on the metabolic conditions in the cell. The purpose of glycolysis is to produce ATP and substrate for the tricarboxylic acid (TCA) cycle for subsequent aerobic ATP production. Pyruvate formation is associated with a stoichiometric reduction of nicotinamide adenine dinucleotide (NAD^+) to NADH (Fig. 1.1). To maintain glycolysis, NADH must be continuously reoxidized to NAD^+. This can occur either through oxidation in the mitochondria or through the lactate dehydrogenase reaction.

Lactate accumulation as an index of accelerated glycolysis has long been appreciated, although a lack of increase in lactate does not necessarily mean that the glycolytic rate is not increased. For example, exercise at 40% of maximal oxygen uptake ($\dot{V}O_2max$) results in a 25-fold increase in glycolysis versus rest [71], whereas there is neither an increase in the content of lactate in the contracting muscle [108] nor in its release from the muscle [3, 58]. Thus, under these conditions, the increase in glycolysis is essentially balanced by an equal increase in pyruvate oxidation (Table 1.1). At higher exercise intensities, an increased proportion of the pyruvate produced is reduced to lactate.

1

FIGURE 1.1

Reactions involved in the degradation of glucose/glycogen. PHOS, *phosphorylase;* PGM, *phosphoglucomutase;* PGI, *phosphoglucoisomerase;* HK, *hexokinase;* PFK, *phosphofructokinase-1;* ALD, *aldolase;* TIM, *trioseisomerase;* GPDH, *glyceraldehyde-3-phosphate dehydrogenase;* PGK, *phosphoglycerate kinase;* PHGM, *phosphoglycerate 2,3-mutase;* ENOL, *enolase;* PK, *pyruvate kinase;* GPT, *glutamic-pyruvic transaminase;* LDH, *lactate dehydrogenase;* G 1-P, *glucose 1-phosphate;* GLU, *glucose;* G 6-P, *glucose 6-phosphate;* F 6-P, *fructose 6-phosphate;* ATP, *adenosine triphosphate;* ADP, *adenosine diphosphate;* F 1,6-P$_2$, *fructose 1,6-bisphosphate;* DHAP, *dihydroxyacetone phosphate;* GAP, *glyceraldehyde 3-phosphate;* G 1,3-P$_2$, *glycerate 1,3-bisphosphate;* G 3-P, *glycerate 3-phosphate;* G 2-P, *glycerate 2-phosphate;* PEP, *phosphoenol pyruvate;* ALA, *alanine;* NAD$^+$(H), *nicotinamide adenine dinucleotide oxidized (reduced). Reactions close to equilibrium ($\leftrightarrow$) and removed from equilibrium ($\rightarrow$).*

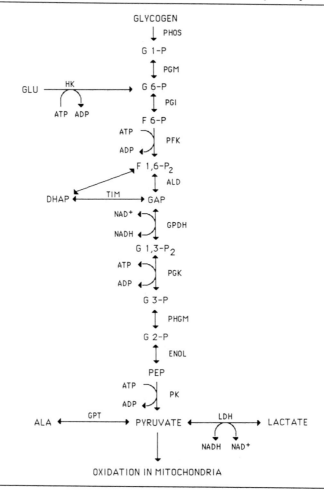

TABLE 1.1
Carbohydrate Metabolism in Human Skeletal Muscle during Dynamic Exercise

	Exercise Intensity ($\%\dot{V}_{O_2}max$)		
	40	*75*	*100*
Rate of lactate accumulation[a]	0	3.1	13.9
Rate of lactate release[b]	0	1.4	4.0
Rate of alanine accumulation[c]	0.3	0.5	0.7
Rate of glycerol 3-P accumulation[d]	0	0.3	0.9
Rate of pyruvate production[e]	4.8	14.1	31.5
Rate of pyruvate oxidation[f]	4.5	9.1	12.9
Pyruvate oxidation/pyruvate production	0.94	0.65	0.41

Values are given in mmol/kg dry wt/min.
[a] Lactate accumulation rates are from Sahlin et al. (108).
[b] Lactate release at 40% $\dot{V}_{O_2}max$ is from Andersen and Saltin (3), at 75% $\dot{V}_{O_2}max$ from Jorfeldt et al. (58), and at 100% $\dot{V}_{O_2}$ from Katz et al. (63). The body weights of the subjects in the latter two studies were ~76 kg. Lactate release was determined from the arterial and femoral venous blood lactate concentrations and the leg blood flows and assuming that the muscle mass of one leg corresponds to 11% of body weight (see Ref. 64).
[c] Alanine accumulation rates are from Katz et al. (63). Value at 40% is actually measured at 50% $\dot{V}_{O_2}max$, whereas value at 75% is a mean of the values at 40 and 100% $\dot{V}_{O_2}max$.
[d] Glycerol 3-P accumulation is from Sahlin et al. (108).
[e] Pyruvate production = 2 × glycolytic rate (71) − rate of glycerol 3-P accumulation.
[f] Pyruvate oxidation = pyruvate production − (lactate accumulation + lactate release and alanine accumulation). The rates of pyruvate accumulation + pyruvate and alanine release are negligible (the sum is never greater than ~0.1 mmol/kg dry wt/min during short-term exercise [63, 108]) and therefore are excluded in the calculation of pyruvate oxidation.

An increase in lactate production is observed at ~50–70% $\dot{V}_{O_2}max$, well before the aerobic capacity is fully utilized. However, the mechanism for the increase in lactate production is not fully understood. The classical explanation has been that the contracting muscle is O_2 deficient and, therefore, part of the energy requirement must be supplemented through increased anaerobically derived ATP [45].

During short-term circulatory occlusion and isometric contraction, when the muscle is anoxic, lactate production accounts for ~30–60% of the ATP turnover [65, 70] and is thus an important source of energy. On the other hand, during steady-state bicycle exercise, lactate production is of negligible importance in terms of ATP production.

The hypothesis that lactate formation is dependent on the availability of O_2 is supported by numerous studies where exercise under conditions of impaired O_2 supply (e.g., respiratory hypoxia) results in increased lactate concentrations in blood and muscle, whereas exercise under hyperoxic conditions results in decreased lactate concentrations in blood and muscle [72]. Recently, however, the idea that lactate formation during submaximal exercise is due to tissue hypoxia has been questioned [11, 21, 22]. The major criticisms against the presence of tissue hypoxia during submaximal exercise are that: (*a*) the NAD(P)H fluorescence from the surface of the muscle is decreased under conditions of increased lactate production [56]; (*b*) measurements of cytosolic O_2 tension, estimated from the myoglobin saturation, show that relatively high levels of O_2 are present in lactate-producing muscle [21]; and (*c*) at a given work load $\dot{V}o_2$ is not altered by aerobic training nor by changing the fraction of inspired O_2 while lactate production does change [50, 83].

It is the intent of this review to examine the current hypotheses on the regulation of glycolysis and lactate production and to define the role of O_2 availability in these processes.

MEASUREMENT OF GLYCOLYSIS AND LACTATE PRODUCTION IN VIVO

The simplest and most accurate way to quantify glycolysis and lactate production is to use a closed system (i.e., where there is no blood flow and no oxygen). Under these conditions glycolysis and lactate production can be quantified from the accumulation of post-PFK intermediates and lactate in the tissue. The requirements for a closed system are met during circulatory occlusion or isometric contraction at >40% maximal force [27].

In an open system, e.g., during rest or dynamic exercise, where the blood flow is intact, quantification of glycolysis is more complex. At rest, the net glycogenolytic and glycogenic rates are approximately zero [18]. Thus measurements of muscle glucose uptake are sufficient to estimate glycolysis (because all of the glucose is glycolyzed) [70]. During exercise glycogenolysis occurs and most of the hexose phosphates formed are glycolyzed. During submaximal exercise (<75% $\dot{V}o_2$max) glycolysis is simply the sum of muscle glucose uptake and glycogenolysis (correcting for any accumulation of hexose monophosphates), whereas during high intensity exercise (100% $\dot{V}o_2$max) glycolysis is essentially equal to glycogenolysis (correcting for accumulation of hexose monophosphates) [71]. Although muscle glucose uptake rates during maximal dynamic exercise are relatively high, this glucose uptake can be excluded from calculations of glycolysis because essentially none of the glucose is phosphorylated by hexokinase and therefore it cannot be glycolyzed [64]. At steady state, glycolysis can also be quantified from the formation of post-phosphofructokinase intermediates. However, because most of the pyruvate that is formed is oxidized in the mitochondria (Table 1.1), it is necessary to estimate the amount of carbohydrate oxidized from the O_2 uptake and CO_2 formation across the muscle. In addition, accumulation and release of metabolites derived from pyruvate (e.g., lactate and alanine) must be determined. This technique is thus limited by the practical difficulties of accurately estimating all of the relevant components.

The measurement of lactate production in an open system is complicated by the fiber heterogeneity of human muscle. Lactate produced in one fiber may diffuse into an adjacent fiber and be oxidized. Measurement of the release and accumulation of lactate would not include the oxidized portion, and thereby result in an underestimation of true lactate production. It has been argued that the use of carbon-labeled lactate tracers would enable measurement of the total lactate production [11]. However, it was recently demonstrated that an apparent uptake of [^{14}C]lactate may occur in the absence of net lactate utilization and thus $^{14}CO_2$ production does not provide a measure of true lactate oxidation [75]. This is probably due to an exchange mechanism where [^{14}C]lactate will exchange with intracellular lactate and pyruvate [107, 126]. Consequently the tracer techniques using labeled lactate cannot distinguish between pyruvate and lactate metabolism [107]. Hence the major part of the "lactate production" and "lactate oxidation" observed with the tracer method at rest and during low intensity exercise is probably due to formation and oxidation of pyruvate. Therefore, it can be concluded that usage of carbon-labeled lactate tracers is not valid for quantifying lactate production. The amount of lactate produced in one fiber and oxidized in another fiber during contraction remains unknown. It is, however, likely that the amount of lactate oxidized relative to that produced decreases with increasing exercise intensity. Under most conditions the accumulation of lactate in blood and muscle can be used as a good qualitative measure of lactate production during short-term exercise.

CELLULAR O$_2$ TENSION: CRITICAL VALUES FOR RESPIRATION AND FOR METABOLIC REGULATION

O_2 is essential for mitochondrial ATP production, but at O_2 tensions only slightly higher than those at which cells function O_2 becomes toxic [33], probably due to the formation of free radicals. The cellular O_2 tension is probably a compromise between maintenance of a complete aerobic metabolism and the necessity of diminishing the toxicity of O_2.

There is little doubt that contracting muscle is hypoxic during exercise at work loads exceeding the $\dot{V}O_2$max or during sustained static contractions where the intramuscular pressure impairs the local blood flow. It is, however, controversial whether the lactate formation during submaximal exercise is due to hypoxia. Part of the controversy exists because hypoxia at the cellular level can be defined in at least two ways: (*a*) cellular respiration is affected by PO_2 and (*b*) cellular metabolism is affected by PO_2. Many investigators have explicitly stated or implied that, if cellular respiration is not impaired, then cellular metabolism (including lactate formation) would not be dependent on O_2. In our view this is a misconception, which probably stems from the idea that the main function of glycolysis is to supplement the production of ATP when oxidative processes do not meet the energetic demand. An alternative view is that the imbalance between the formation and oxidation of pyruvate is a consequence of the stimulation of aerobic energy production and that the availability of O_2 plays a major role in this process.

The critical intracellular Po_2 (Po_2 crit) for respiration is usually defined as the Po_2 at which O_2 availability limits electron transport and oxidative phosphorylation. Po_2 crit is dependent on the rate of cellular respiration [15]. At high rates of O_2 consumption, the O_2 tension where respiration is impaired occurs at a higher value than during low rates of O_2 consumption (i.e., the value during maximal respiration determines the upper limit for Po_2 crit). From experiments on isolated mitochondria during state 3 respiration, it has been concluded that Po_2 crit is ~0.1 torr [54]. In studies on dog gracilis muscle (a red muscle with high aerobic capacity) measurements have been made of the O_2 saturation of myoglobin in freeze-clamped contracting muscle [32]. This technique enables calculations of the tissue Po_2 with a subcellular resolution. The median Po_2 values of these muscles during near maximal rates of O_2 consumption were between 0.6 and 11 torr. Despite the variation in median Po_2, there was no difference in $\dot{V}o_2$ between muscles, and because the glycolytic flux supplied less than 1% of the ATP demand it was concluded that an upper limit for Po_2 crit was 0.5 torr at $\dot{V}o_2$max [32]. The same group has in a series of papers also argued that lactate formation during submaximal contractions, when the minimal Po_2 is about 2–3 torr, cannot be due to an O_2 limitation of respiration or metabolism and that the concept of anaerobic threshold does not apply to red muscle [21, 22].

In contrast to these data where Po_2 crit appears to be similar in isolated mitochondria and intact tissue, studies by Jones and coworkers [57] have shown that the Po_2 crit is quite different in isolated mitochondria and in hepatocytes. Half-maximal reduction of cytochrome c occurred at about 0.5 torr in isolated mitochondria but at 4 torr in intact hepatocytes. The major reason for this difference was considered to be the clustering and uneven distribution of mitochondria [57]. Similarly, studies of the O_2 dependence of isolated cardiac myocytes have shown that intact cells required about 1 order of magnitude higher O_2 concentration (11 torr) than isolated mitochondria (0.6 torr) to obtain the same reduction state of cytochrome a_3 [76]. An important difference between the studies on myoglobin saturation in contracting dog muscle [21, 22, 32] and the work by Jones and coworkers [57] is that the former group defined Po_2 crit as the O_2 tension where respiration was affected, whereas Jones and coworkers studied the O_2 dependence of the redox state of the respiratory chain.

In human studies it has been shown that the Po_2 of femoral venous blood during bicycle exercise at $\dot{V}o_2$max decreases to about 17 torr [96].

In human gastrocnemius muscle, Po_2 decreases to about 7 torr during exercise to fatigue [12]. Due to O_2 gradients between the capillaries and the mitochondria and due to a lack of homogeneity within the muscle, Po_2 can probably reach lower values in certain intracellular loci [57]. However, it seems unlikely that muscle Po_2 could decrease below 1 torr during submaximal exercise and it is therefore unlikely that cellular respiration is limited by Po_2 under these conditions. On the other hand, the O_2 tension observed in human muscle [12] is within the region where an effect on the redox state of the respiratory chain in intact cells has been observed [76].

There is abundant evidence that alterations of the O_2 availability affect the cellular metabolism during submaximal exercise. A diminished O_2 supply during submaximal exercise results in elevated lactate concentrations in blood [52, 67, 78, 83, 86, 99, 122, 127] and in muscle [67, 83]. There is therefore an apparent paradox in that cellular respiration is not limited by, and thus not dependent on, Po_2 during submaximal exercise, whereas cellular metabolism (e.g., lactate formation) shows a clear O_2 dependency. This paradox could, however, be resolved if the regulation of cellular respiration is considered.

Cellular respiration is, in addition to Po_2, dependent upon the cytosolic phosphorylation potential ($ATP/(ADP \times P_i)$) and the mitochondrial redox state [79, 125]. Thus during high rates of respiration, aerobic metabolism may be O_2 dependent at a relatively high Po_2, but due to adaptive changes in the mitochondrial redox state (increase in $NADH/NAD^+$) and the cytosolic phosphorylation potential (or ADP), cellular respiration during steady state is maintained. Furthermore, it is likely that these cellular adaptations to a decreased Po_2, or to an increased energy demand, result in enhanced breakdown of phosphocreatine (PCr) and activation of glycolysis (see below).

The link between relative hypoxia and accelerated lactate production is, however, more involved than being simply a function of accelerated glycolysis. As has already been noted, an accelerated glycolysis, per se, is not always associated with increased lactate production (see Introduction). An increase in mitochondrial NADH is expected to decrease the capacity of the malate-aspartate shuttle to transport reducing equivalents into the mitochondria [72, 108]. This, coupled with a constant or accelerated glycolysis, is expected to result in an increase in cytosolic NADH, which will enhance the reduction of pyruvate to lactate (see below). The strong relationship between the lactate/pyruvate ratio (which is proportional to the cytosolic $NADH/NAD^+$ ratio) and the muscle lactate content after short-term dynamic exercise supports this view [72]. According to this view, the increased lactate production during submaximal exercise should be regarded more as a regulatory phenomenon rather than a necessary supplementation of ATP production.

REGULATION OF PHOSPHOFRUCTOKINASE

PFK is a key regulatory enzyme for glycolysis [93] and is apparently of major importance for the control of glycolysis during muscle contraction [95]. The maximal in vitro activity of human muscle PFK is ~280 mmol/kg dry wt/min (corrected to 35°C assuming a Q_{10} of 2) [8], which is ~3-fold higher than the maximal in vivo activity (see Table 1.2).

To study the regulation of glycolysis in human skeletal muscle, investigators have traditionally challenged the system with various stimuli (Table 1.2). The most striking observation in Table 1.2 is that most challenges are unable to elicit increases in glycolysis of the magnitude seen during intense contraction. The regulation of PFK under in vivo conditions is poorly understood. Under in vitro conditions PFK is subject to complex regulation, being activated (or deinhibited) by AMP, ADP, P_i, fructose 6-P, fructose 1,6-P_2, fructose 2,6-P_2, glucose 1,6-P_2, and cyclic AMP, and inhibited by H^+, ATP, and citrate [25, 85, 87, 93]. There are numerous other regulators, e.g., ribose 1,5-P_2 [37], ammonia (NH_3) [119], and F-actin [81], but their in vivo roles in mammalian skeletal muscle are unclear. Numerous hypotheses have been proposed to explain the in vivo regulation of PFK. Under many conditions where glycolysis is stimulated to a relatively minor extent (e.g., circulatory occlusion, hyperinsulinemia, and hyperadrenalinemia) the activation of PFK can be explained by increased substrate availability and allosteric regulation. The steady-state levels of these activators, however, are unlikely to explain the high glycolytic rate during muscle contraction (see below).

Other hypotheses have been proposed to explain contraction-mediated glycolysis. It has been suggested that catecholamine-induced substrate cycling results in increased sensitivity of PFK to activators [93]. Indeed, in vitro studies have shown that in the presence of insulin, epinephrine increased the rate of substrate cycling by ~10-fold [14].

TABLE 1.2
Glycolysis in Human Skeletal Muscle

Condition	Glycolytic Rate[a]	Reference	Suggested Mechanism of Activation
Rest	~0.05	4, 64	
Circulatory occlusion (30 min)	~0.2	70	AMP, P_i, fructose 6-P
Euglycemic hyperinsulinemia (350–450 min)	~0.2	73, 74	Glucose 1,6-P_2, fructose 2,6-P_2 (?)
Hyperadrenalinemia	~5[b]	19	Fructose 6-P, fructose 2,6-P_2,[c] cAMP
Maximal isometric contraction	~100	1	AMP, fructose 6-P[d]

[a] Values are in mmol/kg dry wt/min.
[b] Estimated from glycogenolysis minus the accumulation of hexose monophosphates.
[c] The increase in fructose 2,6-P_2 in response to adrenaline was observed in the perfused rat hindlimb (51).
[d] See Katz et al. (66).

However, recent studies have demonstrated that infusion of epinephrine, which resulted in an increase of the mole fraction of phosphorylase *a* from 25 to 80% and a 2-fold increase in fructose 6-P immediately before contraction had no effect on the glycolytic rate during isometric contraction to fatigue [20]. These results offer no support for the quantitative significance of substrate cycling on contraction-mediated glycolysis in vivo.

It has also been suggested that phosphorylation of PFK may be important for activation of glycolysis [48]. Consistent with this view is the finding that 2 min of electrical stimulation is associated with an 80% increase in the phosphate content of muscle PFK [48]. However, the relationship between phosphate incorporation and glycolysis during contraction is not known. Moreover, when resting muscle is exposed to epinephrine, phosphorylation of PFK is decreased by ~25% [48], while glycolysis is accelerated [19]. Indeed there is considerable evidence that phosphorylation of PFK results in increased sensitivity to inhibition by ATP and citrate and decreased sensitivity to activation by AMP, glucose 1,6-P_2, and fructose 6-P [30, 77]. These observations are inconsistent with the notion that phosphorylation of PFK is a major mechanism whereby contraction results in the activation of glycolysis.

It is generally accepted that, during contraction, changes in adenine nucleotides and hexose phosphates, although pH is decreasing, are responsible for activating PFK (e.g., see Refs. 25, 93, and 116). It is clear, however, that this approach is too simplistic, and inadequate to satisfactorily explain contraction-induced glycolysis. For example, the glycolytic rate in human skeletal muscle increases to about 50 mmol/kg dry wt./min during isometric contraction at two-thirds maximal force [1]. This rate remains constant throughout contraction until the point of fatigue although pH is continuously decreasing [82, 103, 115]. At fatigue, ATP is markedly decreased (~20%), PCr is depleted, fructose 6-P is increased ~20-fold, fructose 1,6-P_2 is increased ~3-fold, and inorganic phosphate (P_i), free ADP, and free AMP (see below for discussion) are markedly elevated [24, 41, 82]. Clearly the greatest stimulus for glycolysis is present at fatigue. If, however, the circulation to the leg is occluded for 4 min after termination of contraction, then the metabolite contents are virtually identical to the values at fatigue [41, 42]. If the major stimulus for glycolysis is the concentration of the above mentioned metabolites, then lactate during the 4-min occlusion should have increased at the same rate as during contraction. The lactate content in the muscle 4 min after occlusion is, however, similar to the value at fatigue [41]. At least two conclusions can be drawn from these findings. First, no hypothesis presented thus far can satisfactorily explain a 1000–2000-fold increase in the glycolytic rate during contraction. Second, it is clear that glycolysis is intimately linked to the contraction process, an observation made earlier by Karpatkin et al. [62].

Because Ca^{2+} release into the cytosol initiates contraction and after contraction it is rapidly pumped back into the sarcoplasmic reticulum, Ca^{2+} would seem to be an attractive candidate to explain contraction-mediated glycolysis. Indeed, Dawson and Wilkie have suggested this to be the case [24, 124]. Consistent with this explanation is the finding that in vitro Ca^{2+}-calmodulin inhibits PFK under conditions associated with low glycolytic flux, but activates PFK under conditions associated with high glycolytic flux [89]. However, at in vivo concentrations of metabolites (e.g., fructose 6-P and Mg-ATP), the effects of Ca^{2+}-calmodulin are not apparent, or are at best only minor [89]. Others have shown that at physiological concentrations Ca^{2+} had no effect on PFK, whereas at high concentrations it is inhibitory to PFK [120]. These findings, in addition to others, served as a basis for concluding that Ca^{2+}, per se, does not control PFK in muscle [120]. Thus, convincing evidence that Ca^{2+} is the agent that is directly responsible for contraction-mediated glycolysis is as yet lacking.

In attempting to account for the regulation of glycolysis, at least one more factor should be considered, i.e., the structural constraints of the cell. For example, many assume that the cytosol is a homogeneous sap with respect to glycolytic enzymes (and metabolites). There is, however, good evidence that this is not so. It seems likely that multienzyme complexes exist to facilitate transfer of substrate and product through a metabolic pathway. In addition to experimental evidence for the existence of multienzyme complexes, there are also theoretical considerations to support this notion. This is illustrated by estimating the transit time (the time taken for the product of one enzyme to bind to the next enzyme in a metabolic pathway) of glycolytic intermediates. Such estimates show that if transit were to occur by diffusion alone it would not be possible to achieve the observed flux through PFK. Consequently, it has been inferred that some glycolytic enzymes must be organized to reduce transit time (see Ref. 94). This is in a sense comparable to the transfer of electrons along the respiratory chain in the mitochondria.

Lastly, it has been demonstrated that tetanic stimulation increases the extent of binding of some glycolytic enzymes (PFK, aldolase, and glyceraldehyde-3-phosphate dehydrogenase) in skeletal muscle (presumably to contractile proteins) [88]. Moreover, binding has been shown to shift the kinetics of PFK from sigmoidal to Michaelis-Menten (i.e., the affinity for fructose 6-P increases) [88]. Although contraction-induced binding may be of importance in the regulation of PFK, it should be noted that the percentage of PFK bound increased by only ~2-fold and the increase in affinity for fructose 6-P was only ~5-fold. Thus, other factors must be involved to explain the ~2,000-fold increase in glycolysis that occurs during the transition from rest to maximal force production (see Table 1.2). A further test of the functional significance of binding would be to follow the time course of changes in binding during contraction and recovery and to compare this with the glycolytic rates.

It has been proposed that the activation of PFK can in part be attributed to increases in free ADP and free AMP [90]. It should be noted, however, that the free forms of ADP and AMP are considered to represent only a minor fraction of the total tissue contents [121]. Moreover, measurements of total tissue ADP and AMP contents, as well as other metabolites (e.g., PCr) contents, represent the average tissue contents at the time of freezing, which is approximately 5–10 s after contraction, whereas the relevant species are the free forms in the immediate vicinity of the enzyme (PFK) during the contraction. In fact, because the increase of ADP after activation of myosin ATPase has a half-time of <25 ms and can be complete within 50 ms [29], not even the most rapid method of freeze clamping (~80 ms) [80] is adequate to detect the relevant changes in free ADP and free AMP. Due to the high activities of the enzymes responsible for the removal of ADP (creatine kinase) and AMP (adenylate kinase), as soon as contraction is terminated, the levels of ADP and AMP at the relevant sites may decrease markedly (within milliseconds). The implication then is that there are gradients for adenine nucleotides within the cell. Based on mathematical models, however, it was suggested that diffusion gradients for ATP and ADP were minimal in a system containing creatine kinase [91]. Nevertheless, Meyer et al. [91] did not rule out the possibility of such gradients in vivo, especially at low levels of PCr. On the other hand, based on studies of single fibers, and known nucleotide diffusion rates and kinetic constants, marked differences in the concentrations of adenine nucleotides within a fiber were calculated to exist [23]. Moreover, direct measurements of metabolites along the length of stimulated single muscle fibers also showed differences in concentrations [46]. Further evidence for the likelihood of different concentrations of metabolites within a compartment lies in the finding that usage of injection of ^{3}H-labeled precursors into frog muscle resulted in the estimation that the PCr concentration near the edges of the I-bands is ~160 mM [94], which should be compared with an averaged concentration of ~25 mM.

Methodological problems are apparent when rapid and localized changes of the adenine nucleotides should be measured in contracting muscle. A potential way to overcome this problem would be to utilize an intracellular sensor of increased levels of ADP and AMP. AMP deaminase catalyzes the deamination of AMP to IMP and NH_3 [84]. The complete sequence of reactions is as follows:

$$ATP \xrightarrow{\text{myosin ATPase}} ADP + P_i + H^+ \qquad (1)$$

$$2ADP \xleftarrow{\text{adenylate kinase}} AMP + ATP \qquad (2)$$

$$AMP \xrightarrow{\text{AMP deaminase}} IMP + NH_3 \qquad (3)$$

Because total tissue contents of ADP and AMP remain fairly constant during contraction, the increase in IMP during contraction is essentially stoichiometric to the decrease in ATP [10, 92, 104]. ADP and AMP are potent activators of PFK and AMP deaminase [93, 123]. And because the removal of IMP is a slow process [109], we have suggested that the observed increases in IMP (and NH_3) during intense exercise and hypoxia reflect the transient increases in ADP and AMP during the contraction [10, 66, 109]. It should be noted that a similar argument could be made for the regulation of phosphorylase, because AMP is also a potent activator of this enzyme [93]. Such a mechanism could explain how both phosphorylase and PFK are regulated together during contraction. A more in-depth discussion of the regulation of AMP deaminase in vivo is provided elsewhere [109].

Interestingly, during low intensity exercise (e.g., 40% $\dot{V}o_2$max) there is no loss of adenine nucleotides, nor any increase in IMP [108, 110], although a 25-fold increase in the rate of glycolysis versus rest is observed [71]. In our opinion, this should not be viewed as evidence against the concept that AMP and ADP are the major activators of PFK in vivo even at low exercise intensities. This is because, even at this low exercise intensity, there is a significant decrease in PCr [108], which indicates (via the equilibra of the creatine kinase and adenylate kinase reactions) that free ADP and free AMP are increased. The reason, however, that IMP is not increased may be that the PCr content is still sufficiently high to rapidly rephosphorylate ADP, thereby limiting the availability of substrate (and activator) for AMP deaminase, which has a relatively high K_a for ADP and K_m for AMP [123]. Only when the PCr content reaches a critical level (~40 mmol/kg dry wt), which occurs at higher energy turnover rates (~60–70% $\dot{V}o_2$max), does IMP accumulation become evident [110, 111].

It is recognized, however, that increases in IMP do not conclusively prove the existence of the ADP and AMP transients, but they are consistent with the hypothesis. Unfortunately, a direct test (i.e., measurements of concentrations of ADP and AMP at the relevant site during contraction) is, to our knowledge, currently unavailable.

The importance of O_2 availability for glucose utilization and lactate production was demonstrated over 100 years ago by Pasteur, who showed that the admittance of O_2 to anaerobic cells rapidly shut off glycolysis. If the blood supply to human skeletal muscle is occluded, the local O_2 store is depleted after about 5–10 min [9, 39, 105] and lactate starts to accumulate after about 15 min. The rate of glycolysis is, however, very low and only a small fraction of that occurring in contracting muscle (Table 1.2). The reason for the low glycolytic rate is probably that the rate of energy turnover in resting muscle is low. This is also demonstrated by the finding that hypoxemia to a level where arterial Po_2 decreases to 50% of the control value has no effect on muscle and blood lactate at rest [67]. Stimulation of glycolysis in anoxic muscle at rest is probably achieved through increases in free ADP and AMP and in fructose 6-P [70].

During short-term submaximal dynamic exercise, hypoxemia results in a greater production of lactate, P_i, and IMP and greater decreases in PCr while not measurably affecting the $\dot{V}_{O_2}$ [67, 83, 111]. These data suggest that acute hypoxia accelerates glycolysis during exercise and that the increase is due to higher levels of P_i and free AMP (as judged by the increase in IMP) in the contracting muscles. It appears likely that these metabolic changes reflect adaptive responses necessary to stimulate oxygen consumption when O_2 availability decreases (see above).

REGULATION OF LACTATE PRODUCTION DURING EXERCISE

Lactate dehydrogenase (LDH) catalyzes the reduction of pyruvate to lactate: pyruvate + NADH + H^+ ↔ lactate + NAD^+. The LDH reaction is generally considered to be close to equilibrium under most conditions [2, 48, 93]. The high activity of LDH in skeletal muscle compared with other glycolytic enzymes [93] supports the idea that the reaction is close to equilibrium, although the presence of LDH isozymes [114] suggests that kinetic regulation could be of importance under some conditions. Due to the law of mass-action an increase in lactate will occur whenever an increase occurs in the concentration of pyruvate, H^+, or cytosolic NADH. Based on the equilibrium of LDH the lactate/pyruvate ratio in a tissue is an index of the cytosolic redox state.

A decreased availability of O_2 may theoretically be related to an increased lactate production through two mechanisms: (*a*) an increased pyruvate concentration resulting from an increased rate of glycolysis (for a discussion of the effect of hypoxia on glycolysis, see above), and (*b*) an increased concentration of cytosolic NADH (NADHc) occurring secondarily to an increased mitochondrial NADH induced by hypoxia [72, 108].

An increase in the rate of glycolysis resulting in an increased concentration of pyruvate (and lactate) could also occur by stimuli other than O_2 deficiency. Such potential stimuli are (*a*) transformation of phosphorylase *b* to *a* either through increased levels of epinephrine or through contraction-induced increases in Ca^{2+} resulting in subsequent activation of glycogenolysis, and (*b*) increased uptake of blood-borne glucose induced by insulin or contraction. However, these mechanisms are of relatively minor importance in terms of achieving high glycolytic rates (cf. Table 1.2) and, consequently, high rates of lactate production.

Pyruvate formation results in an equimolar formation of NADH in the cytosol. At low work loads, the formation of pyruvate is balanced by an equal rate of pyruvate oxidation and thus reducing equivalents are transported into the mitochondria and oxidized in the respiratory chain at the same rate as their formation. The mitochondrial membrane is, however, impermeable to NADH and the reducing equivalents are transported via shuttle systems, of which the malate-asparate shuttle is considered to be the most important in skeletal muscle [93]. A potential mechanism for increased lactate formation is a limitation in the transport of reducing equivalents from the cytosol into the mitochondria during conditions of high respiratory rates (resulting in increases in NADHc).

It has been shown in several studies that the lactate/pyruvate ratio in muscle increases during conditions of increased lactate formation [12, 108] demonstrating that an increased concentration of cytosolic NADH does occur. It has been suggested that the increases in cytosolic NADH and lactate formation are due to an inability of the NADH shuttles to transport reducing equivalents into the mitochondria at a sufficient rate [113]. The hypothesis is indirectly supported by the finding that the activity of the enzymes involved in the malate-aspartate shuttle is increased after aerobic training [49, 113] and that this is associated with a decrease in the formation of lactate during submaximal exercise [43, 49, 61, 112]. If the increase in cytosolic NADH associated with increased lactate formation is due to a limitation in the malate-aspartate shuttle independent of O_2 availability, one would expect an unchanged mitochondrial redox state at this time. However, recent data indicate that increased lactate formation is associated with an increased mitochondrial NADH [108] and related to a decreased availability of O_2. If lactate formation was due to a limitation of the NADH shuttle enzymes, one would also expect that the rate of pyruvate formation (and NADHc formation) would be an important determinant of lactate formation. However, during one-legged exercise the muscle can reach a higher rate of O_2 consumption and formation of pyruvate and NADHc than during two-legged exercise before a significant lactate formation occurs [3]. This finding suggests that the NADH shuttles are not limiting the rate of transport of reducing equivalents from the cytosol to the mitochondria, and it is conceivable that a decrease of Po_2 to a level where metabolism is affected would result in a reduction of mitochondrial NAD^+ to NADH. Increases in mitochondrial NADH have been suggested to be a sensitive index of O_2 deficiency (i.e., tissue hypoxia [16]).

A study that is frequently cited to provide evidence that lactate production in contracting muscle is not due to a hypoxia is that of Jöbsis and Stainsby [56], who used surface fluorometry to monitor the redox state in dog skeletal muscle at rest and during contraction. It was shown that the fluorescence (i.e., NAD(P)H) decreased during contraction, even during anoxia, when lactate production was reported to occur. However, subsequent studies using laser fluorometry have shown a reduction (i.e., increase in NAD(P)H) of both slow-twitch and fast-twitch muscles during tetanic contractions [26]).

Recently, muscle NADH has been measured in a series of studies by a quantitative method [105]. During ischemia, muscle NADH increased rapidly and reached a plateau after about 10 min at about 2–3-fold the initial value. The increase in NADH during the first 5 min of ischemia occurred despite unchanged values of lactate or lactate/pyruvate, suggesting that the increase occurred not in the cytosol, but within the mitochondria. Recent studies of the oxygenation of human skeletal muscle during ischemia by near infrared monitoring [39] and by usage of O_2 probes [9] have shown that the local O_2 store is depleted after 4–5 min of ischemia. These observations are consistent with the observed changes in muscle NADH. Isometric contraction results in a 2-fold increase in NADH within 5 s [44], which is consistent with a rapid depletion of the O_2 store. When the contraction is sustained to fatigue muscle, lactate and lactate/pyruvate ratio increase indicating an increase in the concentration of cytosolic NADH. Muscle NADH, however, is not significantly different at fatigue compared with the value after a 5-s contraction, which indicates that changes in cytosolic NADH are too small to markedly affect muscle NADH. This is also expected on the basis of estimated cytosolic NADH from the LDH reaction [100]. We have concluded, on the basis of these and other experiments [68, 101], that changes in muscle NADH primarily reflect the changes in the mitochondrial compartment and could be used as a marker of tissue O_2 availability [72].

To further investigate the relationship between O_2 availability, muscle NADH, and lactate, subjects performed incremental bicycle exercise [108]. At low exercise intensities (40% $\dot{V}o_2$max) muscle NADH decreased, whereas at higher intensities (75 and 100% $\dot{V}o_2$max) NADH increased above the value at rest (Fig. 1.2), which suggests that the O_2 availability was limiting for the respiratory chain. The increase in NADH coincided with lactate accumulation in both muscle and blood. The decrease in NADH during submaximal exercise was not accompanied by changes in either muscle or blood lactate and is consistent with data from isolated mitochondria, where an increase of ADP in the presence of sufficient substrate and O_2 results in an oxidation of mitochondrial NADH [17].

An alternative method that has been used to estimate the mitochonrial redox state is to assume that the glutamate dehydrogenase (GDH) reaction is close to equilibrium and use the total tissue contents of ammonia, glutamate, and oxoglutarate. From the data obtained by this method it was concluded that mitochondrial NADH in human muscle was oxidized during exercise at both 70 and 100% of $\dot{V}o_2$max [36], a conclusion opposite from that stated above. Utilization of the GDH reaction to estimate the mitochondrial redox state is, however, based on a number of assumptions with questionable validity [69]. It is generally accepted

FIGURE 1.2

Muscle content of NADH and lactate during cycling at different intensities (40, 75, and 100% of $\dot{V}_{O_2}max$). Values are from 10 subjects and are presented as mean ± SE. Statistical significance versus rest: *p < 0.05, **p < 0.01, ***p < 0.001. (The top of the figure and the lactate values are from Sahlin K, Katz A, Henriksson J: Redox state and lactate accumulation in human skeletal muscle during dynamic exercise. Biochem J *245:551–556, 1987.)*

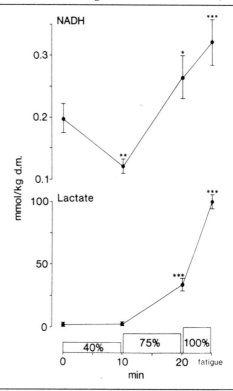

that $\dot{V}_{O_2}max$ during exercise with a large muscle mass (two-leg exercise) is limited primarily by the cardiac output, i.e., the O_2 transport capacity [3]. A limitation of $\dot{V}_{O_2}$ by the O_2 transport would result in O_2 deficiency at the cellular level and in an expected increase of mitochondrial NADH/NAD, which is observed with direct measurements of NADH (Fig. 1.2). The decrease in estimated mitochondrial NADH/NAD during exercise at 100% $\dot{V}_{O_2}$ [36] is, however, not compatible with this idea. We have recently demonstrated that usage of the total tissue contents of ammonia, glutamate, and oxoglutarate did not result in estimation of a reduction of mitochondrial NAD^+ in anoxic human skeletal muscle (induced by circulatory occlusion and isometric contraction at 2/3 maximal force to fatigue) (Katz, Spencer, and Sahlin, unpublished observations). In fact, during isometric contraction a marked oxidation of mitochondrial NADH was estimated. It is apparent that the GDH method is not appropriate for estimating the mitochondrial redox state in human skeletal muscle.

Human muscle is composed of different fiber types with different metabolic characteristics. The possibility of fiber-type heterogeneity in the pattern of NADH changes during exercise was investigated by analysis of NADH in single fibers [97]. During low intensity exercise (40% $\dot{V}o_2$max) NADH decreased only in type I fibers, whereas at higher intensities (75 and 100% $\dot{V}o_2$max) NADH increased above the preexercise value in both fiber types, suggesting that the availability of O_2 was restricted in both fiber types.

The effect of decreased O_2 availability on muscle metabolism at a constant energy demand was investigated in subjects exercising at a submaximal work load (50% of $\dot{V}o_2$max during control; 120 W) while breathing air (control) or a gas mixture poor in O_2 (11% O_2; respiratory hypoxia [67]). The $\dot{V}o_2$ during exercise was similar under both conditions, but the muscle lactate content was increased 4-fold and PCr was significantly lower during respiratory hypoxia versus control (Fig. 1.3). Muscle NADH was significantly higher after exercise during respiratory hypoxia than during control. These results suggest that the decrease in Po_2 affected muscle metabolism (lactate, NADH, and PCr) although cellular respiration was not measurably altered. These data are consistent with the idea that a decrease in tissue Po_2 results in adaptive changes in the mitochondrial redox state and the cytosolic phosphorylation potential, thereby maintaining a constant cellular respiration [125]. Similar findings have been obtained in studies on isolated perfused rabbit heart where a decrease in arterial Po_2 resulted in increased tissue NADH and lactate release. It is therefore likely that hypoxia-mediated increases in lactate production and NADH are occurring within the same muscle fibers [68].

These studies demonstrate that lactate formation during both maximal and submaximal exercise is related to an increased muscle NADH and that the availability of O_2 is restricted to a point where metabolism is affected. The amount of energy derived from the anaerobic processes (i.e., PCr breakdown and lactate formation) can be estimated from the incurred O_2 deficit and amounts to more than 50% of the total energy requirement during the first minute of exercise [102]. This is also emphasized by the rapid decline in PCr, which occurs during the first minute of submaximal exercise [53]. Thereafter PCr reaches a steady state that is related to the work load and maintained throughout the remaining period of short-term exercise [53]. Muscle lactate increases rapidly during the initial period of submaximal exercise and is thereafter maintained constant or decreases [58]. During steady-state exercise it

FIGURE 1.3

*Muscle content of NADH and lactate at rest and after bicycle exercise at 120 ±
6 W, which corresponds to 50% of the normoxic $\dot{V}o_2max$. The subjects exercised
during inspiration of air (normoxia) or 11% O_2 in N_2 (Resp Hx). Statistical
significance versus normoxia: **p < 0.01; n.s., not significant. (From Katz A,
Sahlin K: Effect of decreased oxygen availability on NADH and lactate contents
in human skeletal muscle during exercise. Acta Physiol Scand 131:119–128,
1987.)*

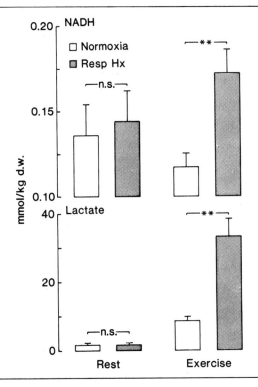

can be calculated (based on lactate release at 71% of $\dot{V}o_2max$ [58]) that
the formation of lactate contributes only about 2% of the total ATP
production. Thus, ATP production from anaerobic processes (PCr
breakdown and lactate formation) is relatively low during steady-state
submaximal exercise.

It is well documented that the measured $\dot{V}o_2$ at a given exercise intensity is similar before and after training [38, 61] or between normoxic and
hypoxic conditions [67, 83] although lactate production is altered. The
constant $\dot{V}o_2$ during these conditions has been used as an argument that
lactate production is not O_2 dependent [11]. From the above discussion,
however, it is clear that the amount of O_2 corresponding to the lactate

production during steady state is small and less than the methodological error in determining $\dot{V}o_2$ during submaximal exercise (coefficient of variation is about 4%, [5]), and consequently the expected increase in $\dot{V}o_2$ due to training or decrease in $\dot{V}o_2$ during respiratory hypoxia is too small to be detected.

ALTERNATIVE EXPLANATIONS FOR THE INCREASED LACTATE PRODUCTION DURING SUBMAXIMAL EXERCISE

The rate of lactate production is determined by the relative kinetics of glycolysis, LDH, and mitochondrial respiration. In the preceding section we have presented evidence that the availability of O_2 is an important factor for regulation of lactate production during exercise. It is, however, clear that enhanced glycolysis and lactate production can be achieved through stimuli other than hypoxia. Some of these factors will be discussed below.

The rate of glycogen utilization and the concentration of lactate in blood has been shown to be dependent on the glycogen level [7, 98]. This was further emphasized in a study of Gollnick et al. [35] where subjects cycled with both legs where one leg had a normal glycogen content and one had a reduced glycogen content. Despite similar amounts of work the leg with normal glycogen released lactate while the glycogen-depleted leg extracted lactate [35]. From their data it could be estimated that the glycolytic rate was markedly reduced in the glycogen-depleted state. These studies demonstrate that factors other than the O_2 availability (i.e., the availability of glycogen) are of importance for glycolysis and lactate formation.

It recently has been argued that the increase in lactate during submaximal exercise is due to a limitation in the activity of pyruvate dehydrogenase (PDH) rather than to tissue hypoxia [13]. The evidence for this conclusion was that plasma lactate was lower during incremental exercise with prior administration of dichloroacetate (DCA) (an activator of PDH). However, in the basal state, plasma lactate was lower in the DCA condition, and thus the exercise-induced increase in lactate was similar during DCA and control conditions. Moreover, the plasma lactate concentrations at fatigue were similar between DCA and control conditions, and the rate of decline in plasma lactate was greater during recovery from exercise in the DCA condition. Because it is likely that the glycolytic rates in muscle were similar during recovery in the two conditions, the lower plasma lactate during DCA treatment can be attributed to enhanced removal, possibly by the liver [13]. Similarly it can be argued that the small absolute difference in plasma lactate (<0.5 mmol/liter) during exercise is due to increased removal from blood during DCA rather than decreased lactate production.

Catecholamines also can increase glycolysis and lactate production. This is demonstrated by the increased muscle and blood lactate at rest during infusions of epinephrine [19]. The effect is mediated through an increased in cAMP, which induces a transformation of phosphorylase *b* to *a* [19].

It has been argued that the increased lactate production during exercise is a consequence of the rise in plasma epinephrine [118]. The scenario suggested by Stainsby et al. [118] is that the epinephrine-mediated increase in adenosine $3',5'$-cyclic monophosphate will activate glycogen phosphorylase in excess of what is required for oxidative function and that an imbalance occurs between formation and oxidation of pyruvate, resulting in increased lactate production. Indeed there are data that may appear to be consistent with this hypothesis. The exponential increase in muscle lactate production with increasing work loads (>50% $\dot{V}o_2max$) is associated with a similar profile in plasma catecholamines [31]. Furthermore, the decreased lactate production during respiratory hyperoxia is also associated with a decreased catecholamine response, whereas the converse occurs during respiratory hypoxia (see Ref. 31). Infusion of epinephrine during prolonged intermittent muscle contractions has been found to temporarily increase the muscle lactate concentration from 26 to 34 mmol/kg dry wt, whereas continuation of the stimulation for another 15 min resulted in a similar muscle lactate level with and without epinephrine [117]. Jansson et al. [55] infused epinephrine into one femoral artery (resulting in a high femoral venous epinephrine concentration) during two-leg bicycle exercise at 50% $\dot{V}o_2max$. From the arteriovenous differences of both legs, it was found that on average the epinephrine-infused leg released twice as much lactate as the control leg did (assuming similar blood flows), although the muscle lactate contents after exercise were similar in the two legs. Similarly, infusion of propranolol (a nonselective β-adrenoceptor blocker, βB) into one femoral artery during bicycle exercise (50% of $\dot{V}o_2max$) resulted in a reduced release of lactate despite unchanged muscle blood flow [59]. However, because treatment with βB does not decrease the exercise-induced increase in muscle lactate [10, 60], it was concluded that the reduced release of lactate during βB was due to a decreased transport rate rather than to a decreased production [59].

Furthermore, it is well recognized that lactate production decreases as exercise duration increases (e.g., see Refs. 6 and 43), while plasma epinephrine levels increase continuously (see Ref. 31). Moreover, bilaterally adrenalectomized subjects, whose plasma epinephrine concentration during exercise at 60% $\dot{V}o_2max$ is <50% of the plasma epinephrine concentration in normal subjects at rest, achieve the same blood lactate concentration (if not slightly higher) during submaximal exercise as do normal subjects [47]. These findings indicate that an elevation of plasma epinephrine during exercise can enhance lactate formation but only to a minor extent.

Human muscle is composed of different fiber types with different metabolic characteristics: type I or slow-twitch fibers, which have high aerobic capacity, and type II or fast-twitch fibers, which have high glycolytic capacity. The pattern of glycogen depletion has been used to identify the fiber type recruitment during different types of exercise. From such measurements it has been concluded that during low intensity exercise type I fibers are predominantly recruited, whereas both fiber types are used at higher intensities [34]. It has been suggested that the increased lactate production at the lactate threshold is related to an increased recruitment of type II fibers [11], which have a higher glycogenolytic and glycolytic potential. The finding that NADH increases above the preexercise value in both type I and II fibers during exercise at or above the lactate threshold [97] suggests that the availability of O_2 is restricted in both fiber types. This finding however, does not rule out the possibility that an increased recruitment of type II fibers is an important factor for the augmented lactate formation during submaximal exercise. As type II fibers have a lower aerobic capacity, one would expect a more pronounced increase in $NADH/NAD^+$ and $(ADP \times P_i)/ATP$ to obtain a certain degree of cellular respiration. This, in combination with the higher glycogenolytic [40] and glycolytic [28] capacity of type II fibers should result in a higher rate of lactate production in type II fibers. The increased NADH content in both fiber types does, however, suggest that a decreased availability of O_2 plays an important role in this process.

CONCLUSIONS

Within the last decade numerous reviews on lactate metabolism have been published. In many of these reviews it has been argued that lactate production during submaximal exercise is not due to tissue hypoxia. In the present review we have shown that the existing experimental findings can be interpreted in an alternative manner and that the increased lactate formation during submaximal exercise is indeed due to a restricted availability of O_2 in the mitochondria. Part of the apparent controversy exists because hypoxia at the cellular level can be defined in at least two ways: (*a*) cellular respiration is affected by Po_2 and (*b*) cellular metabolism is affected by Po_2. Many investigators have explicitly stated or implied that if cellular respiration is not impaired then cellular metabolism (including lactate formation) would not be dependent on O_2. This misconception probably stems from the idea that the main function of glycolysis is to supplement ATP production when the oxidative processes are insufficient to meet the energy demand.

In the present review we have summarized a series of recent papers where the NADH and lactate contents in human and animal muscle have been determined under a variety of conditions. In contrast to the study by Jöbsis and Stainsby [56], where redox changes were monitored by surface fluorescence, we have shown that submaximal exercise (>50% $\dot{V}o_2$max) and decreased O_2 availability result in increases in NADH that occur in parallel with increased lactate production. Thus there are both experimental data and theoretical reasons to support the idea that cellular metabolism is affected by the O_2 availability long before respiration is compromised. It is proposed that under conditions of restricted O_2 availability mitochondrial respiration is stimulated by increases in ADP, P_i, and NADH. These changes in the adenine nucleotides and P_i will favor stimulation of glycolysis. The increased rate of glycolysis and thereby cytosolic NADH formation will, together with the increase in mitochondrial NADH, result in an increased cytosolic NADH, which will shift the LDH equilibrium toward increased lactate production.

However, it is not likely that the availability of O_2 is the sole determinant or a prerequisite for glycolysis and lactate production during exercise or any other condition. The rate of lactate production is determined by the relative kinetics of glycolysis, LDH, and mitochondrial respiration. It is apparent that many factors affect lactate levels in body fluids. These factors indicate the complexity of the regulation of lactate metabolism. However, from the data presented in this review, it is clear that O_2 availability is of major importance for the regulation of lactate production during exercise.

ACKNOWLEDGMENTS

The authors acknowledge the support of the: Arizona Department of Health Services, Karolinska Institute, Swedish Institute, Swedish Medical Research Council, and Swedish Sport Research Council.

The authors are grateful to Deb Shilts and Eva Brimark for excellent secretarial assistance.

REFERENCES

1. Ahlborg B, Bergström J, Ekelund LG, Guarnieri G, Harris RC, Hultman E, Nordesjö LO: Muscle metabolism during isometric exercise performed at constant force. *J Appl Physiol* 33:224–228, 1972.
2. Akerboom TPM, Van Der Meer R, Tager JM: Techniques for the investigation of intracellular compartmentation. In *Techniques in the Life Sciences. Biochemistry. Techniques in Metabolic Research.* Amsterdam, Elsevier, B2 (Part 1)(B205):1–33, 1979.

3. Andersen P, Saltin B: Maximal perfusion of skeletal muscle in man. *J Physiol* 366:233–249, 1985.

4. Andres R, Cader G, Zierler KL: The quantitatively minor role of carbohydrate in oxidative metabolism by skeletal muscle in intact man in the basal state. Measurements of oxygen and glucose uptake and carbon dioxide and lactate production in the forearm. *J Clin Invest* 34:671–682, 1956.

5. Armstrong LE, Costill DL, Wright GA: Day-to-day variation in respiratory exchange data during cycling and running (Abstract). *Med Sci Sports Exerc* 15:141–142, 1983.

6. Bang O: The lactate content of blood during and after muscular exercise in man. *Scand Arch Physiol Suppl* 74:51–82, 1936.

7. Bergström J, Hermansen L, Hultman E, Saltin B: Diet, muscle glycogen and physical performance. *Acta Physiol Scand* 71:140–150, 1967.

8. Blomstrand E, Ekblom B, Newsholme EA: Maximum activities of key glycolytic and oxidative enzymes in human muscle from differently trained individuals. *J Physiol* 381:111–118, 1986.

9. Bonde-Petersen F, Lundgaard JS: Gas tensions (O_2, CO_2, Ar and N_2) in human muscle during static exercise and occlusion. In Knuttgen HG, Vogel JA, Poortmans J (eds): *Biochemistry of Exercise*. Champaign, IL, Human Kinetics, 1983, pp 781–786.

10. Broberg S, Katz A, Sahlin K: Propranolol enhances adenine nucleotide degradation in human skeletal muscle during exercise. *J Appl Physiol* 65:2478–2483, 1988.

11. Brooks GA: Anaerobic threshold; review of the concept and directions for future research. *Med Sci Sports Exerc* 17:22–31, 1985.

12. Bylund-Fellenius A-C, Walker PM, Elander A, Holm S, Holm J, Schersten T: Energy metabolism in relation to oxygen partial pressure in human skeletal muscle during exercise. *Biochem J* 200:247–255, 1981.

13. Carraro F, Klein S, Rosenblatt JI, Wolfe RR: Effect of dichloroacetate on lactate concentration in exercising humans. *J Appl Physiol* 66:591–597, 1989.

14. Challis RAJ, Arch JRS, Newsholme EA: The rate of substrate cycling between fructose 6-phosphate and fructose 1,6-bisphosphate in skeletal muscle. *Biochem J* 221:153–161, 1984.

15. Chance B: Reaction of oxygen with the respiratory chain in cells and tissues. *J Gen Physiol* 49:163–188, 1965.

16. Chance B: Pyridine nucleotide as an indicator of the oxygen requirements for energy-linked functions of mitochondria. *Circ Res* 38 (Suppl I):I31–I38, 1976.

17. Chance B, Williams GR: Respiratory enzymes in oxidative phosphorylation. III. The steady state. *J Biol Chem* 217:409–427, 1955.

18. Chasiotis D, Hultman E: The effect of circulatory occlusion on the glycogen phosphorylase-synthetase system in human skeletal muscle. *J Physiol* 345:167–173, 1983.

19. Chastiotis D, Sahlin K, Hultman E: Regulation of glycogenolysis in human muscle in response to epinephrine infusion. *J Appl Physiol* 54:45–50, 1983.

20. Chasiotis D, Hultman E: The effect of adrenaline infusion on the regulation of glycogenolysis in human muscle during isometric contraction. *Acta Physiol Scand* 123:55–60, 1985.

21. Connett RJ, Gayeski TEJ, Honig CR: Lactate accumulation in fully aerobic, working dog gracilis muscle. *Am J Physiol* 246:H120–H128, 1984.

22. Connett RJ, Gayeski TEJ, Honig CR: Lactate efflux is unrelated to intracellular PO_2 in a working red muscle in situ. *Am J Physiol* 61:H402–H408, 1986.

23. Cooke R, Pate E: The effects of ADP and phosphate on the contraction of muscle fibers. *Biophys J* 48:789–798, 1985.

24. Dawson MJ, Gadian DG, Wilkie DR: Muscular fatigue investigated by phosphorus nuclear magnetic resonance. *Nature* 274:861–866, 1978.

25. Dobson GF, Yamamoto E, Hochachka PW: Phosphofructokinase control in muscle: nature and reversal of pH-dependent ATP inhibition. *Am J Physiol* 250:R71–R76, 1986.

26. Duboc D, Muffat-Joly M, Renault G, Degeorges M, Toussaint M, Pocidalo J-J: In situ NADH laser fluorimetry of rat fast- and slow-twitch muscles during tetanus. *J Appl Physiol* 64:2692–2695, 1988.

27. Edwards RHT, Hill DK, McDonnell M: Myothermal and intramuscular pressure measurements during isometric contractions of the human quadriceps muscle. *J Physiol* 224:58P–59P, 1972.

28. Essen B, Jansson E, Henriksson J, Taylor AW, Saltin B: Metabolic characteristics of fibre types in human skeletal muscle. *Acta Physiol Scand* 95:153–165, 1974.

29. Ferenzci MA, Homsher E, Trentham DR: The kinetics of magnesium adenosine triphosphate cleavage in skinned muscle fibres of the rabbit. *J Physiol* 352:575–599, 1984.

30. Foe LG, Kemp RG: Properties of phospho and dephospho forms of muscle phosphofructokinase. *J Biol Chem* 257:6368–6372, 1982.

31. Galbo H: *Hormonal and Metabolic Adaptation to Exercise.* Stuttgart, Georg Thieme, 1983.

32. Gayeski TEJ, Connett RJ, Honig CR: Minimum intracellular PO_2 for maximum cytochrome turnover in red muscle in situ. *Am J Physiol* 252:H906–H915, 1987.

33. Gerschman R: Biological effects of oxygen. In Dickens F, Neil E (eds): *Oxygen in the Animal Organism.* Oxford, Pergamon Press, 1964, pp 475–494.

34. Gollnick PD, Piehl K, Saltin B: Selective glycogen depletion pattern in human muscle fibers after exercise of varying intensity and at varying pedalling rates. *J Physiol* 241:45–57, 1974.

35. Gollnick PD, Pernow B, Essen B, Jansson E, Saltin B: Availability of glycogen and plasma FFA for substrate utilization in leg muscle of man during exercise. *Clin Physiol* 1:27–42, 1981.

36. Graham TE, Saltin B: Estimation of the mitochondrial redox state in human skeletal muscle during exercise. *J Appl Physiol* 66:561–566, 1989.

37. Guha SK, Rose ZB: The enzymatic synthesis of ribose 1,5-bisphosphate: studies on its role in metabolism. *Arch Biochem Biophys* 250:513–518, 1986.

38. Hagberg JM, Hickson RC, Ehsani AA, Holloszy JO: Faster adjustment to and recovery from submaximal exercise in the trained state. *J Appl Physiol* 48:218–224, 1980.

39. Hampson NB, Piantadosi CA: Near infrared monitoring of human skeletal muscle oxygenation during forearm ischemia. *J Appl Physiol* 64:2449–2457, 1988.

40. Harris RC, Essen B, Hultman E: Glycogen phosphorylase activity in biopsy samples and single muscle fibres of musculus quadriceps femoris of man at rest. *Scand J Clin Lab Invest* 36:521–526, 1976.

41. Harris RC, Hultman E, Sahlin K: Glycolytic intermediates in human muscle after isometric contraction. *Pflugers Arch* 389:277–282, 1981.

42. Harris RC, Edwards RHT, Hultman E, Nordesjö LO, Nylind B, Sahlin K: The time course of phosphorylcreatine resynthesis during recovery of the quadriceps muscle in man. *Pflugers Arch* 367:137–142, 1976.

43. Henriksson J: Training induced adaptation of skeletal muscle and metabolism during submaximal exercise. *J. Physiol* 270:661–675, 1977.

44. Henriksson J, Katz A, Sahlin K: Redox state changes in human skeletal muscle after isometric contraction. *J Physiol* 380:441–451, 1986.

45. Hill AV, Long CNH, Lupton H: Muscular exercise, lactate acid, and the supply and utilization of oxygen. VI. The oxygen debt at the end of exercise. *Proc R Soc Lond (Biol)* B97:127–137, 1924.

46. Hintz CS, Chi MMY, Lowry OH: Heterogeneity in regard to enzymes and metabolites within individual muscle fibers. *Am J Physiol* 246:C288–C292, 1984.

47. Hoelzer DR, Dalsky GP, Schwartz NS, Clutter WE, Shah SD, Holloszy JO, Cryer PE: Epinephrine is not critical to prevention of hypoglycemia during exercise in humans. *Am J Physiol* 251:E104–E110, 1986.

48. Hofer HW: Phosphorylation of phosphofructokinase—the possible role of covalent modification in the regulation of glycolysis. In Beitner R (ed): *Regulation of Carbohydrate Metabolism.* Boca Raton, FL, CRC Press, 1985, pp 105–141.
49. Holloszy JO: Adaptations of skeletal muscle to endurance exercise. *Med Sci Sports Exerc* 7:155–164, 1975.
50. Holloszy JO, Coyle EF: Adaptations of skeletal muscle to endurance exercise and their metabolic consequences. *J Appl Physiol* 56:831–838, 1984.
51. Hue L, Blackmore PF, Shikama H, Robinson-Steiner A, Exton JH: Regulation of fructose-2,6-bisphosphate content in rat hepatocytes, perfused hearts, and perfused hindlimbs. *J Biol Chem* 257:4308–4313, 1982.
52. Hughes RL, Clode M, Edwards RHT, Goodwin TJ, Jones NL: Effect of inspired O_2 on cardiopulmonary and metabolic responses to exercise. *J Appl Physiol* 24:336–347, 1968.
53. Hultman E, Bergström J, McLennan Anderson N: Breakdown and resynthesis of phosphorylcreatine and adenosine triphosphate in connection with muscular work in man. *Scand J Clin Lab Invest* 19:56–66, 1967.
54. Idström J-P, Harihara Subramanian V, Chance B, Schersten T, Bylund-Fellenius A-C: Oxygen dependence of energy metabolism in contracting and recovering rat skeletal muscle. *Am J Physiol* 248:H40–H48, 1985.
55. Jansson E, Hjemdahl P, Kaijser L: Epinephrine-induced changes in muscle carbohydrate metabolism during exercise in male subjects. *J Appl Physiol* 60:1466–1470, 1986.
56. Jöbsis FF, Stainsby WN: Oxidation of NADH during contractions of circulated mammalian skeletal muscle. *Respir Physiol* 4:292–300, 1968.
57. Jones DP: Intracellular diffusion gradients of O_2 and ATP. *Am J Physiol* 250:C663–C675, 1986.
58. Jorfeldt L, Juhlin-Dannfelt A, Karlsson J: Lactate release in relation to tissue lactate in human skeletal muscle during exercise *J Appl Physiol* 44:350–352, 1978.
59. Juhlin-Dannfelt A, Aström H: Influence of β-adrenoceptor blockade on leg blood flow and lactate release in man. *Scand J Clin Lab Invest* 39:179–183, 1979.
60. Kaiser P, Tesch PA: Muscle lactate accumulation during exercise following β-adrenergic blockade. *Acta Physiol Scand* 117:149–151. 1983.
61. Karlsson J, Nordesjö LO, Jorfeldt L, Saltin B: Muscle lactate, ATP and CP levels during exercise after physical training in man. *J Appl Physiol* 33:199–203, 1972.
62. Karpatkin S, Helmreich E, Cori CF: Regulation of glycolysis in muscle. II. Effect of stimulation and epinephrine in isolated frog sartorius muscle. *J Biol Chem* 234:3139–3145, 1964.
63. Katz A, Broberg S, Sahlin K, Wahren J: Muscle ammonia and amino acid metabolism during dynamic exercise in man. *Clin Physiol* 6:365–379, 1986.
64. Katz A, Broberg S, Sahlin K, Wahren J: Leg glucose uptake during maximal dynamic exercise in humans. *Am J Physiol* 251:E65–E70, 1986.
65. Katz A, Sahlin K, Henriksson J: Muscle ATP turnover data during isometric contraction in humans. *J Appl Physiol* 60:1839–1842, 1986.
66. Katz A, Sahlin K, Henriksson J: Muscle ammonia metabolism during isometric contraction in humans. *Am J Physiol* 250:C834–C840, 1986.
67. Katz A, Sahlin K: Effect of decreased oxygen availability on NADH and lactate contents in human skeletal muscle during exercise. *Acta Physiol Scand* 131:119–128, 1987.
68. Katz A, Edlund A, Sahlin K: NADH content and lactate production in the perfused rabbit heart. *Acta Physiol Scand* 130:193–200, 1987.
69. Katz A: Mitochondrial redox state in skeletal muscle cannot be estimated with glutamate dehydrogenase system. *Am J Physiol* 254:C587–C588, 1988.

70. Katz A: G-1,6-P₂, glycolysis, and energy metabolism during circulatory occlusion in human skeletal muscle. *Am J Physiol* 255:C140–C144, 1988.
71. Katz A, Sahlin K, Henriksson J: Carbohydrate metabolism in human skeletal muscle during exercise is not regulated by G-1,6-P₂. *J Appl Physiol* 65:487–489, 1988.
72. Katz A, Sahlin K: Regulation of lactic acid production during exercise. *J Appl Physiol* 65:509–518, 1988.
73. Katz A, Nyomba BL: Mechanism of insulin-mediated glycolysis in human skeletal muscle (Abstract). *Diabetes* 37 (Suppl 1):72A, 1988.
74. Katz A, Bogardus C: Role of glucose 1,6-P₂ in mediating insulin-stimulated glycolysis in human skeletal muscle (Abstract). *FASEB J* 3:A540, 1989.
75. Katz J: The application of isotopes to the study of lactate metabolism. *Med Sci Sports Exerc* 18:353–359, 1985.
76. Kennedy FG, Jones DP: Oxygen dependence of mitochondrial function in isolated cardiac myocytes. *Am J Physiol* 250:C374–C383, 1986.
77. Kitajima S, Sakakibara R, Uyeda K: Significance of phosphorylation of phosphofructokinase. *J Biol Chem* 258:13292–13298, 1983.
78. Knuttgen HG, Saltin B: Oxygen uptake, muscle high-energy phosphates, and lactate in exercise under acute hypoxic conditions in man. *Acta Physiol Scand* 87:368–376, 1973.
79. Koretsky AP, Balaban RS: Changes in pyridine nucleotide levels alter oxygen consumption and extramitochondrial phosphates in isolated mitochondria: a ³¹P-NMR and NAD(P)H fluorescence study. *Biochim Biophys Acta* 893:398–408, 1987.
80. Kretzschmar KM, Wilkie DR: A new approach to freezing tissues rapidly (Abstract). *J Physiol* 202:66P–67P, 1969.
81. Kuo HJ, Malencik DA, Liou RS, Anderson SR: Factors affecting the activation of rabbit muscle phosphofructokinase by actin. *Biochemistry* 25:1278–1286, 1986.
82. Lee AD, Katz A: Transient increase in glucose 1,6-bisphosphate in human skeletal muscle during isometric contraction. *Biochem J* 258:915–918, 1989.
83. Linnarsson D, Karlsson J, Fagraeus L, Saltin B: Muscle metabolites and oxygen deficit with exercise in hypoxia and hyperoxia. *J Appl Physiol* 36:399–402, 1974.
84. Lowenstein JM: Ammonia production in muscle and other tissues: the purine nucleotide cycle. *Physiol Rev* 52:382–414, 1972.
85. Lowry OH, Passonneau JV: Kinetic evidence for multiple binding sites on phosphofructokinase. *J Biol Chem* 241:2268–2279, 1966.
86. Lundin G, Ström G: The concentration of blood lactic acid in man during muscular work in relation to the partial pressure of oxygen of the inspired air. *Acta Physiol Scand* 13:253–266, 1947.
87. Mansour TE: Phosphofructokinase activity in skeletal muscle extracts following administration of epinephrine. *J Biol Chem* 247:6059–6066, 1972.
88. Masters C: Interactions between glycolytic enzymes and components of the cytomatrix. *J Cell Biol* 99:222S–225S, 1984.
89. Mayr GW: Interaction of calmodulin with muscle phosphofructokinase. Interplay with metabolic effectors of the enzyme under physiological conditions. *Eur J Biochem* 143:521–529, 1984.
90. McGilvery RW, Murray TM: Calculated equilibria of phosphocreatine and adenosine phosphates during utilization of high energy phosphate by muscle. *J Biol Chem* 249:5845–5850, 1974.
91. Meyer RA, Sweeney HL, Kushmerick MJ: A simple analysis of the "phosphocreatine shuttle." *Am J Physiol* 246:C365–C377, 1984.
92. Meyer RA, Dudley GA, Terjung RL: Ammonia and IMP in different skeletal muscle fibers after exercise in rats. *J Appl Physiol* 49:1037–1041, 1989.
93. Newsholme E, Start C: *Regulation in Metabolism.* London, Wiles, 1974.
94. Ottaway JH, Mowbray J: The role of compartmentation in the control of glycolysis. *Curr Top Cell Regul* 12:107–208, 1977.

95. Özand P, Narahara HT: Regulation of glycolysis in muscle. III. Influence of insulin, epinephrine and contraction on phosphofructokinase activity in frog skeletal muscle. *J Biol Chem* 239:3146–3152, 1964.

96. Pirnay F, Lamy M, Dujardin J, Deroanne R, Petit JM: Analysis of femoral venous blood during maximum muscular exercise. *J Appl Physiol* 33:289–292, 1972.

97. Ren JM, Henriksson J, Katz A, Sahlin K: NADH content in type I and type II human muscle fibres after dynamic exercise. *Biochem J* 251:183–187, 1988.

98. Richter EA, Galbo H: High glycogen levels enhance glycogen breakdown in isolated contracting muscle. *J Appl Physiol* 61:827–831, 1987.

99. Rowell LB, Blackmon JR, Kenny MA, Escourrou P: Splanchnic vasomotor and metabolic adjustments to hypoxia and exercise in humans. *Am J Physiol* 247:H251–H258, 1984.

100. Sahlin K: NADH and lactate in human skeletal muscle during short-term intense exercise. *Pflugers Arch* 403:193–196, 1985.

101. Sahlin K, Katz A: The content of NADH in rat skeletal muscle at rest and after cyanide poisoning. *Biochem J* 239:245–248, 1986.

102. Sahlin K, Ren JM, Broberg S: Oxygen deficit at the onset of submaximal exercise is not due to a delayed oxygen transport. *Acta Physiol Scand* 134:175–180, 1988.

103. Sahlin K, Harris RC, Hultman E: Creatine kinase equilibrium and lactate content compared with muscle pH in tissue samples obtained after isometric exercise. *Biochem J* 152:173–180, 1975.

104. Sahlin K, Palmskog G, Hultman E: Adenine nucleotide and IMP contents of the quadriceps muscle in man after exercise. *Pflugers Arch* 374:193–198, 1978.

105. Sahlin K: NADH and NADPH in human skeletal muscle at rest and during ischaemia. *Clin Physiol* 3:477–485, 1983.

106. Sahlin K: Metabolic changes limiting muscle performance. In Saltin B (ed): *Biochemistry of Exercise VI.* Champaign, IL, Human Kinetics, 1986, pp 323–343.

107. Sahlin K: Lactate production cannot be measured with tracer techniques. *Am J Physiol* 252:E439–E440, 1987.

108. Sahlin K, Katz A, Henriksson J: Redox state and lactate accumulation in human skeletal muscle during dynamic exercise. *Biochem J* 245:551–556, 1987.

109. Sahlin K, Katz A: Purine nucleotide metabolism. In Poortmans JR (ed): *Principles of Exercise Biochemistry,* Med. Sport Sci., Basel, Karger 27:120–139, 1988.

110. Sahlin K, Broberg S, Ren JM: Formation of inosine monophosphate (IMP) in human skeletal muscle during incremental dynamic exercise. *Acta Physiol Scand* 136:195–200.

111. Sahlin K, Katz A: Hypoxaemia increases the accumulation of inosine monophosphate (IMP) in human skeletal muscle during submaximal exercise. *Acta Physiol Scand* 136:199–203.

112. Saltin B, Nazar K, Costill DL, Stein E, Jansson E, Essen B, Gollnick P: The nature of the training response; peripheral and central adaptations to one-legged exercise. *Acta Physiol Scand* 96:289–305, 1976.

113. Schantz P: Plasticity of human skeletal muscle. *Acta Physiol Scand Suppl* 558, 1986.

114. Sjödin B: Lactate dehydrogenase in human skeletal muscle. *Acta Physiol Scand Suppl* 436, 1976.

115. Sjöholm H, Sahlin K, Edström L, Hultman E: Quantitative estimation of anaerobic and oxidative energy metabolism and contraction characteristics in intact human skeletal muscle in response to electrical stimulation. *Clin Physiol* 3:227–239, 1983.

116. Spriet LL, Söderlund K, Bergström M, Hultman E: Skeletal muscle glycogenolysis, glycolysis, and pH during electrical stimulation in men. *J Appl Physiol* 62:616–621, 1987.

117. Spriet LL, Ren JM, Hultman E: Epinephrine infusion enhances muscle glycogenolysis during prolonged electrical stimulation. *J Appl Physiol* 64:1439–1444, 1988.

118. Stainsby WN, Sumners C, Eitzman PD: Effects of catecholamines on lactic acid output during progressive working contractions. *J Appl Physiol* 59:1809–1814, 1985.
119. Sugden PH, Newsholme EA: The effects of ammonia, inorganic phosphate and potassium ions on the activity of phosphofructokinases from muscle and nervous tissues of vertebrates and invertebrates. *Biochem J* 150:113–122, 1975.
120. Vaughan H, Thornton SD, Newsholme EA: The effects of calcium ions on the activities of trehalase, hexokinase, phosphofructokinase, fructose diphosphatase and pyruvate kinase from various muscles. *Biochem J* 132:527–535, 1973.
121. Veech RL, Lawson JWR, Cornell NW, Krebs HA: Cytosolic phosphorylation potential. *J Biol Chem* 254:6538–6547, 1979.
122. Vogel JA, Gleser MA: Effect of carbon monoxide on oxygen transport during exercise. *J Appl Physiol* 32:234–239, 1972.
123. Wheeler TJ, Lowenstein JM: Adenylate deaminase from rat muscle. Regulation by purine nucleotides and orthophosphate in the presence of 150 mM KCl. *J Biol Chem* 254:8894–8899, 1979.
124. Wilkie DR, Dawson MJ, Edwards RHT, Gordon RE, Shaw D: ^{31}P NMR studies of resting muscle in normal human subjects. In Pollack GM, Suai H (eds): *Contractile Mechanisms in Muscle.* England, Plenum, 1984, pp 333–346.
125. Wilson DF, Erecinska M, Drown C, Silver IA: Effect of oxygen tension on cellular energetics. *Am J Physiol* 233:C135–C140, 1977.
126. Wolfe RR, Jahoor F, Miyoshi M: Evaluation of the isotopic equilibration between lactate and pyruvate. *Am J Physiol* 254:532–535, 1988.
127. Woodson RD, Wills RE, Lenfant C: Effect of acute and established anemia on O_2 transport at rest, submaximal, and maximal work. *J Appl Physiol* 44:36–43, 1978.

2
Control of Lactic Acid Metabolism in Contracting Muscles and during Exercise

WENDELL N. STAINSBY, Sc.D.
GEORGE A. BROOKS, Ph.D

INTRODUCTION

When we were invited to write this review we asked the question, why write another review on the control of lactic acid production and removal during exercise now? There is no doubt that the issue is controversial. Scientific meetings and journals concerned with the physiology of exercise have repeatedly included this issue for years. Why not wait for new data to clarify the issue? The concluding argument was that the discussion lately was unfocussed and confusing. Therefore, the goal of this review is to gather what we see as the most relevant data on the issue. This review is not intended to be exhaustive. With a few digressions the context is normoxia and normal blood flow. We shall take selected data from contracting muscle and exercising whole animals, particularly humans, and try to weave it into a clear picture regarding the most relevant facts that are available at this time, and we will try to point out the best current hypotheses concerning the production and removal of lactate in contracting muscle and in exercising humans.

Terminology

As mentioned above, in this review we shall be discussing the metabolism of lactic acid, an end product of the glycolytic (Embden-Meyerhof) pathway. Because it is a strong organic acid ($pK = 3.8$), at physiological pH values, lactic acid will dissociate to a proton (H^+) and an anion ($C_3H_5O_3^-$). Thus, when the metabolite of interest is formed via glycolysis, or removed via direct oxidation, conversion to glucose, or other pathways chemical balance requires that the metabolism of lactic acid ($C_3H_6O_3$) be considered. However, during the interim between production and removal, the proton and anion exist separately, each exerting different influences, and, perhaps, ultimately taking different pathways of metabolism.

Origin of the Controversy

The concepts of this issue held by some investigators appear to be based on the studies by Hill and associates [50–52]. It was noted by these authors that, as exercise intensity increased, lactate concentration in the blood rose slowly at first, but at higher work levels and $\dot{V}o_2$, blood lactate rose rapidly. From this they proposed that at low work rates O_2 delivery to the muscle by the blood ($Cao_2 \times \dot{Q}$) was adequate. At higher work rates O_2 delivery was inadequate to meet metabolic demand by the muscles, and anaerobic metabolism, with conversion of glycogen to lactic acid, was used to supplement energy supply. This interpretation of the data was based on general information available at the time. Cells and tissues, including muscle, exposed to low O_2 produce lactic acid, the Pasteur effect. The logic of this interpretation was so good it has persisted for many years. The work rate or Vo_2 at which lactate in the blood began to rise has been called the anaerobic threshold [119, 121], and it has generally been assumed that the source of the lactic acid that appeared in the blood was mainly or exclusively the working muscles.

The "oxygen debt" concept of Hill and associates [50–52] was that lactate produced in contracting muscle as the result of insufficient oxygen supply during exercise was converted back to glycogen in situ during recovery. Because such a process would require extra oxygen consumption during recovery, it was reasoned that the postexercise "O_2 debt" supported the the energy transduction necessary to accomplish glycogen restitution from lactate. It is now known, however, that the postexercise fate of lactate is mainly to oxidation [14], and that a variety of factors explain the recovery oxygen consumption seen in excess of a resting baseline (EPOC) [36, 37, 99].

The report of Margaria et al. [78] recognized differences in the kinematics (rate of change in concentration) of the postexercise blood lactate and the kinetics (mass rate of change) of the postexercise O_2 consumption. Margaria *et al.* ascribed the first, fast phase of the recovery O_2 curve to the restoration of the then recently discovered phosphagen (later found to represent ATP and creatine phosphate), and the second, slow phase to glycogen restoration. As just noted, a variety of factors explain the EPOC. In the 1920s and 1930s, the appearance of lactate during exercise was taken to represent insufficient oxygen supply, a situation that was compensated for in recovery. As reviewed recently [11], attempts at identifying a muscle anaerobic threshold from changes in pulmonary ventilation were unsuccessful because the fundamental assumption of muscle oxygen insufficiency during submaximal exercise could not be substantiated.

Investigation of this issue using muscles in situ with isolated or partly isolated circulation was originally directed only at quantifying the lactic acid output of working muscles. Concern for the cause of lactic acid was engendered by the data obtained. The in situ preparations permitted direct application of the relation popularized by Fick. The early studies showed that during repetitive twitch contractions net lactic acid output

(L̇), was transient. It rose to a peak in 3–7 min and then declined to near zero in 10–20 min, where it remained [4, 19, 97, 115, 126]. Although the peak L̇ rises in slightly more than a direct proportion to the twitch frequency and $\dot{V}o_2$, the later steady level of L̇ was not related to twitch frequency or $\dot{V}o_2$. It was near zero at all $\dot{V}o_2$ levels. These data were interpreted as suggesting that if there was a lack of O_2 in the muscles it only occurred immediately after the initiation of contractions and was not present at any twitch rate studied (0.5–10 twitches/s), under steady-level condition with spontaneous flow and normoxia.

These early experiments also showed where $\dot{V}o_2$ became limited in dog muscle at higher twitch frequencies. $\dot{V}o_2$ rose in close direct relation to twitch frequency up to about 2.5 twitches/s. As twitch rate was increased further, $\dot{V}o_2$ rose less with each increment in twitch rate to 4–5 twitches/s. From 4 to 7 twitches/s there was little change in $\dot{V}o_2$. At 10 twitches/s $\dot{V}o_2$ was reduced below the levels seen at 4–7 twitches/s [126]. This relationship between contraction frequency and $\dot{V}o_2$ with no net L under steady-level conditions reinforced questions regarding O_2 as a determinant of maximal oxygen consumption ($\dot{V}o_2$max).

To assess the role of O_2 in lactic acid production directly, a new method was applied to the muscle [64]. This method measured the fluorescence of mitochondrial NADH as an indicator of mitochondrial oxidation/reduction state. Fluorescence was relatively high at rest. It decreased during both twitch and tetanic contractions. The twitch frequencies were 0.5–5/s and the tetanic frequency was 50/s limited to 3–5 s duration. The twitch contractions were followed for up to 20 min. The responses were the same: contraction with free flow and normoxia always resulted in an immediate decrease of fluorescence, oxidation, of mitochondrial NAD/NADH, compared to rest. These data fit the relevant categories of metabolic control previously established by Chance and Williams [18]. At rest, state 4 conditions were present. Substrate availability was high but $ATP/ADP \cdot P_i$ was also high. The low $ADP \cdot P_i$ limited reducing equivalent flux through the mitochondrial electron transport system, and mitochondrial NAD/NADH was low. Contractions caused a fall in $ATP/ADP \cdot P_i$, state 3. The rise in $ADP \cdot P_i$ reduced the block of electron transport relative to substrate availability and mitochondrial NAD/NADH rose. This rise also indicated that the other substrate for electron transport, O_2, was also adequate. Therefore, there was no lack of O_2 in the mitochondria at any time during the contractions. The simple conclusion from this study of mitochondrial NADH was that the transient production and release of lactic acid by muscle during contractions with normoxic conditions and free flow was not related to lack of O_2 in the mitochondria. This simple conclusion was not accepted by all muscle or exercise physiologists. From this the current controversy seems to have developed.

MUSCLE LACTATE PRODUCTION AND RELEASE

Caveats for in Situ Muscle Studies

The metabolic patterns of skeletal muscle in situ form a base for under-standing the metabolism of the active muscles in exercise. Study of me-tabolism of contracting skeletal muscle is not a direct study of exercise. The activity of a single muscle or muscle group does not generate the whole body response to exercise. The hormonal and neural influences of exercise are not present. From the base of in situ muscle the effects of the hormonal and neural influences of exercise can be determined. The goal of the in situ preparations is to make accurate measurements under conditions that represent normal physiology as closely as possible. Some simple clues to the quality of the preparation are needed. One sensitive indicator of quality of the preparations is the presence of the transient responses of autoregulation of blood flow [104]. Artificial perfusates and excess trauma abolish these transients and probably abolish capillary flow regulation [103]. Loss of capillary flow control raises the minimal critical Pvo_2 and lowers the maximal $\dot{V}o_2$. It is also necessary that the flow isolation be done carefully. Interference with normal flow will bias the results.

REVIEW OF LACTATE EXCHANGE BY MUSCLE

Lactic Acid Output during Repetitive Contractions

Lactic acid net output, $\dot{L}$, measurements during repetitive contractions using dog muscle showed $\dot{L}$ to be transient at all twitch rates from 0.5 to 10 twitches/s [98, 126]. The most commonly studied frequency was 4 twitches/s. Data obtained over the years has remained unchanged [4, 19, 88, 98, 101, 102, 115, 126]. The $\dot{L}$ pattern is characterized by a rapid rise to a maximal value at 3–7 min followed by a decline to near zero in 10–20 min. Frequently there was a modest uptake of lactic acid under steady-level conditions after 10–20 min of contractions. The $\dot{L}$ in repeti-tive tetanic contractions, which produced a similar $\dot{V}o_2$ as in twitch con-tractions at 4/s, was similar [100, 109]. Recent studies with higher stimu-lation frequencies have shown a slightly greater than proportional increase in $\dot{L}$. [106]. These studies also showed the same pattern in isometric and isotonic contractions. The preparations all showed normal autoregulation transients. When similar measurements were made using cat muscles, the $\dot{V}o_2$ maximum was approximately one-eighth that of the dog muscle. Nevertheless, the peak $\dot{L}$ for a given twitch frequency was approximately the same as that for dog muscle [101]. The peak $\dot{L}$ was achieved somewhat later, at about 10 min, and the decline toward zero was slower. A study of $\dot{L}$ during static contractions of cat muscle also showed similar $\dot{L}$ values for high and low aerobic capacity muscles [88]. These studies suggested that $\dot{L}$ during contractions was not strongly affected by fiber type.

Lactic Acid Output during Progressively Intense Contractions

Progressively intense tetanic contractions to maximal work are more analogous to the actions of the working muscles in a progressive exercise test than repetitive contractions. During progressive, tetanic contractions $\dot{L}$ rose with stimulation voltage (to recruit more fibers), work, and $\dot{V}o_2$. The relation of $\dot{L}$ to work and $\dot{V}o_2$ was direct and curvilinear, rising as work and $\dot{V}o_2$ increased [21, 107]. The rise of $\dot{L}$ was continuous and there was no sign of a break or threshold for $\dot{L}$ in the relation, and maximal $\dot{L}$ was relatively low. When the maximal $\dot{L}/g \cdot min$ of muscle was scaled up to a likely mass of working muscle in exercise, and given a conservative distribution volume of plasma and only part of the interstitial space, the $\dot{L}$ could not account for the rise of blood lactate seen in a progressive exercise above the anaerobic threshold of humans. It was concluded that there was additional stimulation of $\dot{L}$ during exercise that was not present during contractions of muscle in situ.

Effect of Catecholamines on Lactate Exchange

Epinephrine infusion has been shown to increase $\dot{L}$ transiently during repetitive twitch contractions [98]. When epinephrine and norepinephrine were infused together in a progressive manner during increasingly intense tetanic contractions, to mimic the rise of these agents in blood during exercise, the infusion increased $\dot{L}$ in a pattern suggesting a threshold at higher work rates and $\dot{V}o_2$ [100, 107, 110]. During repetitive tetanic contractions, strongly β-adrenergic agonists such as epinephrine and isoproterenol increased $\dot{L}$ while strongly α-adrenergic agonists such as norepinephrine and phenylephrine did not [100]. α receptor antagonists increased $\dot{L}$ during epinephrine infusion while β receptor antagonists reduced $\dot{L}$ during epinephrine infusion. These data suggest epinephrine is an effector of $\dot{L}$ by muscle, which should be considered as significant in exercise.

Effect of Flow on $\dot{V}o_2$ and $\dot{L}$

The $\dot{V}o_2$ during 4/s repetitive twitch contractions is significantly dependent upon blood flow. Raising and lowering flow relative to the control, free flow level, raised and lowered $\dot{V}o_2$ respectively [5]. In a complicated experimental paradigm in which O_2 delivered to the muscle ($Cao_2 \times Q$) was kept constant, the rate of fatigue development and decline of $\dot{V}o_2$ during twitch contractions were inversely related to flow through the muscle [6]. This finding implies flow rather than O_2 transport per se is an important determinant of $\dot{V}o_2$. A step decrease in flow to reduce O_2 transport to muscle during repetitive 4/s twitch contractions caused a quick decrease in tension development and $\dot{V}o_2$ with only a small decrease in Pvo_2 and no change in tension/$\dot{V}o_2$ [43]. These data also suggest a specific effect of flow on $\dot{V}o_2$. The $\dot{L}$ was not measured in these studies. To fill this gap in knowledge, the $\dot{L}$ was measured in similar recent studies using tetanic contractions [105]. A 25% reduction in flow reduced $\dot{V}o_2$ about 22% but $\dot{L}$ was not increased compared to controls. Apparently ischemia reduces $\dot{V}o_2$ during contractions without increasing $\dot{L}$. Once again there is an implied effect of flow that is not mediated directly by O_2 transport.

Effect of Raising Blood Lactate Concentration

Raising the concentration of lactate by intravenous infusion of lactate has a very significant effect on muscle $\dot{L}$ during contractions. The net exchange of lactate during twitch contractions was always uptake when blood concentrations were elevated [40–42], and the uptake was increased when the frequency of twitches was increased. This would be difficult to explain if the origin of $\dot{L}$ as an output during contractions was O_2 lack.

Effect of Hypoxia on $\dot{V}o_2$ and $\dot{L}$

Modest hypoxia produced by breathing 13% O_2 in N_2 did not significantly affect $\dot{V}o_2$ or tension development, during repetitive tetanic contractions, while $\dot{L}$ was increased [56]. More severe hypoxia, during twitch contractions, lowered $\dot{V}o_2$ but had no consistent effect on $\dot{L}$ [55, 57]. In another report, modest hypoxia alone did not decrease $\dot{V}o_2$, but $\dot{V}o_2$ was decreased when hypercapnia was induced at the same time [83]. Hypoxia from breathing 9% O_2 did not reduce $\dot{V}o_2$ at 1 twitch/s, but did decrease $\dot{V}o_2$ during 4 twitch/s contractions [72]. Severe hypoxia in a study utilizing pump perfusion to maintain O_2 delivery ($Cao_2 \times \dot{Q}$) constant showed again $\dot{V}o_2$ was decreased by hypoxia compared to normoxia. In this study $\dot{L}$ was increased by the hypoxia [55]. In a recent study lowering Cao_2 by hypoxia enough to reduce $\dot{V}o_2$ during contractions about 50% increased $\dot{L}$, but the $\dot{L}$ decreased with time almost to the control level by 30 min of contractions [106]. These data suggest metabolic arrest occurs (62), perhaps to prevent lethal lactacidosis. The data also suggest $\dot{L}$ may not always be a suitable indicator of O_2 lack even when hypoxia is severe.

Effect of Hyperoxia on $\dot{V}o_2$ and $\dot{L}$

Raising the arterial Po_2 by breathing 100% O_2 had no effect on $\dot{V}o_2$ or contraction performance during repetitive twitches [56, 128], and $\dot{L}$ was not affected [56]. The respiratory exchange ratio, $\dot{V}co_2/\dot{V}o_2$, was decreased by breathing 100% O_2 during twitch contractions compared to breathing room air [128].

Assessment of Mitochondrial O/R State

The first assessment of the oxidation-reduction state of the mitochondria in muscles during contractions utilized a fluorescence measurement [64]. The fluorescence measured was mainly from mitochondrial NADH and, therefore, indicated mitochondrial NAD/NADH inversely. Fluorescence was relatively high in resting muscle, indicating that NAD/NADH was low (Fig. 2.1). After the onset of repetitive twitch contractions at frequencies from 1 to 5/s and during 50/s tetanic stimulation, up to 5 s duration, fluorescence decreased; NAD/NADH increased. It was concluded that in resting muscle electron transport was blocked by lack of ADP and/or P_i, state 4 [18]. During contractions, ADP and P_i were adequate and NAD/NADH rose; the block by lack of ADP and P_i was relieved. It must also be true that O_2 was adequate, because the rise in the ratio must mean no block of electron transport was present. The major test of the responsiveness of the system was intraarterial infusion of Amytal which blocks electron transport downstream from NAD/NADH. Amytal caused a maximal increase in fluorescence, a maximal decrease in mitochondrial NAD/NADH. During contractions, ischemia produced by an arterial clamp (which probably decreased flow 50–60% and hypoxia produced by breathing nitrogen 3–4 min did not cause maximal increase in fluorescence to the Amytal level. In fact, these maneuvers did not increase fluorescence to the resting level. These findings were not understood at the time. Some have used them to suggest the method was generally not valid (e.g., see Ref. 71). The recent studies suggest that there are more control components in the system that so far have not been included in the analysis. There may be flow-related mechanical shutdown with ischemia [43, 47] and metabolic arrest with hypoxia [54, 77]. In the case of severe hypoxia, O_2 lack may be present but metabolic arrest may reduce substrate availability and preclude production of lactic acid. Hypoxia increased $\dot{L}$ only transiently whereas ischemia did not increase it [106]. Control responses such as these may also occur in mitochondria.

The criticism of the original NADH studies has not been substantiated by any other valid experimental test. A study of the same type, some 20 years later has been applied to the interior muscle cells and has confirmed the original observation; there was oxidation of NADH and no indication of O_2 lack in the mitochondria during contractions under free flow, normoxic conditions [86]. An entirely different method of O_2 supply assessment in muscle has lead to a similar conclusion. Measurements of muscle myoglobin saturation during repetitive twitch contractions have shown O_2 to be low, but adequate in muscle and unrelated to $\dot{L}$ [22,

FIGURE 2.1

Reflectance (top trace) *and fluorescence changes* (lower trace) *in the dog's gastrocnemius.* **A,** *Responses to twitch activity at 5 contractions/s. Note the pen reset 30 s after the start of the stimulation.* **B,** *The first stage of recovery after 20 min of contractile activity. About 16 min of recording has been deleted between* **A** *and* **B.** *The* broken line *indicates the florescence baseline after the several pen resets during the activity.* **C,** *Effect of nitrogen breathing during another period of continued contractions at 5/s. Apnea occurred and a few puffs of artificial respiration were administered at the* second arrow. **D,** *Effect of partial ischemia during continued contractions.* **E,** *Amytal effect and its washout during continued contractile activity at 5 contractions/s. The Amytal was dissolved in 20 ml of whole blood and administered by injection in the femoral artery. The washout was never complete, thus indicating a significant Amytal concentration after dilution in the body. (From Jöbsis FF, Stainsby WN: Oxidation of NADH during contractions of circulated skeletal muscle.* Respir Physiol *4:292–300, 1968.)*

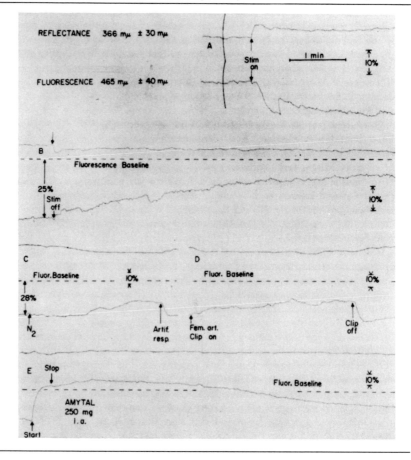

23]. Another direct assessment of mitochondrial O/R state assessing the glutamate dehydrogenase reaction has lead to the same conclusion; mitochondria are relatively oxidized during contractions under normoxic conditions [131]. Finally, a recent direct near-infrared spectrophotometric assessment of the O/R state of cytochrome oxidase, a-a_3, has shown it to become more oxidized than the resting state during repetitive twitch and tetanic contractions [105]. Net $\dot{L}$ was the same in this study as seen previously. This finding should lay to rest any arguments suggesting O_2 lack occurs under normoxic free-flow conditions.

In summary, the data agree and are consistent with the hypothesis that O_2 lack in the mitochondria does not occur and is not related to $\dot{L}$ during repetitive contractions under free flow, normoxic conditions. Both $\dot{L}$ and the limitation of $\dot{V}o_2$ at high stimulation frequencies that reach maximal $\dot{V}o_2$ values during both twitch and tetanic contractions originate via one or more other mechanisms. New data, which have yet to be tested by others, suggest that even when O_2 lack may be assumed to be present, ischemia and hypoxia, there are grounds for suggesting other mechanisms participate in the reduction of $\dot{V}o_2$. During ischemia, $\dot{L}$ was not increased. During hypoxia, $\dot{L}$ was increased only transiently. Muscle $\dot{V}o_2$ and mechanical performance are significantly affected by the blood flow through contracting muscles, and epinephrine profoundly affects $\dot{L}$.

BLOOD AND MUSCLE LACTATE CONCENTRATIONS DURING EXERCISE

Blood and Muscle Lactate Levels as the Resultant of Lactate Appearance and Removal Rates

Metabolites such as lactate and glucose are continuously formed and enter the circulation. Because this entry into the circulation is balanced by a simultaneous removal, metabolites such as lactate and glucose are said to turn over in the blood. In a metabolic steady state, the rates of appearance (R_a) and disappearance (R_d) of a metabolite will be equal, so turnover, appearance and disappearance rates will be equivalent ($R_t = R_a = R_d$). In a nonsteady state, R_a and R_d are not equal, and blood concentration rises, or falls, at a rate dependent on the pool size and the extent of imbalance between R_a and R_d (e.g., see Fig. 2.2).

The rate of turnover (R_t) in the blood can be measured by means of injecting or infusing isotopically labeled tracers and observing the dilution of isotope in the endogenous pool: $R_t = I/SAv$, where I is the isotope infusion rate and SAv is the specific activity (isotopic enrichment) in mixed venous blood. In the case of glucose, it is possible to fix hydrogen

FIGURE 2.2

Arterial lactate concentration, rate of appearance (RaL), and lactate metabolic clearance rate (MCR) as a function of time during rest and exercise at 40% of Vo₂ max in two subjects. Subject 8 was a trained endurance cyclist and subject 5 was a competitive rower. The rower shows an increase in blood lactate due to an increase in RaL. The cyclist shows a fall in arterial lactate concentration during exercise despite an increase in RaL. This is because the MCR increased approximately three times during exercise as compared to rest. (From Stanley WC, Wisneski JA, Gertz ED, Neese RA, Brooks GA: Glucose and lactate interactions during moderate intensity exercise in humans. Metabolism *37:850–858, 1988.)*

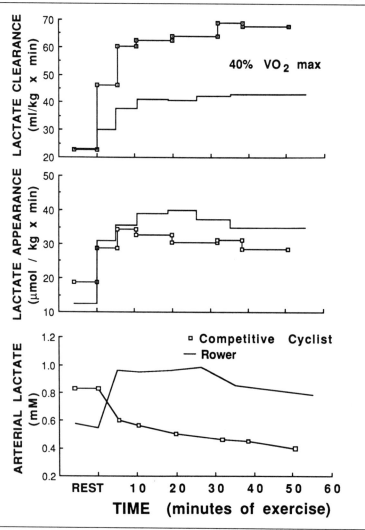

tracer atoms to glucose molecules such that when they are degraded the hydrogen atoms are unlikely to again be fixed to glucose molecules in vivo. Such atoms are said to be lost "irreversibly" and [^{3}H]glucose is an example of an "irreversible" tracer. Unfortunately, it is not possible to use hydrogen-labeled lactate to estimate lactate turnover in vivo [31, 80, 95]. In contrast to the case for hydrogen atoms, isotopes of carbon are less likely to be disposed of irreversibly in vivo. Such tracers are said to be "reversible," and their use will underestimate the "true" turnover rate. For this reason of isotopic carbon recycling, when blood lactate turnover is estimated using carbon-labeled tracer, the term "disposal rate" (R_i) is used. Because the use of isotopic tracers allows calculation of specific rates of parameters related to blood turnover, it is said that the use of tracers allows the measurement of blood metabolite "kinetics." The term "flux" is also used to describe the rate of metabolite turnover in the blood.

Inspection of the literature will reveal reports on isotope tracer studies of lactate turnover using isotopic tracers on dogs [30, 61, 62], rats [15, 31], fish [82, 124], seals [47], eels [25], lizards [48], horses [123, 125], and humans [58, 74, 75, 80, 93, 111, 113]. Tracers have been used to study not only the metabolic response to exercise, but also the responses to endotoxin shock, cancer, obesity, and hemorrhage.

Recognition of the difference between lactate accumulation and lactic acid production as afforded by isotope tracer techniques allows physiological interpretations not otherwise possible. For instance, with hemorrhagic dogs Eldridge [32] showed that elevated blood lactate was not entirely due to enhanced lactic acid production, but rather lactic acidosis was in large part due to a failure of blood lactate clearance mechanisms. Similarly, Spitzer and associates [127, 130] showed that a major factor in lactic acidosis associated with endotoxin shock was failure of blood lactate clearance mechanisms.

In a recent report Stanley et al. [111] determined parameters of blood lactate kinetics in response to submaximal leg cycling exercise in two individuals of different athletic histories (Fig. 2.2). In one individual, a trained rower, arterial lactate rose in the transition from rest to submaximal exercise. In contrast, however, blood lactate fell in the trained bicyclist during the rest-exercise transition. Use of isotopic tracers allowed the observation that exercise caused similar increments in blood lactate appearance in both individuals but that the difference in blood lactate concentration was due to greater clearance capacity in the trained cyclist. Differences in blood lactic acid clearance during exercise due to training have previously been noted in rats [31] and humans [80, 113]. As in the cases of interpreting the blood lactate response to hemorrhage and endotoxin shock, interpretation of the blood lactate response to exercise benefits from an evaluation of the balance of entry (appearance) and removal (disappearance) rates that use of isotopes can afford. Sometimes, as illustrated by the cases of shock and exercise training, the conclusions reached with tracers are, in fact, opposite those reached based on blood concentration alone.

TISSUE SITES OF LACTIC ACID PRODUCTION

Skeletal Muscle as the Major Site of Lactic Acid Production

Since the work of Fletcher and Hopkins [33] it has become recognized that contracting skeletal muscle is a site of lactic acid production. It is now routinely observed that intense exercise causes lactate accumulation in skeletal muscle and that significant quantities are released into the vasculature [69].

Figure 2.3 is from Welch and Stainsby [126], who measured lactate exchange across dog gastrocnemius muscle in situ. The following are apparent. Resting skeletal muscle releases lactate on a net basis. In some cases, however, resting skeletal muscle can take up lactate on a net basis. Regardless of the uptake-removal status at rest, when contractions commence, muscle becomes a site of net lactate release. However, if contractions continue, and if there is an absence of β-adrenergic stimulation (see below), over time contracting muscles stop being net producers of lactic acid and become net consumers even if net release occurred at rest.

For comparison Figure 2.4 is from the recent work of Richter et al. [90], who studied lactate exchange across human quadriceps muscle. During rest as well as contractions, the quadriceps released lactate (Fig. 2.4**A**). However, when arm exercise was added to leg exercise, arterial lactate rises and the quadriceps switched from net release to net lactate uptake (Fig. 2.4**B**). Similar observations were made by Gladden [40–42], who studied dog gastrocnemius in situ. Moreover, results of isotopic tracer studies on dogs [61] and humans [113] show that blood lactate disposal is concentration dependent.

Beyond demonstrating that contracting human skeletal muscle is capable of taking up lactate on a net basis, the results of Richter et al. [90] show also that lactic acid production and removal occur simultaneously. When arm exercise is added to leg exercise, it is probable that lactic acid production in the contracting quadriceps was as great as when there was leg exercise alone. Unfortunately, without benefit of a tracer it is impossible to calculate the absolute rates of lactic acid production and removal within a tissue bed. For this reason, we know that the net quadriceps release demonstrated in Figure 2.4**A** likely concealed simultaneous lactate removal. Net lactate uptake by contracting human quadriceps did, however, suppress glucose uptake.

FIGURE 2.3

Net lactate release (L) from dog gastrocnemius-plantaris preparations at rest and during contractions at 1 twitch/s. At rest, most preparations release lactate. Contractions cause a transient increase in lactate release, but most muscle switch to net uptake as exercise continues. (From Welch HG, Stainsby WN: Oxygen debt in contracting dog skeletal muscle in situ. Resp Physiol 3:229–242, 1967.)

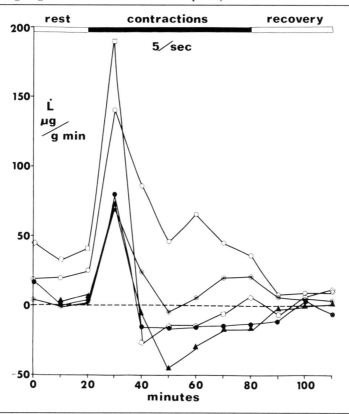

The Glucose Paradox

Studies in contemporary biochemistry and regulation of intermediary metabolism are concerned with pathways of hepatic glycogen synthesis during refeeding after a fast. These studies are important because they illustrate that significant lactic acid production can occur in non-muscular tissues during rest. From several sets of data [35, 85], it has become apparent that significant liver glycogen synthesis may occur from the "indirect pathway" whereby dietary carbohydrate is digested to glucose, and glucose is catabolized to lactic acid, which then serves as the precursor for liver glycogen synthesis. The indirect pathway complements the

FIGURE 2.4

Glucose uptake and lactate exchange in left and right thighs at rest and during six different work bouts. The order of work bouts is indicated in the cartoon. During right thigh exercise (second column), *glucose uptake and lactate release are greater in the active muscle. When arm exercise is added* (third column), *arterial lactate level rises and the active thigh switches to net lactate uptake. At the same time glucose uptake is suppressed. During arm exercise, the inactive (left) thigh consumes more lactate than when arterial lactate was low. Substitution of lactate for glucose and simultaneous lactate production and consumption in the active thigh are indicated. (From Richter EA, Kienes B, Saltin B, Christensen NJ, Savard G: Skeletal muscle glucose uptake during dynamic exercise in humans: role of muscle mass. Am J Physiol 254:E555-E561, 1988.)*

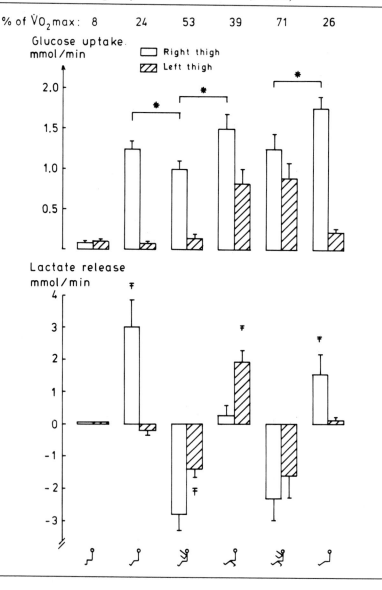

"direct pathway" in which portal blood glucose is taken up by the liver, phosphorylated to UDP glucose, and synthesized to glycogen. Because liver glycogen is paradoxically formed by the indirect, as opposed to the direct pathway, this phenomenon is alternatively referred to as the "glucose paradox." Not only are peripheral tissues such as skeletal muscle and skin implicated as anatomical sites of glucose conversion to lactic acid, but also studies in this area have revealed that intestinal mucosa [96, 129] as well as specific anatomical zones in the liver [7, 85] convert glucose to lactic acid. Even though at this time it is difficult to know with certainty the relative contributions of the "direct" and "indirect" pathways of liver glycogen synthesis, an important lesson of these studies is that muscle as well as non-muscle tissues are capable of releasing significant amounts of lactate into the systemic circulation under resting conditions. The relevance of the existence of an indirect pathway of liver glycogen synthesis after eating is that tissue hypoxia can not be regarded as the sole cause of lactic acid production.

Intestine as a Site of Lactic Acid Production

Over 30 years ago, Wilson [129] observed that cells of the intestinal wall convert dietary glucose to lactic acid. Recently, this observation has been confirmed [96]. Conversion of some of a carbohydrate load to lactate in the intestinal wall would facilitate operation of a glucose paradox because the necessity of converting glucose to lactic acid peripherally (i.e., in skeletal muscle) is reduced. The presence of a glucose paradox with a component of intestinal conversion of glucose to lactic acid is facilitated by the presence of an intestinal lactate transporter [49, 116] and by metabolic zonation of the liver (see below). Therefore, the rise in portal vein lactate in dogs after feeding observed by Davis et al. [27] was likely due to glycolysis in intestinal wall cells. Moreover, because net hepatic lactate release occurred in dogs after feeding, maintenance of stable arterial lactate levels meant that extrahepatic sites were responsible for blood lactate clearance.

Liver as a Site of Lactic Acid Production

The net hepatic lactate release in dogs observed by Davis et al. [28] was shown to be associated with glucagon stimulation. Apparently, glucagon-induced hepatic glycogenolysis can result in net releases of both glucose and lactic acid. In their work on exercising dogs, Wasserman et al. [118, 120] also attributed net hepatic release to the action of glucagon.

That the liver can be capable of both net lactate release [28, 118,120] and gluconeogenesis from lactate may be explained by segregation of function into different metabolic zones. There now exists extensive evidence (see Ref. 8 for review) that periportal regions of the liver are gluconeogenic via the indirect pathway (i.e., glycogen synthesis from 3-C precursors), whereas perivenous regions deal with glucose and are glycolytic as well as synthesize glycogen via the direct (glucose → G6P → UDPG → glycogen) pathway. This arrangement would appear to facilitate function of the glucose paradox and lactate shuttle pathways.

Skin as a Site of Lactic Acid Production

Epidermal cells of the skin are capable of taking up glucose and releasing lactate. In their review in 1972, Johnson and Fusaro [66] made a remarkable attempt to interpret this observation within the then contemporary context of skeletal muscle as the predominant site of lactic acid production and liver as the tissue responsible for lactic acid removal. To the extent that skin converts glucose to lactic acid, the action of the glucose paradox is facilitated. During exercise, glycolysis in the skin can complicate obtaining a representative blood sample when an arm vein, or similar superficial location, is the sampling site. The presence of significant glycolysis and lactic acid production in human skin during rest is, however, extremely useful in evaluating the proposition that lactic acid is formed exclusively as the result of oxygen-limited metabolism.

TISSUE SITES OF LACTIC ACID REMOVAL

Liver as a Site of Lactic Acid Removal

Since the classic work up to Himwich et al. in 1930 [53], the liver has been generally accepted to be the tissue responsible for lactic acid removal, gluconeogenesis from lactic acid, and glycogen synthesis. These classic observations have been repeatedly confirmed (e.g., see Refs. 2 and 3). However, it is becoming increasingly apparent that the liver regulates not only blood glucose homeostasis, but also overall carbohydrate substrate supply. As described immediately above and reviewed separately [12, 37], the liver can either take up lactate and release glucose or store glycogen, but also the liver can release lactate in an effort to maintain substrate supply. For our purposes in the present review, it is important to recognize that the liver is not the exclusive, or even a major, site of blood lactate clearance during exercise.

Heart as a Site of Lactate Removal

The heart is well-known as a site of net blood lactate removal [38]. However, as demonstrated by Gertz et al. [39], lactic acid production and removal occur simultaneously in the heart. As described by them, this phenomenon could not have been observed without benefit of tracers.

Carbon tracer glucose entering the coronary artery appears as lactate in the coronary sinus. Additionally, when carbon-labeled lactate enters the coronary circulation, the label appears mainly as CO_2 in the coronary sinus. For our purposes, however, the existence of simultaneous lactic acid production and net removal by healthy, beating human hearts also refutes the proposition that lactic acid production occurs exclusively because of oxygen-limited metabolism.

Skeletal Muscle as the Major Site of Lactate Removal during Exercise

In addition to the beating heart, contracting skeletal muscle is another tissue capable of taking up lactate on a net basis. The net uptake of lactate by dog skeletal muscle in situ was shown by Welch and Stainsby [126] (Fig. 2.3). During continual, phasic contractions lactate was released into the vasculature upon the initiation of contractions and was taken up as exercise continued. Some muscle preparations that released lactate during rest switched over to net lactate consumption during exercise. With similar dog muscle preparations, Gladden et al. [40–42] have shown that elevations in arterial lactate caused the uptake of lactate by contracting skeletal muscle to increase. Also with dog muscle preparations in situ, Corsi et al. [26] and Granata et al. [45] showed that tracer lactate was taken up and converted to CO_2 during contractions. To date the literature contains two reports [68, 112] using carbon tracers to show lactate and lactate tracer uptake by contracting human skeletal muscle in vivo. Because in their study Stanley et al. [112] had measures of vascular lactate appearance and disappearance rates as well as arterial-venous difference measurements across active and inactive skeletal muscle beds, they were able to show that the equivalent of approximately half the lactic acid formed during sustained, submaximal exercise was removed by oxidation in contracting skeletal muscle. As has already been discussed with regard to net lactate release by liver and other tissues during exercise onset, and as will be discussed below with regard to lactate release from noncontracting skeletal muscle due to β-adrenergic stimulation, blood lactate taken up by contracting skeletal muscle could have been produced at several anatomical sites.

Additional evidence that skeletal muscle is the major site of blood lactate removal during exercise comes from the studies of Wasserman et al. [118, 120]. In their studies on dogs during exercise, the liver released lactate at exercise onset and for an extended time thereafter. Thus, depending on the balanced effects of insulin, glucagon, and the catecholamines, it is possible that extrahepatic sites can become completely responsible for lactate removal during exercise.

As reviewed above, lactic acid is produced in the intestinal wall, liver, skin, and even healthy heart under resting conditions when there is no data to indicate, and no reason to suspect, the presence of oxygen-limited metabolism. Similarly, there is no reason to believe that lactic acid is produced in resting or even contracting skeletal muscle exclusively because of an oxygen lack.

BLOOD LACTATE KINETICS IN HUMANS DURING SUSTAINED EXERCISE

Lactate Turnover and Oxidation as Functions of Metabolic Rate

Lactate disposal has been studied during sustained, submaximal exercise in rats [31], dogs [30, 60, 61), and humans [80, 112, 113). Every study that has determined lactate disposal during exercise has reported a direct relationship between lactate disposal rate and metabolic rate as given by the oxygen consumption ($\dot{V}o_2$). Those studies that have determined lactic acid oxidation during exercise have reported that the rate of lactic acid oxidation is related to $\dot{V}o_2$, and, further, that the relative removal through oxidation increases during exercise.

In their study, Mazzeo et al. [80] reported data on six men studied at rest and during continuous exercise at 50 and 75% of $\dot{V}o_2$max (Fig. 2.5). At rest, approximately 50% of the lactate disposal was by direct oxidation. During exercise at 50% of $\dot{V}o_2$max, lactate disposal and oxidation increased compared to rest but the relative removal through oxidation increased to approximately 90%.

Stanley et al. [113] assessed the rate of lactate appearance (R_a) during graded exercise using a continuous infusion of [^{14}C]lactate in humans in an attempt to describe the mechanism of the sudden rise in arterial lactate level. The lactate R_a and rate of disappearance (R_d) were both exponential functions of the rate of oxygen consumption. Arterial lactate concentration increased during graded exercised because the rise in R_a overwhelmed the rise in R_d. The inflection point in arterial lactate concentration as a function of increments in exercise power output was not due to a sudden increase in lactate R_a without a change in R_d. Stanley et al. [113] reported the relationship between blood lactate appearance rate and oxygen consumption rate to be:

$$R_a = 1.09^{\dot{V}o_2} \text{ (9.7)}$$

where R_a is in μmol/kg·min, and $\dot{V}o_2$ is in ml/kg·min.

Under conditions of sustained moderate-intensity exercise, arterial lactate levels may increase slightly, remain the same, or decrease compared to rest [61, 111, 113]. During exercise for a given constant blood lactate level, the rate of lactic acid appearance may exceed that during

FIGURE 2.5

Blood lactate disposal (R$_i$, turnover measured with reversible carbon tracer) and oxidation (R$_{ox}$) in six men as functions of metabolic rate ($\dot{V}_{O_2}$). Direct relationships between lactate turnover and oxidation and metabolic rate are indicated. (From Mazzeo RS, Brooks GA, Schoeller DA, Budinger TF: Disposal of [1-^{13}C] lactate in humans during rest and exercise. J Appl Physiol 60:232–241, 1986.)

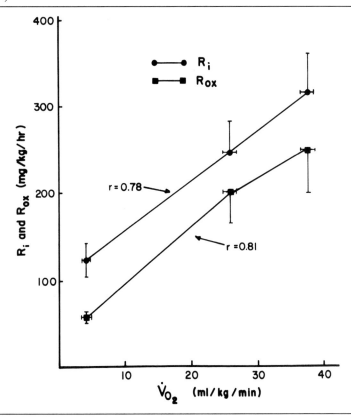

rest by 3–5-fold [69]. This is because the lactate metabolic clearance rate (MCR = Rd/[lact], and = Ri/[lact] in the steady state) increases tremendously in the transition from rest to exercise. Consequently, it is impossible to estimate lactic acid production rates during exercise from measurements of blood lactate levels, or to interpret the blood lactate inflection point solely in terms of a sudden increase in glycolysis due to oxygen-limited metabolism in skeletal muscle.

Interpretation of data on blood lactate kinetics during exercise is dependent upon validity of isotope tracer techniques. Challenges to validity of isotope dilution techniques for studies of lactate metabolism (e.g., see Ref. 71) have resulted in several approaches to assessing their validity. Literature reports using tracer [58, 74, 75, 80, 93, 111, 113] and nontracer techniques [24] provide similar values on resting humans. Moreover, simultaneous determinations of blood lactate kinetics obtained using bolus injections of labeled and unlabeled lactate [94] provide excellent agreement, particularly at elevated lactate levels. Based on recent results it is possible to conclude that under resting conditions tracer-measured blood lactate disposal (R_i) underestimates "true" lactate turnover (by approximately 20%). However, during exercise when cardiac output and arterial lactate concentration rise, the error in underestimating blood lactate turnover by tracer methods becomes only a few percent.

Human Muscle Lactate Release in Hypoxemia

In a recent report Rowell et al. [92], using graded exercise, hypoxemia (breathing 10–11% O_2), and an ergometer-measurement system, performed an extremely important experiment on the regulation of vascular resistance in active skeletal muscle. These results are relevant to our discussion of the role of oxygen limitation as a cause of muscle lactic acid production during exercise and the value of blood lactate measurements.

In the experiments of Rowell et al. [92] subjects performed graded quadriceps muscle (knee extension exercise) up to maximum while breathing air or hypoxic gas. Results indicated that quadriceps blood flow increased and (a-v)O_2 decreased during submaximal exercise so that muscle $\dot{V}O_2$ was maintained during hypoxemia. Moreover, muscle net efficiency (=caloric equivalent of work/caloric equivalent of $\dot{V}O_2$ above resting) remained at 23% during hypoxemic exercise, as it was during normoxic exercise. In contrast to the constancy of $\dot{V}O_2$ and muscular efficiency, net lactate release increased dramatically during hypoxemia. During hypoxic exercise at a submaximal power output of 38 W, the (a-v) lactate increased from approximately 0.5 to approximately 1.4 mmol/liter. Moreover, at the same time, quadriceps flow increased from 5.4 to 6.4 liters/min. Thus, the net quadriceps release almost tripled from 2.5 to 7 mmol/min. In such a circumstance there are data from which to argue that exaggerated lactate release was not due to oxygen-limited metabolism. Oxygen consumption and muscular efficiency were unchanged. Rather, the results support the conclusion that there is a change in the intramuscular lactic acid production-removal relationship that originates elsewhere. The authors observed a 3–4-fold increase in arterial epinephrine levels during exercise with hypoxia. Accordingly it is possible to suggest that the increased quadriceps lactate outflow was, in part, due to a β-adrenergic stimulation of muscle glycogenolysis.

Lactate Accumulation as a Consequence of β-Adrenergic Stimulation

We believe that the literature supports the conclusion that β-adrenergic stimulation of skeletal muscle causes an acceleration in the rate of glycogenolysis, whether the muscle is contracting or not. As already noted above, in the experiments of Rowell et al. [92], elevated lactate release was observed during hypoxic exercise when arterial epinephrine was elevated. This result is consistent with that of Stainsby et al. [98, 100, 107, 109, 110], who observed with dog muscle preparations that epinephrine stimulation exaggerated lactate release. With intact dogs Issekutz and associates [60, 62] have observed that epinephrine infusion increased tracer-measured blood lactate appearance, whereas β-adrenergic blockade reduces blood lactate appearance during exercise [60]. Most recently, Gregg et al. [46] have obtained a correlation of 0.97 (Fig. 2.6) between tracer-measured blood lactate appearance and arterial epinephrine over a wide range of epinephrine levels and lactate appearance rates in running rats.

Beyond an acceleration of glycogenolysis and muscle lactic acid pro-

FIGURE 2.6.
*Correlation between blood lactate disposal (**RiLac**) and arterial epinephrine concentration in resting and exercising anemic and control rats; r = 0.97. (From Gregg SG, Mazzeo RS, Budinger TF, Brooks GA: Acute anemia increases lactate production and decreases clearance during exercise.* J Appl Physiol *67:756– 764, 1989.)*

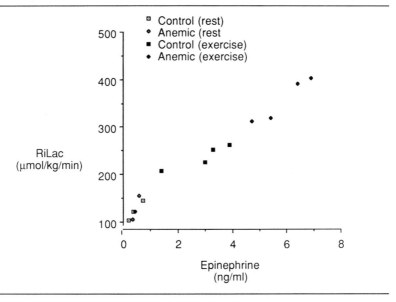

duction by stimulation of phosphorylase, epinephrine could raise blood lactate by decreasing flow through splanchnic areas of removal. In their experiment on exercising rats Gregg et al. [46] observed that elevated catecholamines were associated with shunting of blood away from liver and kidneys and decreased lactate clearance.

Not only does epinephrine stimulate glycogenolysis and lactic acid production in active skeletal muscle, but the epinephrine response is global [89]. In the recent work of Rowell et al. [92] increased arterial lactate levels during hypoxemic exercise could not be explained by muscle lactate release. In their experiments Ahlborg [1] and Ahlborg et al. [2, 3] showed that epinephrine stimulation caused lactate release from inactive skeletal muscle. Additionally, Spriet et al. [97] have provided data to show that epinephrine stimulation accelerates glycogenolysis in contracting skeletal muscle. A reasonable interpretation of this literature leads to the conclusion that with constant O_2 supply epinephrine raises blood lactate by elevating production as well as decreasing clearance.

The Lactate Shuttle Hypothesis

It is possible to extend the Cori cycle and glucose paradox concepts to form a hypothesis (the "lactate shuttle") about the role of lactate in the overall distribution of oxidizable substrate during rest and exercise. According to this hypothesis [10–12], the formation and distribution of fuel in the form of lactate provides a central means by which the coordination of intermediary metabolism in diverse tissues and different cells within the tissues is accomplished. Lactate formed in some muscle cells with high rates of glycogenolysis and glycolysis becomes an energy source not only in adjacent cells with high cellular respiratory rates, but also in anatomically remote tissues with high respiratory rates, heart (e.g., see Refs. 30 and 39), and skeletal muscle [90, 112]. The production and release of lactate also provide for distribution of the major gluconeogenic precursor [65, 117]. Support for the lactate shuttle hypothesis comes from several sources that have been reviewed previously [10]. Lactate can be exchanged between muscle and blood (e.g., see Refs. 98 and 115), between blood and muscle [68], between active and inactive muscles [112], between inactive and active muscles [1], between active and active muscles [90], between blood and heart [38], between active muscle and liver [117, 118], between liver and other tissues such as exercising muscle [118], between skin and blood [66], between intestine and portal blood [29], between portal blood and liver [7], and along pH and concentration gradients within muscle tissue [16, 91]. During exercise blood lactate turnover equals or exceeds that of glucose [31, 111, 113].

The lactate shuttle concept can be applied to the interior of cells such as muscle. Jones [67] reminds us that in the extramitochondrial space there are gradients of metabolites between sources and sinks. For example the source of both pyruvic acid and NADH is in the extramitochondrial space. The primary sink for both is the mitochondria. The pyruvate and NADH concentrations will be greatest at the center (or midline) of the extramitochondrial space and be lowest adjacent to the mitochondria. Lactic acid production and lactate concentrations should also be highest in the middle of the extramitochondrial space because that is its greatest source, because the reactants that produce it are highest there. One sink for lactate is the extracellular space. However, as pyruvate and NADH concentrations fall toward the mitochondria, there will be a place where lactic acid production, on a net basis, will be zero. Closer to the mitochondria lactic acid may go to pyruvic acid and NADH. Thus, the lactate shuttle occurs intracellularly in the extramitochondrial space. Only a minor fraction of the lactic acid formed may diffuse to the cell membrane for transport to the extracellular space, and that may be dominated by the extramitochondrial space near the cell membrane. This scene raises questions about the relation between net cell membrane exchange and lactic acid turnover far from the cell membrane and reinforces the concept that blood lactate kinetics may not reflect clearly deep intracellular activity.

The Cell Membrane Lactate Transporter

A small fraction of lactate moves across cell membranes via simple diffusion. However, most lactate appears to move across cell membranes in conjunction with a cation (Na^+ or H^+) via facilitated transport. Lactate transporters have been established to exist in erythrocytes, intestinal brush-border cells [49], and kidney [116]. More recent studies on isolated muscles [63] have led to verification of a sarcolemmal lactate transporter [16, 91]. Thus, the exchange of lactate between cells and tissues is affected by both lactate concentration and proton gradients and is thus not solely reflective of the rate of glycolysis.

Mitochondrial Lactate Dehydrogenase (LDH)

Kline and associates [73] have recognized that presence of lactic dehydrogenase (LDH) in the mitochondrial piroplasmic space facilitates the flux of reducing equivalents between the cytoplasm and mitochondrial TCA cycle and electron transport chain. Brandt and Kline have corroborated the finding of Molé et al. [84] that isolated mitochondria oxidize exogenous lactate at the same or greater rate than pyruvate. In each tissue studied to date by Brandt and Kline the mitochondrial LDH obtained appears to be isophoretically distinct from that in the surrounding cytoplasm. Thus, mitochondrial contamination with cytoplasmic components during isolation does not appear to be responsible for their results.

Muscle Mitochondrial Redox during Exercise

The importance of knowing the status of muscle mitochondrial oxygenation during exercise has produced several approaches to addressing this technically difficult problem. One approach has been to use measures of blood lactate and pyruvate [59]. This approach requires assumptions about equilibria between lactate and pyruvate in the central circulation and contracting muscles. Further, assumptions about the equilibrium between cytoplasmic and mitochondrial redox are required. We conclude that the circulatory lactate/pyruvate is of little value in assessing the status of mitochondrial redox and oxygenation in contracting muscles.

Another approach has been to measure NADH and NAD^+ in biopsy samples taken from exercising muscles. Such measurements have led to the conclusion that lactic acid formation in contracting skeletal muscle is caused by oxygen-limited metabolism [71]. Validity of the NADH/NAD^+ measurements as representative of mitochondrial redox status has been challenged on the basis that the technical approach could not distinguish between intra- and extra-mitochondrial NADH/NAD^+, and between free and bound NADH and NAD^+. Most recently, Graham and Saltin [44] evaluated the effect of exercise on human muscle mitochondrial redox from the mass-action ratio for the glutamate dehydrogenase (GDH) reaction. This enzyme was used because it is located only in the mitochondrial compartment and because it has sufficient activity to reach equilibrium in vivo. This system has been used by numerous investigators to study the mitochondrial redox state of liver, heart, brain, and skeletal muscle (see Graham and Saltin [44] for details). Despite large increases in muscle and blood lactate during submaximal and maximal exercise, they observed an increase in the mass-action ratio for the GDH reaction, which should be reflective of a rise in the mitochondrial NAD/NADH. As a result of their observations, Graham and Saltin concluded that the mitochondrial electron transport chain of skeletal muscle is more oxidized during exercise than during rest. In this regard, the results of Graham and Saltin are consistent with similar measurements in muscle [131], and with those of Jobsis and Stainsby [64], Olgin et al. [86], and Connett et al. [22, 23] obtained on dog skeletal muscle contracting in situ, and are contradictory to the conclusions based on measurements of NAD/NADH in biopsy specimens [71].

SUMMARY, CONCLUSIONS, AND INTEGRATION

The Role of O_2 in Lactic Acid Production

In muscles in situ, self perfused with the animal's blood during repetitive (or phasic) contractions and normoxic conditions, there is no clear evidence that lack of O_2 limits $\dot{V}O_2$ at any level or has any direct role in the production or removal of lactic acid. The valid assessments of mitochondrial oxidation/reduction state all indicate that the mitochondria are relatively oxidized. Mitochondrial NAD/NADH was always relatively oxidized during contractions. The measurements of intracellular Po_2 via myoglobin saturation showed it to be low but adequate for oxidative phosphorylation, and cytochrome oxidase became more oxidized during contractions. The only assessment of mitochondrial O/R state that implied reduction of the mitochondria is the indirect assessment based on chemical measurements of muscle NAD, NADH, lactate, and pyruvate. There are several assumptions in the analysis, some of which are indefensible. The most critical is the assumption of a relationship between cytoplasmic and mitochondrial NAD/NADH. Since reducing equivalent transport across the inner mitochondrial membrane is active transport [29], dependent upon the mitochondrial membrane potential and other unmeasured factors, this assumption is not likely to be valid.

Exercise

The evidence available in exercise is less extensive than that for muscles in situ, but the conclusion from that evidence is the same; O_2 lack per se does not limit $\dot{V}O_2max$ and has no direct role in the muscles on the production or removal of lactic acid. The assessment of mitochondrial O/R state by the mitochondrial glutamate dehydrogenase reaction showed the same response in active muscles during exercise as it did in muscles in situ, oxidation. The assessment based on chemically measured NAD, NADH, lactate, and pyruvate suggested the opposite, but the assumptions of that assessment are probably not valid. Therefore, the assessment is probably not valid.

THE ORIGINS OF LACTIC ACID

In Situ Muscle

Why then do muscles in situ produce lactic acid during contractions? It is important to note that in muscles in situ stimulated to contract phasically without other perturbations, net lactic acid output, reflecting the balance of the intracellular lactate production and removal, is a transient event [34, 126]. It occurs during the transition from rest to steady activity. When a steady level is reached after 10–20 min of contractions, the net lactic acid output is nearly zero at all levels of $\dot{V}O_2$. In fact, the average $\dot{L}$ within the usual range of arterial lactate concentrations, between 1.0 and 2.0 μmol/ml, is a small uptake. When the arterial lactate concentration is elevated this uptake increases and the increase appears to be greater the higher the $\dot{V}O_2$.

The origin of the net lactic acid output during the rest-to-activity transition has been presented previously [108]. Since then no contrary proposal has been promulgated. Briefly, the proposal suggested that the origin of the net lactic acid output was an imbalance between the production of the products of glycolysis, pyruvic acid and NADH, and the removal of these products into the mitochondria for oxidative phosphorylation. Initially glycogenolysis is stimulated by the same rise in cytoplasmic Ca^{2+} that initiates the contractions. This is supplemented later by rising cytoplasmic P_i and other factors. The removal of the products into the mitochondria is delayed as the pyruvate dehydrogenase reaction is activated by Ca^{2+} and pyruvate, and by a slight delay in activation of the TCA cycle and the electron transport chain. Mitochondrial NAD/NADH reached full oxidation from the relatively reduced resting state after 1–2 min. Transport of high energy phosphates to and from the mitochondria is restricted until the concentration of Cr is elevated for operation of the creatine-creatine kinase shuttle [8, 81]. During the transition the balance favors net lactic acid production and intracellular lactate rises. The mechanisms for transport of lactic acid out of the muscle cells as pointed out above is currently under intensive investigation. It is complicated. For this summary it may be sufficient to say that the transport is restricted, equilibrium is not achieved, significant cell-to-blood gradients do exist, and the net output may be delayed significantly relative to net production. Thus 10–20 min are required to establish the steady level.

It should follow from this proposal to explain lactic acid production during the rest-to-activity transition that any stimulus for glycolysis should increase net lactic acid output. A well-known group of stimulators of glycolysis are the β-adrenergic agonists. Epinephrine and isoproterenol increase net lactic acid output of contracting muscles transiently. This action of these agonists is blocked by β-adrenergic-antagonists and appears to be inhibited by α-adrenergic agonists. It is not yet known why the stimulation of net lactic acid output by β-adrenergic agonists is transient. Either the stimulatory actions are inherently brief or there are control reactions in the cells that inhibit the response over time. The β-adrenergic stimulation does not appear to be restricted to the rest-to-activity transition phase. Although not studied systematically, it has been shown to occur during the steady-level phase [98].

Exercise

In exercise the major focus has been on the blood lactate concentration and how much and when it changes during progressive and steady-level conditions. The blood concentration of lactate and changes in blood lactate concentrations are the resultant of additions of lactic acid to the blood by some tissues or parts of tissues and removal of lactic acid from the blood by others. This is complicated and not yet systematically quantified during exercise for many tissues. Therefore, the discussion must be relatively general.

In exercise of short duration up to 15 min, the contribution of lactic acid from the active muscles will be derived from net muscle lactate exchange during the rest-to-activity transition phase. The contribution will be directly related to the mass of active muscles and the number of stimulatory impulses delivered to the muscles to activate them. The latter relation is extrapolated from the cat-dog muscle comparison [79, 101]. The net $\dot{L}$ for both was similar for the same stimulation frequencies regardless of $\dot{V}o_2$, and the proportionality constant seems to increase as activation rises. In general terms this means that the net release of lactic acid from muscle to blood is determined by the mass of active muscle and the intensity of the activation of these muscles. There will be fine-point variations in this generality related to fiber types, blood flow and its distribution, and effectors of membrane lactic acid transport that are beyond the scope of this review. How high the blood lactate rises for a given mass and intensity of stimulation will also be directly related to the duration of the activity within the limits of the proposed time frame. The contribution of muscle-derived lactic acid will be significantly modified if effectors of muscle glycolysis or glycogenolysis change. For example, if the epinephrine concentration of the blood is elevated the net output of lactic acid by the active muscles will be increased.

The basic determinants of lactic acid removal from the blood by active muscle appear to be the concentration of lactate in the blood and the activity level. The higher the blood lactate concentration and activity level, the greater the net removal of lactate from the blood will be. Precise quantification of the removal by inactive muscle compared to skin, liver, heart, or other tissues is not yet possible. This removal of lactic acid from the blood will also be significantly affected by effectors of glycolysis, glycogenolysis, and gluconeogenesis. Two of these effectors are epinephrine and glucagon. Epinephrine will reduce lactate removal and in some tissues convert removal from the blood to addition to the blood.

Putting together the basic determinants of addition of lactic acid to the blood with the basic determinants of removal from the blood provides the following scenario for a progressive exercise test. Lactic acid addition to the blood by muscle rises in increasing proportion to the increasing number of muscle motor fibers recruited and the intensity of activation. Thus the blood lactate concentration would be expected to rise in a curvilinear manner as work and $\dot{V}o_2$ increase. At the same time the removal of lactic acid from the blood should rise as blood lactate concentration and activity rise. As a result, the rate of rise of blood lactate will be slow during this stage of the test. However, when blood epinephrine begins to rise during the progress of the test, the contribution of lactic acid by the active muscles will be increased while the removal by other tissues will be decreased or switched to addition to the blood. From these considerations it is easy to envision a pattern of blood lactate like that actually seen in a progressive exercise test. Blood lactate rises slowly at the lower work rates and then rises progressively more rapidly as work rate and $\dot{V}o_2$ rise to $\dot{V}o_2$max.

During long duration, steady-level exercise blood lactate concentration appears to be relatively stable. Apparently, a balance is achieved between production and removal. Because active muscle would be predicted to remove lactic acid from the blood during the steady-level phase, other tissues must contribute significant lactic acid to the blood. Further investigation under these conditions is needed.

Blood Flow

There are other complicating interacting factors in exercise that are not present during contractions of muscles in situ. One of these that seems to be of significant importance, which was alluded to earlier, may be generalized as competition for blood flow. Rowell et al. [92] have pointed out that the blood flow through the leg extensor group is greater when it works alone than when a large additional muscle mass is active at the same time. The exact mechanisms by which this occurs are complicated and not clearly established, but the generalities seem to go as follows. As exercise intensity and the mass of active muscle increases, central command in concert with assorted peripheral chemoreceptor and mechanoreceptor afferent inputs increases sympathetic vasoconstrictor activity to muscle and other tissues. In the active muscles this constrictor activity is opposed by local vasodilator mechanisms, which are linked by unknown mechanisms to the metabolic rate of the muscle. In muscles in situ the vasodilation is roughly proportional to $\dot{V}o_2$ but, as would be expected for proportional control systems, the system does not fully compensate. As a result, flow does not rise as much as $\dot{V}o_2$, and extraction of O_2 increases to aid in the elevation of $\dot{V}o_2$. During exercise, flow would rise even less as extrinsic constrictor activity increases, and a further increase in extraction, compared to muscles in situ, would be predicted. However, there is something unique about the effects of reduced flow or ischemia in muscle. In muscles contracting in situ, reduction of arterial inflow causes a rapid decrease in contractile activity [43]. Immediately after a sudden modest (20–30%) reduction in flow the force of contraction decreases with little increase in extraction. As a result, $\dot{V}o_2$ decreases almost as much as the flow. Recent studies [106] have confirmed this flow effect during isotonic contractions and have shown that $\dot{L}$ was not significantly increased. These findings indicate that contracting muscle performance and $\dot{V}o_2$ are very sensitive to changes in blood flow and suggest that the effect is not mediated via O_2 limitation in the mitochondria. The mechanism is unknown. Whatever the mechanism, flow is a significant effector of $\dot{V}o_2$, and when it is changed $\dot{V}o_2$ may be changed. Because of competition for flow, the maximal $\dot{V}o_2$ of a given muscle will be reduced, compared to that when working alone, when a large mass of muscle is active at the same time.

Speculating further along this line we propose that mild hypoxia, which itself should not be sufficient to decrease $\dot{V}o_2$ of muscles in situ, may reduce $\dot{V}o_2$max in exercise via a reduction in flow through the muscles. Chemoreceptor responses to the hypoxia may increase sympathetic vasoconstriction and reduce muscle flow and $\dot{V}o_2$. If blood epinephrine also rises, blood lactate concentration will rise. But at no time need the muscle be so hypoxic that O_2 transport per se limits oxidative phosphorylation in the muscles. This flow effect on muscle $\dot{V}o_2$ may be the final path of other effectors of $\dot{V}o_2$max, from decreased cardiac function and blood volume changes to blood doping, and suggests that none of them is mediated directly via O_2 transport changes.

CONCLUSION

Causes of muscle and whole-body lactic acid production are several. At the level of isolated muscle tissue, factors such as contraction pattern, duration of contraction, substrate availability, hypoxia, and β-adrenergic stimulation play pivotal roles. Recent findings suggest that metabolic control systems in the cells produce significant modulator effects, and that ischemia is a unique issue. At the whole-body level, circulating lactate levels depend on the balance of release and uptake of lactate from diverse tissues, which can, depending on the conditions, change from net producers to consumers or vice versa. An oxygen limitation to metabolism can increase muscle lactate production and raise circulating levels, but hypoxia is only one of the causes of elevated lactate production and accumulation. Usually, oxygen-limited metabolism is not a cause of lactate production. A major effector of blood lactate is the β-adrenergic receptor system. From our reading of the literature, we conclude that it is a mistake to interpret lactate accumulation solely on the basis of increased production. Rather, lactate is a metabolic intermediate that can be formed, shared, and utilized within and among cells and tissues.

ACKNOWLEDGMENTS

This work was supported in part by National Institutes of Health Grant AR 39378-02 and American Heart Association Grant 860879. We gratefully acknowledge the tireless efforts of Pia Jacobs and Janine Balcom in preparing the manuscript.

REFERENCES

1. Ahlborg G: Mechanism of glycogenolysis in nonexercising human muscle during and after exercise. *Am J Physiol* 248:E540–E545, 1985.
2. Ahlborg G, Felig P: Lactate and glucose exchange across the forearm, legs and splanchnic bed during and after prolonged leg exercise. *J Clin Invest* 69:45–54, 1982.
3. Ahlborg G, Wahren J, Felig P: Splanchnic and peripheral glucose and lactate metabolism during and after prolonged arm exercise. *J Clin Invest* 77:690–699, 1986.
4. Barbee RW, Stainsby WN, Chirtel SJ: Dynamics of O_2, CO_2, lactate, and acid exchange during contractions and recovery. *J Appl* Physiol 54:1687–1692, 1978.
5. Barclay JK, Stainsby WN: The role of blood flow in limiting maximal metabolic rate in muscle. *Med Sci Sports* 7:116–119, 1975.
6. Barclay JK: A delivery-independent blood flow effect on skeletal muscle fatigue. *J Appl Physiol* 61:1084–1090, 1986.
7. Bartels H, Vogt B, Jungerman K: Glycogen synthesis via the indirect pathway in periportal and via the direct glucose utilizing pathway in the perivenous zone of perfused rat liver. *Histochemistry* 89:253–260, 1988.
8. Bessman SP, Geiger PJ: Transport of energy in muscle: the phosphorylcreatine shuttle. *Science* 211:448–452, 1981.
9. Brandt RB, Laux JE, Spainhour SE, Kline ES: Lactate dehydrogenase in rat mitochondria. *Arch Biochem Biophys* 259:412–422, 1987.
10. Brooks GA: Lactate, glycolytic end product and oxidative substrate during exercise in mammals: "The Lactate Shuttle." In Gilles R (ed): *Comparative Physiology and Biochemistry: Current Topics and Trends,* vol A, *Respiration Metabolism—Circulation.* New York, Springer-Verlag, 1985.
11. Brooks GA: The lactate shuttle during exercise and recovery. *Med Sci Sports Exerc* 18:360–368, 1986.
12. Brooks GA: Lactate production under fully aerobic conditions: the lactate shuttle during rest and exercise. *Fed Proc* 45:2924–2929, 1986.
13. Brooks GA, Donovan CM: Effect of endurance training on glucose kinetics during exercise. *Am J Physiol* 244:E505–E512, 1983.
14. Brooks GA, Gaesser GA: End points of lactate and glucose metabolism after exhausting exercise. *J Appl Physiol* 49:1057–1069, 1980.
15. Brooks GA, Henderson SA, Dallman PR: Increased glucose dependence in resting, iron-deficient rats. *Am J Physiol* 253:E461–E466, 1987.
16. Brooks GA, Roth DA: Characterization of the lactate transporter in muscle. *Med Sci Sports Exerc* 21:S35, 1989.
17. Brooks GA, Stanley WC: Measuring lactate production. *Am J Physiol* 253:E472–E473, 1987.
18. Chance B, Williams GR: Respiratory enzymes in oxidative phosphorylation. I–III. *J Biol Chem* 217:383–427, 1955.
19. Chapler CK, Stainsby WN: Carbohydrate metabolism in contracting dog skeletal muscle *in situ. Am J Physiol* 215:995–1004, 1968.
20. Chirtel SJ, Barbee RW, Stainsby WN: Net O_2, CO_2, lactate, and acid exchange by muscle during progressive working contractions. *J Appl Physiol* 56:161–165, 1984.
21. Connett RJ, Gayeski TEJ, Honig CR, Brooks GA: Defining hypoxia: a systems view of Vo_2 glycolysis, energetics and intracellular Po_2. *J Appl Physiol* (in press).
22. Connett RJ, Gayeski TEJ, Honig CR: Lactate accumulation in fully aerobic, working, dog gracilis muscle. *Am J Physiol* 246:H120–H128, 1984.

23. Connett RJ, Gayeski TEJ, Honig CR: Lactate efflux is unrelated to intracellular P_{O_2} in a working red skeletal muscle *in situ. J Appl Physiol* 61:402–408, 1986.
24. Connor H, Woods HF, Lindingham JGG: A model of L(+)-lactate metabolism in normal man. *Ann Nutr Metab* 216:254–263, 1982.
25. Cornish I, Moon TW: Glucose and lactate kinetics in American eel *Anguilla rostata. Am J Physiol* 249:R67–R72, 1985.
26. Corsi A, Midrio M, Granata AL, Corgnati A, Wolf D: Lactate oxidation by skeletal muscle *in vivo* after denervation. *Am J Physiol* 223:219–222, 1972.
27. Davis MA, Williams PE, Cherrington AD: Effect of a mixed meal on hepatic lactate and gluconeogenic precursor metabolism in dogs. *Am J Physiol* 247:E362–E369, 1984.
28. Davis MA, Williams PE, Cherrington AD: Effect of glucagon on hepatic lactate metabolism in the conscious dog. *Am J Physiol* 248:E463–E470, 1985.
29. Davis EJ, Bremer J, Akerman KE: Thermodynamic aspects of translocation of reducing equivalents by mitochondria. *J Biol Chem* 255:2277–2283, 1980.
30. Depocas F, Minaire Y, Chatonnet J: Rates of formation and oxidation of lactic acid in dogs at rest and during moderate exercise. *Can J Physiol Pharmocol* 47:603–610, 1969.
31. Donovan CM, Brooks GA: Training affects lactate clearance not lactate production. *Am J Physiol* 244:E83–E92, 1983.
32. Eldridge FL: Relationship between lactate turnover rate and blood concentration in hemorrhagic shock. *J Appl Physiol* 37:321–323, 1974.
33. Fletcher WH, Hopkins FG: Lactic acid in amphibian muscle. *J Physiol* 35:247–309, 1907.
34. Flock EV, Ingle DJ, Bollman JL: Formation of lactic acid, an initial process in working muscle. *J Biol Chem* 129:99–110, 1939.
35. Foster DW: From glycogen to ketones—and back. *Diabetes* 33:1188–1199, 1984.
36. Gaesser GA, Brooks GA: Glycogen repletion following continuous and intermittent exercise to exhaustion. *J Appl Physiol* 49:722–728, 1980.
37. Gaesser GA, Brooks GA: Metabolic bases of excess post-exercise oxygen consumption. *Med Sci Sports Exerc* 16:29–43, 1984.
38. Gertz EW, Wisneski JA, Stanley WC, Neese RA: Myocardial substrate utilization during exercise in humans: dual carbon-labeled carbohydrate isotope experiments. *J Clin Invest* 82:2017–2025, 1988.
39. Gertz EW, Wisneski JA, Neese R, Bristow JD, Searle GL, Hanlon JT: Myocardial lactate metabolism: evidence of lactate release during net chemical extraction in man. *Circulation* 63:1273–1279, 1981.
40. Gladden LB, Yates JW: Lactic acid infusion in dogs: effects of varying infusate pH. *J Appl Physiol* 54:1254–1260, 1983.
41. Gladden LB: Blood flow and A-V lactate difference during lactate uptake by *in situ* canine skeletal muscle. *Med Sci Sports Exerc* 21:S35, 1989.
42. Gladden LB: Lactate uptake by skeletal muscle. In Pandolf KB (ed): *Exercise and Sport Sciences Review.* Baltimore, Williams & Wilkins, 1989, pp 115–155.
43. Gorman MW, Barclay JK, Sparks HV: Effects of ischemia on $\dot{V}_{O_2}$, tension, and vascular resistance in contracting canine skeletal muscle. *J Appl Physiol* 65:1075–1081, 1988.
44. Graham TE, Saltin B: Estimation of mitochondrial redox state in human skeletal muscle during exercise. *J Appl Physiol* 66:561–566, 1989.
45. Granata AL, Midrio M, Corsi A: Lactate oxidation by skeletal muscle during contractions *in vivo. Pflugers Arch* 366:247–250, 1976.
46. Gregg SG, Mazzeo RS, Budinger TF, Brooks GA: Acute anemia increases lactate production and decreases clearance during exercise. *J Appl Physiol* 67:756–764, 1989.
47. Guppy M, Hill RD, Schneider RC, Qvist J, Liggins GC, Zapol WM, Hochachka PW: Microcomputer-assisted metabolic studies of voluntary diving Weddell seals. *Am J Physiol* 250:R175–R187, 1986.

48. Guppy M, Bradshaw SD, Fergusson B, Hansen IA, Atwood C: Metabolism in lizards: low lactate turnover and advantages of heterothermy. *Am J Physiol* 253:R77–R82, 1987.

49. Hildman B, Storelli C, Haase W, Barac-Nieto M, Murer H: Sodium ion/lactate co-transport in rabbit small intestinal brush-border-membrane vesicles. *Biochem J* 186:169–176, 1980.

50. Hill AV, Lupton H: Muscular exercise, lactic acid and the supply and utilization of oxygen. *Q J Med* 16:135–171, 1923.

51. Hill AV, Long CNH, Lupton H: Muscular exercise, lactic acid, and the supply and utilization of oxygen. IV–VIII. *Proc R Soc Lond (Biol)* 97:84–176, 1924.

52. Hill AV, Long CNH, Lupton H: Muscular exercise, lactic acid and the supply and utilization of oxygen. I–III. *Proc R Soc Lond (Biol)* 96:438, 1924; 97:176, 1924.

53. Himwich HE, Koskoff YD, Nahlum LH: Studies in carbohydrate metabolism. I. A glucose-lactic acid cycle involving muscle and liver. *J Biol Chem* 85:571–584, 1930.

54. Hochachka PW, Guppy M: *Metabolic Arrest and the Control of Biological Time.* Cambridge, MA, Harvard University Press, 1987.

55. Hogan MC, Roca J, West JB, Wagner PD: Dissociation of maximal O_2 uptake from O_2 delivery in canine gastrocnemius *in situ. J Appl Physiol* 66:1219–1226, 1989.

56. Hogan MC, Welch HG: Effect of altered arterial O_2 tensions on muscle metabolism in dog skeletal muscle during fatiguing work. *Am J Physiol* 251:C216–C222, 1986.

57. Hogan MC, Roca J, Wagner FD, West JB: Limitation of maximal O_2 uptake and performance by acute hypoxia in dog muscle *in situ. J Appl Physiol* 65:815–821, 1988.

58. Holyrod CP, Axelrod RS, Skutches CL, Haff AC, Paul P, Reichard GA: Lactate metabolism in patients with metastatic colorectal cancer. *Cancer Res* 39:4900–4904, 1979

59. Huckabee WE: Relationship of pyruvate and lactate during anaerobic metabolism. II. Exercise and the formation of oxygen debt. *J Clin Invest* 37:255–263, 1958.

60. Issekutz B: Effect of beta-adrenergic blockade on lactate turnover in exercising dogs. *J Appl Physiol* 57:1754–1759, 1984.

61. Issekutz B, Shaw WAS, Issekutz AC: Lactate metabolism in resting and exercising dogs. *J Appl Physiol* 40:312–319, 1976.

62. Issekutz B, Allen M: Effect of catecholamine and methylprednisolone on carbohydrate metabolism in dogs. *Metobolism* 21:48–59, 1972.

63. Jeul C: Intracellular pH recovery and lactate efflux in mouse soleus muscles stimulated *in vitro:* the involvement of a sodium/proton exchange as a lactate carrier. *Acta Physiol Scand* 132:363–371, 1988.

64. Jöbsis FF, Stainsby WN: Oxidation of NADH during contractions of circulated skeletal muscle. *Respir Physiol* 4:292–300, 1968.

65. John-Alder HB, McAlister RM, Terjung RL: Reduced running endurance in gluconeogenesis-inhibited rats. *Am J Physiol* 251:R137–R142, 1986.

66. Johnson JA, Fusaro RM: The role of skin in carbohydrate metabolism. *Adv Metab Disord* 6:1–55, 1972.

67. Jones DP: Intracellular diffusion gradients of O_2 and ATP. *Am J Physiol* 250:C663–C675, 1986.

68. Jorfeldt L: Metabolism of L-(+)-lactate in human skeletal muscle during exercise. *Acta Physiol Scand (Suppl)* 338:1–67, 1970.

69. Karlsson J, Diamant B, Saltin B: Muscle metabolites during submaximal and maximal exercise in man. *Scand J Clin Lab Invest* 39:179–183, 1971.

70. Katz JF, Okajima F, Chenoweth M, Dunn A: The determination of lactate turnover *in vivo* with ^3H and ^{14}C-labeled lactate. *Biochem J* 194:513–524, 1981.

71. Katz A, Sahlin K: Regulation of lactic acid production during exercise. *J Appl Physiol* 65:509–518, 1988.

72. King CE, Dodd SL, Cain SM: Muscle O_2 deficit during hypoxia and two levels of O_2 demand. *J Appl Physiol* 62:1384–1391, 1987.

73. Kline ES, Brandt RB, Laux JE, Spinhour SE, Higgins E, Rogers KS, Tinsley SB, Walters MG: Location of L-lactate dehydrogenase in mitochondria. *Arch Biochem Biophys* 246:673–680, 1986.
74. Kreisberg RA, Owen WC, Segal AM: Ethanol-induced hyperlacticademia: inhibition of lactate utilization. *J Ciin Invest* 50:166–174, 1971.
75. Kreisberg RA, Fennington LF, Boshell BR: Lactate turnover and gluconeogenesis in normal and obese humans. *Diabetes* 19:53–63, 1977.
76. Lehman SL, Stanley WC: Measuring tracer turnover from tracer specific activity in the steady state. *Am J Physiol* 255:E94–E98, 1988.
77. Lewis SF, Haller RG: The pathophysiology of McArdle's disease: clues to regulation in exercise and fatigue. *J Appl Physiol* 61:391–401, 1986.
78. Margaria R, Edwards HT, Dill DB: Possible mechanisms of contracting and paying oxygen debt and the role of lactic acid in muscular contraction. *Am J Physiol* 106:689–715, 1933.
79. Maxwell LC, Barclay JK, Mohrman DE, Faulkner JA: Physiological characteristics of skeletal muscles of dogs and cats. *Am J Physiol* 233:C14–C18, 1977.
80. Mazzeo RS, Brooks GA, Schoeller DA, Budinger TF: Disposal of (1-^{13}C]lactate in humans during rest and exercise. *J Appl Physiol* 60:232–241, 1986.
81. Meyer RA, Sweeney HL, Kushmerick MJ: A simple analysis of the "phosphocreatine shuttle." *Am J Physiol* 246:C365–C377, 1984.
82. Milligan CL, McDonald DG: *In vivo* lactate kinetics at rest and during recovery from exhaustive exercise in coho salmon (*Oncorhynchus Kisutch*) and starry flounder (*Platichthys stellatus*) . *J Exp Biol* 135:119–131, 1988.
83. Mohrman DE, Regal RR: Relation of blood flow to $\dot{V}o_2$, Po_2, and Pco_2 in dog gastrocnemius muscle. *Am J Physiol* 255:H1004–H1010, 1988.
84. Mole PA, Van Handel PJ, Sandel WR: Extra O_2 consumption attributable to $NADH_2$ during maximum lactate oxidation in the heart. *Biochem Biophys Res Commun* 85:1143–1149, 1978.
85. Newgard CB, Hirsch LJ, Foster DW, McGarry JM: Studies on the mechanism by which exogenous glucose is converted into liver glycogen in the rat: a direct or indirect pathway. *J Biol Chem* 258: 1254–1256, 1983.
86. Olgin J, Connett RJ, Chance B: Mitochondrial redox changes during rest-work transition in dog gracilis muscle. *Adv Exp Biol Med* 200:545–554, 1986.
87. Petrofsky JS, Phillips CA, Sawka MN, Hanpeter D, Stafford D: Blood flow and metabolism during isometric contractions in cat skeletal muscle. *J Appl Physiol* 50:493–502, 1981.
88. Pope A, Scharf SM, Brown R: Diaphragm metabolism during supramaximal phrenic nerve stimulation. *J Appl Physiol* 66:567–572, 1989.
89. Richter EA, Sonne B, Christensen NJ, Galbo H: Role of epinephrine for muscular glycogenolysis and pancreatic hormonal secretion in running rats. *Am J Physiol* 240:E526–E532, 1981.
90. Richter EA, Kienes B, Saltin B, Christensen NJ, Savard G: Skeletal muscle glucose uptake during dynamic exercise in humans: role of muscle mass. *Am J Physiol* 254:E555-E561, 1988.
91. Roth DA, Brooks GA: Facilitated lactate transport across muscle membranes. *Med Sci Sports Exerc* 21:S35, 1989.
92. Rowell LB, Saltin B, Kiens B, Christensen NJ: Is peak quadriceps blood flow in humans even higher during exercise with hypoxemia? *Am J Physiol* 251:H1038–H1044, 1986.
93. Searle GL, Cavalieri RR: Determination of lactate kinetics in the human: analysis of data from single injection and continuous infusion. *Proc Soc Exp Biol Med* 139:1002, 1972.
94. Searle GL, Feingold KR, Hsu FSF, Clark OH, Gertz EW, Stanley WC: Inhibition of endogenous lactate turnover with lactate infusion in humans. *Metabolism* 38:1120–1123, 1989.

95. Shiota M, Golden S, Katz J: Lactate metabolism in the perfused rat hindlimb. *Biochem J* 222:281–292, 1984.
96. Smadja C, Morin J, Ferre P, Girard J: Metabolic fate of a gastric glucose load in unrestrained rats bearing a portal vein catheter. *Am J Physiol* 254:E407–E413, 1988.
97. Spriet L, Ren JM, Hultman E: Epinephrine infusion enhances muscle glycogenolysis during prolonged electrical stimulation. *J Appl Physiol* 64:1439–1444, 1988.
98. Stainsby WN, Welch HG: Lactate metabolism of contracting dog skeletal muscle. *Am J Physiol* 211:177–183, 1966.
99. Stainsby WN, Barclay JK: Exercise metabolism: O_2 deficit, steady level of O_2 uptake and O_2 uptake in recovery. *Med Sci Sports* 2:177–186, 1970.
100. Stainsby WN, Sumners C, Eitzman PD: Effects of adrenergic agonists and antagonists on muscle O_2 uptake and lactate metabolism. *J Appl Physiol* 62:1845–1851, 1987.
101. Stainsby WN, Eitzman PD: Lactic acid output of cat gastrocnemius-plantaris during repetitive twitch contractions. *Med Sci Sports Exerc* 18:668–673, 1986.
102. Stainsby WN, Eitzman PD: Roles of CO_2, O_2, and acid in arteriovenous [H^+] difference during contractions. *J Appl Physiol* 65:1803–1810, 1988.
103. Stainsby WN, Otis AB: Blood flow, blood oxygen tension, oxygen uptake, and oxygen transport in skeletal muscle. *Am J Physiol* 206:858–866, 1964.
104. Stainsby WN: Local control of regional blood flow. *Annu Rev Physiol* 35:151–168, 1973.
105. Stainsby WN, Brechue WF, O'Drobinak DM, Barclay JK: The oxidation/reduction state of cytochrome oxidase during repetitive contractions. *J Appl Physiol* 67:2158–2162, 1989.
106. Stainsby WN, Brechue WF, O'Drobinak DM, Barclay JK: Effects of ischemia and hypoxic hypoxia on $\dot{V}o_2$ and lactic acid output during tetanic contractions. *J Appl Physiol* (in press).
107. Stainsby WN, Sumners C, Eitzman PD: Effects of catecholamines on lactic acid output during progressive working contractions. *J Appl Physiol* 59:1809–1814, 1985.
108. Stainsby WN: Biochemical and physiological bases for lactate production. *Med Sci Sports Exerc* 18:341–343, 1986.
109. Stainsby WN, Sumners C, Eitzman PD: Effects of catecholamines and their effect on blood lactate and muscle lactate output. *J Appl Physiol* 57:321–325, 1984.
110. Stainsby WN, Sumners C, Andrew GM: Plasma catecholamines and their effect on blood lactate and muscle lactate output. *J Appl Physiol* 57:321–325, 1984.
111. Stanley WC, Wisneski JA, Gertz ED, Neese RA, Brooks GA: Glucose and lactate interactions during moderate-intensity exercise in humans. *Metabolism* 37:850–858, 1988.
112. Stanley WC, Gertz EW, Wisneski JA, Neese RA, Morris DL, Brooks GA: Lactate extraction during net lactate release by the exercising legs of man. *J Appl Physiol* 60:1116–1120, 1986.
113. Stanley WC, Gertz EW, Wisneski JA, Neese RA, Brooks GA: Systemic lactate kinetics during graded exercise in man. *Am J Physiol* 249:E595–E602, 1985.
114. Stanley WC, Lehman SJ: A model for measurement of lactate disappearance with isotopic tracers in the steady state. *Biochem J* 256:1035–1038, 1988.
115. Steinhagen C, Hirche HJ, Nestle HW, Bovenkamp U, Hosselmann I: The interstitial pH of the working gastrocnemius muscle of the dog. *Pflugers Arch* 367:151–156, 1976.
116. Storelli C, Corcelli A, Cassano G, Hildman B, Murer M, Lippe C: Polar distribution of sodium-dependent and sodium-independent transport system for L-lactate in plasma membrane of rat enterocytes. *Pflugers Arch* 388:11–16, 1980.
117. Turcotte LP, Brooks GA: Glucose kinetics in MPA-treated rats. *Med Sci Sports Exerc* 20:S62, 1988.
118. Wasserman DH, Lacey DB, Green DR, Williams PE, Cherrington AD: Dynamics of hepatic lactate and glucose balances during prolonged exercise and recovery in the dog. *J Appl Physiol* 63:2411–2417, 1987.

119. Wasserman K, McIlroy MB: Detecting the threshold of anaerobic metabolism. *Am J Cardiol* 14:844–852, 1964.
120. Wasserman DH, Williams PE, Lacy DB, Goldstein RE, Cherrington AD: Exercise-induced fall in insulin and hepatic carbohydrate metabolism during muscular work. *Am J Physiol* 256:E500–E509, 1989.
121. Wasserman K, Whipp BJ, Koyal SN, Beaver WL: Anaerobic threshold and respiratory gas exchange during exercise. *J Appl Phyiol* 35:236–243, 1973.
122. Watt PW, Maclennan PA, Hundal HS, Kuret CM, Rennie MJ: L(+)-lactate transport in perfused skeletal muscle: kinetic characteristics and sensitivity to pH and transport inhibitors. *Biochim Biophys Acta* 944:213–222, 1988.
123. Weber J-M, Parkhouse WS, Dobson GP, Hardman JC, Snow HH, Hochachka PW: Lactate kinetics in exercising thoroughbred horses: regulation of turnover rate in plasma. *Am J Physiol* 253:R896–R903, 1987.
124. Weber J-M, Brill RW, Hochachka PW: Mammalian metabolite flux rates in a teleost: lactate and glucose turnover in tuna. *Am J Physiol* 250:R452–R458, 1986.
125. Weber J-M: Design of exogenous fuel supply systems: adaptive strategies for endurance locomotion. *Can J Zool* 66:1116–1121, 1988.
126. Welch HG, Stainsby WN: Oxygen debt in contracting dog skeletal muscle *in situ. Resp Physiol* 3:229–242, 1967.
127. Wiener R, Spitzer JJ: Lactate metabolism following severe hemorrhage in the conscious dog. *Am J Physiol* 227:58–62, 1974.
128. Wilson BA, Stainsby WN: Effects of O_2 breathing on RQ, blood flow, and developed tension in *in situ* dog muscle. *Med Sci Sports* 10:167–170, 1978.
129. Wilson H: The role of lactic acid production in glucose absorption from the intestine. *J Bioi Chem* 222:751–763, 1956.
130. Wolfe RR, Elahi D, Spitzer JJ: Glucose and lactate kinetics after endotoxin administration in dogs. *Am J Physiol* 232:E180–E185, 1977.
131. Wolfe BR, Graham TE, Barclay JK: Hyperoxia, mitochondrial redox state, and lactate metabolism of *in situ* canine muscle. Am J Physiol 253:C263–C268, 1987.

3
Energy Substrate Utilization during Exercise in Extreme Environments

ANDREW J. YOUNG, Ph.D.

INTRODUCTION

Contracting skeletal muscle requires a continuous source of energy. This energy is supplied by the breakdown of biochemical compounds containing high-energy phosphate bonds. The metabolic processes by which these high-energy phosphate compounds are regenerated in muscle during exercise have been the focus of considerable research, and a number of excellent reviews have been published on this subject [16, 40, 51]. Most of the information concerning human exercise metabolism has been obtained from studies completed in temperate environments at sea level. Exposure to extremes of heat, cold, and high altitude alters physiological responses to exercise and impairs physical performance. While many investigations have addressed the effects of environmental stress on respiratory, cardiovascular, and thermoregulatory responses to exercise, less attention has been directed to energy substrate utilization during exercise in environmental extremes. In this chapter, the information available concerning the effects of heat, cold, and high altitude on human muscle metabolism during exercise will be considered. The focus will be on the effect of the environment on carbohydrate and fat utilization during exercise.

EXERCISE AT HIGH ALTITUDE

Cardiovascular and Respiratory Responses

Persons who reside at low altitudes exhibit a number of physiological responses when they ascend to higher elevations. These responses tend to compensate for the relative lack of oxygen and limit, at least to some degree, performance decrements. Lowlanders who remain at high altitude undergo physiological adaptations with time as the process of acclimatization takes place. Physiological responses to exercise observed under acute hypoxic conditions are changed with acclimatization such that the physiological strain of exercise is lessened, and exercise tolerance at altitude is improved. Cardiovascular and respiratory responses of unacclimatized and acclimatized lowlanders at high altitude have been considered in detail elsewhere [34, 43, 140]; however, a brief review will follow because these responses have metabolic consequences.

Barometric pressure decreases with increasing altitude, resulting in a reduction in the partial pressure of oxygen in inspired air (P_{IO_2}). Acute hypoxia (i.e., $P_{IO_2} < \sim 110$ torr) stimulates ventilation during both rest and exercise [19, 34]. Despite increased ventilation, alveolar and arterial oxygen pressures remain below sea-level values. Tachycardia increases cardiac output of the unacclimatized lowlander at rest or during submaximal exercise at altitude as compared to sea level [43]. The increased cardiac output sustains systemic oxygen transport and enables submaximal oxygen uptake ($\dot{V}_{O_2}$) for a given power output to be maintained the same at altitude as at sea level [43, 140]. Maximal cardiac output, however, is the same initially at altitude as at sea level, but is achieved at a lower exercise intensity, and therefore, maximal oxygen uptake ($\dot{V}_{O_2}$max) is reduced at altitude [34, 43]. The reduction in $\dot{V}_{O_2}$max with acute high-altitude exposure is proportional to the reduction in arterial oxygen content (C_{aO_2}) resulting from arterial desaturation. There is little or no measurable decrement in $\dot{V}_{O_2}$max between sea level and 1000 m, a small and variable decrement between 1000 and 2000 m [112], and above 2000 m the decrement increases linearly with altitude by about 10% for every additional 1000 m ascended [34, 43]. The reduction in $\dot{V}_{O_2}$max with no change in $\dot{V}_{O_2}$ elicited at a submaximal power output means that a given absolute exercise intensity corresponds to a greater relative intensity (i.e., % $\dot{V}_{O_2}$max) at high altitude than at sea level. This effect, depicted in Figure 3.1, has ramifications for metabolism during submaximal exercise at altitude.

If the lowlander remains 8–10 days at high altitude, acclimatization results in an increase in C_{aO_2} as compared to that on arrival at altitude. Two factors contribute to this adaptation. First, a further increase in ventilation raises alveolar and arterial oxygen pressure and arterial saturation over that elicited by acute hypoxia [19]. In addition, hemoconcentration (a decrease in plasma volume with no change in erythrocyte volume) during the first week or so at altitude increases hematocrit [43, 140]. Despite the increased C_{aO_2} with acclimatization, $\dot{V}_{O_2}$max remains about the same as upon arrival at high altitude [43, 135, 140, 141]. This is because, at least at moderate altitudes (<6000 m), maximal cardiac output is reduced due to reduced stroke volume [43]. The hemoconcentration with acclimatization apparently limits stroke volume during exercise at altitude. The failure of $\dot{V}_{O_2}$max to rise with altitude acclimatization has also been attributed to a loss of muscle mass at high altitude and/or a limitation to tissue oxygen delivery during maximal exercise due to a viscosity impairment of muscle microcirculation arising from high hematocrits [14].

FIGURE 3.1

Example of how high altitude affects the relationship between oxygen uptake
($\dot{V}o_2$) for a given submaximal power output and the relative exercise intensity (%
maximum oxygen uptake, % $\dot{V}o_2max$). (From Young AJ, Young PM: Human
acclimatization to high terrestrial altitude. In Pandolf KB, Sawka MN, Gonzalez
RR *(eds):* Human Performance Physiology and Environmental Medicine
at Terrestrial Extremes. *Indianapolis, Benchmark, 1988, pp 497–543.)*

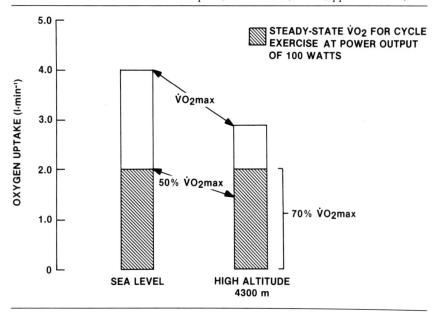

Altitude acclimatization has no effect on $\dot{V}o_2$ during submaximal exercise [43, 140]. As with maximal exercise, cardiac output during submaximal exercise decreases with altitude acclimatization [43, 140]. The
increased Cao_2 with altitude acclimatization enables muscle oxygen delivery to be maintained by increased oxygen extraction (greater arteriovenous oxygen difference) despite decreased muscle blood flow during
submaximal exercise [3]. The importance of these changes for muscle
metabolism is that exercise at a given power output will elicit the same
relative exercise intensity on the 1st day at high altitude as after 3 weeks
of acclimatization, assuming there are no changes in aerobic fitness due
to training or detraining.

Metabolic Responses

Unacclimatized Lowlanders Acutely Exposed to Hypoxia. The
effect of high altitude exposure on blood lactate concentration has at-

tracted considerable research interest. In one of the earliest detailed studies, Edwards [25] of the Harvard Fatigue Laboratory noted that unacclimatized lowlanders exhibited the same resting blood lactate concentration on their 1st day at high altitude (2810 m) as they had at sea level. However, whereas metabolic rate during exercise at a given power output was the same as at sea level, postexercise blood lactate concentrations were higher at altitude than at sea level. Furthermore, Edwards [25] reported that lowlanders who had acclimatized at high altitude for 6 weeks, exhibited similar or lower blood lactate concentrations following exercise than following a comparable exercise bout at sea level. Many subsequent investigations have confirmed and extended these observations.

The increased blood lactate accumulation experienced by unacclimatized lowlanders at high altitude is an effect of the reduction in the P_{IO_2} rather than the other stresses (e.g., hypobaria, cold) associated with the mountainous environment. Acute hypoxia produced in a hypobaric decompression chamber [e.g., see Refs. 33, 45, 68, and 73] or by breathing gas mixtures composed of <21% oxygen under normobaric conditions [e.g., see Refs. 50, 59, and 86] results in the same effect on blood lactate as observed in unacclimatized lowlanders sojourning at high altitude. From a practical standpoint, more reliable data can be obtained from unacclimatized persons acutely exposed to hypoxia by simulating high altitude conditions in a hypobaric chamber as opposed to making measurements in sojourners during the first few days after arrival at a high mountain site.

The increment in blood lactate concentration observed with acute hypoxic exposure is influenced by at least two factors: the altitude ascended and the metabolic rate. Lactate concentration following maximal exercise is the same for unacclimatized persons exposed to hypoxic conditions as at sea level, but because of the reduction in maximal work capacity, maximal lactate concentrations are achieved at lower power outputs at altitude than at sea level [9, 30, 47, 50, 81]. In general, the increment in postexercise blood lactate concentration observed at a particular altitude becomes greater as exercise intensity rises [47, 68], and the altitude-induced increment in postexercise lactate concentration at a particular exercise intensity becomes greater as the elevation increases and the P_{IO_2} falls [47, 72, 73, 86]. Thus at moderate elevations (e.g., 2000 to 4500 m), blood lactate concentrations of unacclimatized lowlanders at rest or during low-intensity exercise are about the same as at sea level, but when $\dot{V}_{O_2}$ exceeds about 1.5 liters·min^{-1} the hypoxia-induced increment in blood lactate concentration is apparent [47, 68, 72]. At altitudes above 4600 m, even resting lactate concentration can be elevated in unacclimatized lowlanders exposed to acute hypoxia [33, 45]. The studies cited above considered the effects of acute hypoxia on blood lactate responses to relatively short-duration (5-min or less) exercise bouts, but similar effects are observed when exercise lasts 40 min or longer [59, 83].

Although postexercise blood lactate concentrations are increased with acute high-altitude exposure compared to sea-level exercise at the same absolute intensity (same $\dot{V}O_2$ and power output), Hermansen and Saltin [47] observed that there were no differences in lactate concentration between altitudes for exercise bouts of the same relative intensity, i.e., at the same % $\dot{V}O_2$max. Similar observations were reported by Knuttgen and Saltin [68]. As shown in Figure 3.2, not only blood, but also muscle lactate concentrations at high altitude were similar if exercise of the same relative intensity was compared [68]. The aforementioned studies [47, 68) considered short-duration (4-min) exercise, but blood lactates after 10–30 min of exercise are also the same with acute altitude exposure as at sea level, when the exercise is of the same relative intensity [76, 82, 135].

The effect of acute hypoxia on blood lactate concentration has also been studied using exercise tests in which power output is increased at regular intervals during exercise until the subject reaches exhaustion. Compared to sea-level normoxic responses, unacclimatized lowlanders exhibited blood lactate accumulation (defined either as an increase in concentration above resting levels or a disproportionate increase in blood lactate concentration relative to the increase in exercise intensity) at a lower power output and $\dot{V}O_2$ at 4200-m simulated altitude [81]. However, expressed as a function of relative exercise intensity, this "threshold" of lactate accumulation was observed to occur at about 50% $\dot{V}O_2$max at both simulated high altitude and sea level [81].

Blood lactate concentration during exercise reflects the balance between net diffusion of lactate from the contracting skeletal muscles to the blood and net removal of lactate from the blood by the liver, heart, and the active and inactive skeletal muscles. The effect of hypoxia on heart or skeletal muscle lactate uptake during exercise has not been reported. However, Rowell et al. [100] have shown that when subjects performing steady-state submaximal exercise were switched from a normoxic to a hypoxic ($P_{IO_2} \sim 11\%$) breathing mixture, hepatic blood flow tended to increase ($\sim 10\%$, nonsignificant) and hepatic lactate extraction (i.e., arterial-hepatic venous lactate difference) showed a 5-fold increase. Furthermore, Bender et al. [3] observed that, during exercise at a $\dot{V}O_2$ of ~ 2.6 liters·min^{-1}, leg muscle lactate release was over 80% greater while breathing hypoxic ($P_{IO_2} = 83$ torr) air mixtures as compared to breathing ambient air at sea level. Thus, lactate uptake by the liver (and probably by inactive skeletal muscle) is greater during exercise under acute hypoxic conditions than during normoxia, and the increased blood lactate accumulation during hypoxic exercise probably reflects increased lactate release from active muscle rather than a decrease in lactate clearance.

FIGURE 3.2

*Effect of acute exposure to simulated high altitude (~4000 m) on blood (**A** and **C**) and muscle (**B** and **D**) lactate accumulation in lowland residents during exercise. Lactate concentrations are expressed as a function of absolute oxygen uptake (**A** and **B**) STPD, standard temperature and pressure-dry and % maximum oxygen uptake (**C** and **D**). (Drawn from data of Knuttgen HG, Saltin B: Oxygen uptake, muscle high-energy phosphates, and lactate in exercise under acute hypoxic conditions in man. Acta Physiol Scand 87:368–376, 1973 and Knuttgen HG, Saltin B: Muscle metabolites and oxygen uptake in short-term submaximal exercise in man. J Appl Physiol 32:690–694, 1972.)*

Muscle as well as blood lactate concentration is greater following exercise under acute hypoxic conditions as compared to normoxic conditions, if the exercise requires the same $\dot{V}o_2$ [62, 68, 72]. When exercise bouts are performed at the same % $\dot{V}o_2$max no difference in muscle lactate concentrations are observed between hypoxic and normoxic environmental conditions [82]. As in blood, muscle lactate concentration reflects the balance between lactate appearance in the muscle and lactate removal from muscle.

Lactate removal from the contracting muscle reflects the summated effects of lactate efflux from the muscle and lactate oxidation within the muscle. Muscle lactate efflux during exercise is increased by acute hypoxia [3], but the effects of acute hypoxic exposure on muscle lactate oxidation have not been evaluated. However, during sea-level exercise, it has been reported that over 50% of the lactate taken up by contracting muscle is immediately oxidized [61], and the amount of lactate taken up by contracting muscle has been estimated to be nearly equal to the amount of lactate released by the contracting muscle [113]. Thus, a substantial amount of lactate oxidation may be taking place in contracting muscle during normoxic exercise, and a decrease in lactate oxidation during hypoxic exercise could contribute to the observed increased muscle lactate concentration.

Lactate appearance in muscle during exercise reflects not only lactic acid production, but also lactate entry from the blood. During exercise at sea level, lactate extraction from the blood by contracting muscle has been reported to be closely correlated with arterial lactate concentration and that data showed no evidence that extraction became limited at high lactate concentrations [113]. The mechanism by which there is net lactate extraction from blood simultaneous with net lactate release into blood (i.e., against a concentration gradient) is not clear, but it is unlikely that the process is facilitated by acute hypoxic exposure. Therefore, changes in lactate appearance in muscle during acute hypoxic exposure most likely reflect changes in the rate of lactic acid production. Lactic acid formation will be influenced by the overall rate of glycolysis (mass-

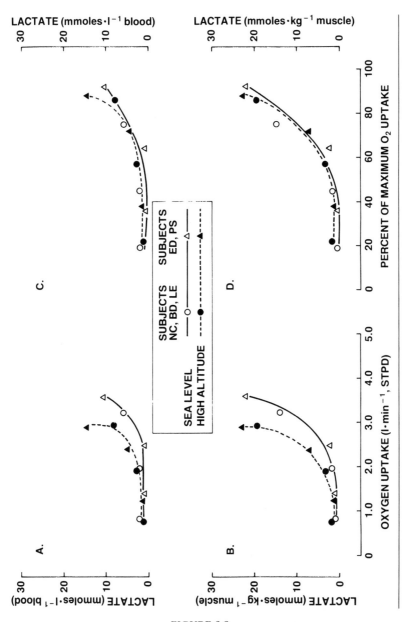

FIGURE 3.2

action effect due to increased pyruvate) as well as by the independent effect of the cytosolic availability of reduced nicotinamide adenine dinucleotide (NADH) on lactate dehydrogenase activity. It has been reported that the concentration of NADH in muscle increases more during exercise with respiratory hypoxia than normoxia [62]. However, there is considerable controversy over whether or not *mitochondrial* hypoxia is responsible for an increase in muscle NADH.

There is evidence that muscle glycolysis is accelerated during exercise with acute hypoxic exposure compared to normoxic exercise. The effect of an acute reduction in P_{IO_2} on muscle glycogen breakdown during exercise has been studied in two investigations. Linnarsson et al. [72] reported that muscle glycogen utilization was similar during submaximal exercise under hypoxic conditions ($P_{IO_2} = 99$ torr) as compared to exercise at the same power output under normoxic conditions. However, in that study [72], the subjects exercised only 4 min at a power output (~147 W) requiring only 50% of $\dot{V}_{O_2}$max. During such short, low-intensity exercise, relatively little muscle glycogen would be utilized, and an effect of hypoxia might be difficult to discern. Young et al. [135] measured muscle glycogen utilization by unacclimatized lowlanders during 30 min of submaximal exercise at sea level and at 4300-m simulated altitude. In that study, both exercise bouts were performed at about 85% $\dot{V}_{O_2}$max; power output was reduced in the hypoxic experiment to offset the measured reduction in $\dot{V}_{O_2}$max and maintain relative intensity constant for both trials [135]. The change in muscle glycogen and blood lactate concentrations were the same during both exercise bouts [135]. It therefore seems reasonable to conclude that if muscle glycogen breakdown had been measured during exercise bouts at the same absolute power output, a greater glycogen utilization would have been seen under acute hypoxic conditions.

The change in muscle adenosine triphosphate (ATP) levels is about the same [62, 68, 72] but the decrease in creatine phosphate (CP) during the first few minutes of exercise is more pronounced in hypoxic as compared to normoxic environments [62, 72]. The rate of ATP hydrolysis by myosin-ATPase is determined by the force and velocity of contraction, which is constant for a given exercise intensity at both sea level and high altitude. Therefore, the greater decrease in muscle CP probably reflects an impairment of the rate of ATP formation.

Reliance on the adenylate kinase reaction for ATP in muscle during exercise may be increased in hypoxic environments. In the adenylate kinase reaction, two adenosine diphosphate (ADP) molecules are used to form one molecule each of ATP and adenosine monophosphate (AMP). Young et al. [141] have shown that plasma ammonia levels are the same following exercise at 75% $\dot{V}_{O_2}$max on the 1st day at 4300 m as at sea level despite the lower absolute exercise intensity at high altitude (see Fig. 3.3). Therefore, greater ammonia accumulation would be expected if

FIGURE 3.3
Changes in plasma ammonia concentration (mean ± SE) in lowland residents during exercise at 75% maximum oxygen uptake at sea level and on days 1 and 13 at high altitude (4300 m). (From Young PM, Rock PB, Fulco CS, Trad LA, Forte VA, Cymerman A: Altitude acclimatization attenuates plasma ammonia accumulation during submaximal exercise. J Appl Physiol *63:758–764, 1987.)*

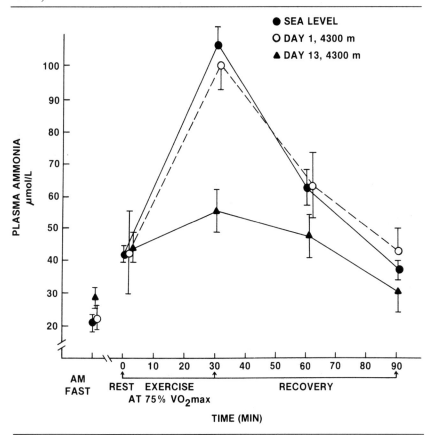

the same absolute intensity had been used at altitude as at sea level. During exercise, ammonia is produced in the muscle by deamination of AMP to inosine monophosphate (IMP) during the purine nucleotide cycle [74, 85]; an increase in plasma ammonia accumulation may represent the mass-action effect of an increased AMP formation via the adenylate kinase reaction. An increased muscle ammonia accumulation during exercise under hypoxic conditions may contribute to the metabolic stimulus for accelerated glycolysis and increased lactate formation because ammonia stimulates phosphofructokinase activity [74, 85] and inhibits pyruvate dehydrogenase and pyruvate carboxylase (85].

The oldest and most commonly advanced explanation for the accelerated glycogenolysis and lactate accumulation at high altitude is that the decreased Cao_2 results in muscle hypoxia. Aerobic energy production is thereby limited, thus forcing an increase in anaerobic metabolism and lactate production [49]. However, in animal experiments it has been shown that oxygen delivery to and uptake by the exercising muscle is unchanged by an acute reduction in Cao_2 due to the offsetting increase in muscle blood flow [54, 63]. Bender et al. [3] recently confirmed this in humans, observing that for a given absolute exercise intensity, oxygen delivery to the exercising leg was the same under acute hypoxic conditions as at sea level, but net lactate release by the muscle was increased. Furthermore, the observation that $\dot{V}o_2$ during exercise at a given power output is the same at high altitude as at sea level has been interpreted as indicating that muscle tissue oxygen levels do not limit aerobic metabolism during exercise in hypoxic environments, the argument being that $\dot{V}o_2$ should be decreased if oxygen availability is limited.

On the other hand, experiments with isolated cell suspensions indicate that when extracellular oxygen tension is falling, cellular ratios of [ATP]/[ADP] and [NAD]/[NADH] decrease at a higher oxygen tension than those at which cellular respiratory rate decreased [131, 132]. This constancy of respiration over a wide range of oxygen tensions was not because the mitochondrial respiratory processes were insensitive to low oxygen levels; rather, compensatory changes in mitochondrial [ATP]/[ADP] $\times$ [P_i] and a progressive reduction in cytochrome *c* enabled respiratory rate to be sustained [131, 132]. In support of this view, Katz and Sahlin [62] observed that, although $\dot{V}o_2$ was the same, skeletal muscle NADH (assumed to reflect mitochondrial NADH) of men exercising during respiratory hypoxia was greater than in normoxic conditions, and they concluded that muscle hypoxia had caused increased muscle lactate production. That interpretation is not universally accepted, and the concept that increases in lactate concentration during exercise reflect and are due to tissue oxygen limitation remains controversial (see Chapters 1 and 2 of this volume).

Muscle glycogen breakdown and lactate accumulation during exercise could be accelerated during acute hypoxic exposure by mechanisms other than tissue oxygen hypoxia. One possibility is that acute high-altitude exposure may affect the responses to exercise of various hormones that modulate energy metabolism [32, 34]. Although resting catecholamine levels are unchanged in unacclimatized lowlanders acutely exposed to hypoxia [34] , circulating epinephrine concentrations during exercise are elevated over levels seen during normoxia [28, 79]. This could result in additional stimulation of muscle glycogenolysis during exercise, particularly in fast-twitch fibers [95]. When unacclimatized lowlanders perform exercise of the same absolute intensity at sea level and in acute hypoxic conditions, plasma cortisol [93] and growth hormone [93, 118] responses are more pronounced in the latter. These endocrine effects could tend to facilitate lipolysis and hepatic gluconeogenesis [118], and perhaps are more important for recovery from exercise, because fatty acid oxidation during exercise does not appear to be enhanced by acute hypoxia [135]. Insulin [118] and glucagon [117] responses to exercise are only slightly or not at all affected by acute hypoxia.

Although speculative, one other alternative deserves mention. Possibly, for a given intensity of submaximal exercise at high altitude, unacclimatized lowlanders recruit more motor units, or perhaps fast-twitch fibers are preferentially recruited at a lower exercise intensity compared to sea-level exercise. A change in recruitment pattern due to acute hypoxia might seem to conflict with the concept that motor-unit and fiber-type recruitment pattern is determined by the force and velocity of muscular contraction [24]. Although those parameters would be expected to be the same for a given exercise intensity at sea level and high altitude, this has never been experimentally verified. A detailed investigation of motor-unit recruitment during exercise at high altitude has not been reported. However, motor unit recruitment might be altered at high altitude via changes in peripheral nerve excitability. Willer et al. [129] reported that acute respiratory hypoxia resulted in a decrease in the threshold stimulus intensity required to elicit the Hoffman (H) reflex in humans. The monosynaptic H reflex indicates the excitability of both muscle spindle afferent neurons and skeletal muscle motor neurons [29]. Results of earlier animal experiments had indicated that the motor neuron was relatively insensitive to hypoxia [23]. Therefore, Willer et al. [129] suggested that the hypoxia-induced lowering of the threshold for stimulation of the H reflex was due to increased excitability of the muscle efferent nerve fibers, the neuromuscular function, the muscle membrane itself, or all three. Thus, there is at least one mechanism by which hypoxia might result in an altered neuromuscular recruitment pattern during exercise. Furthermore, fast-twitch glycolytic muscle fibers, which have a greater capacity for glycolysis and lactic acid production than do slow-twitch fibers, also appear to be the primary source of blood ammonia during exercise [22]. The increased blood ammonia accumulation during exercise with acute hypoxic exposure may indicate increased recruitment of these fibers. The possible effects of hypoxia on neuromuscular recruitment pattern during exercise appears to be an area in need of further study.

ADAPTATIONS WITH ALTITUDE ACCLIMATIZATION. Physical work capacity and endurance of lowlanders are reduced initially after ascent to high altitude. However, after a period of altitude acclimatization, exercise tolerance improves dramatically. Buskirk et al. [13] noted that after

4–5 weeks of living at 4000 m, athletes from low altitudes were able to compete equally in soccer with the athletes who had resided at high altitude since birth. Improvements in endurance have also been documented under more standardized experimental conditions. Maher et al. [76] observed a 45% increase in endurance time for cycle exercise at 75% of $\dot{V}O_2$max on the 12th as compared to the 2nd day that lowlanders had resided at 4300 m. Similarly, Horstman et al. [55] observed a 60% increase in endurance time for treadmill running at 85% $\dot{V}O_2$max on the 16th compared to the 2nd day at 4300 m. Interestingly, in both studies, endurance was found to be the same on day 2 at high altitude as during exercise of the same relative intensity (% $\dot{V}O_2$max) performed at sea level [55, 76].

Sea-level investigations have shown that a major determinant of an individual's endurance during exercise is the relative exercise intensity, expressed as the % $\dot{V}O_2$max. Glesser and Vogel [39] induced acute alterations in $\dot{V}O_2$max by having subjects breathe gas mixtures having 21, 16, and 12% oxygen, and they observed that the size of the decrement in endurance time could be accurately predicted ($r > 0.91$) for each subject by measuring the change in $\dot{V}O_2$max (and thus the % $\dot{V}O_2$max required for the submaximal endurance tests) induced by the hypoxic breathing mixtures. The observation that endurance time was the same on the 2nd day at high altitude as sea level when exercise at the same relative intensity [55, 76] agrees with the concept that relative exercise intensity is an important determinant of endurance time.

By comparing endurance times of different individuals at a variety of different absolute and relative exercise intensities, Glesser and Vogel [38] empirically derived an equation to predict endurance time:

$$\log(t) = A{\cdot}L_r + B$$

where L_r is the absolute power output divided by the $\dot{V}O_2$max. The constants A and B vary between individuals, and the values are the slope and intercept of the line generated by plotting an individual's endurance time at different relative exercise intensities. Glesser and Vogel [38, 39] speculated that the parameters A and B reflected individual characteristics related to muscle glycogenolysis. Parameter A related to the amount that muscle glycolytic rate increased for a given increase in relative intensity, and parameter B related to the amount of glycogen stored in the muscle before exercise and the basal glycolytic rate. Thus, the overall rate of muscle glycolysis would vary with the relative exercise intensity as indicated by the term $A{\cdot}L_r$ in the above equation.

Muscle glycogen availability is well known to be one of the determinants of exercise endurance, especially at higher intensities [16]. Although the explanation for Glesser's and Vogel's [38, 39] empirically derived equation was entirely theoretical, there are experimental results supporting the importance of relative exercise intensity in determining muscle glycolytic rate. Cross-sectional comparisons of trained and untrained subjects have shown that individuals exercising at different power outputs but at the same relative intensity experienced a similar amount of glycogen depletion [102]. Furthermore, in a longitudinal training study, increases in an individual's $\dot{V}o_2$max were associated with a reduction in muscle glycogen utilization during steady-state exercise, despite the fact that pre- and posttraining exercise tests were performed at the same power output and $\dot{V}o_2$ [102]. That unacclimatized lowlanders exercising at the same relative intensity at sea level and high altitude utilize similar amounts of muscle glycogen [135] and accumulate similar amounts of blood lactate [76, 135] further supports the importance of relative intensity as a determinant of muscle glycolysis during exercise.

From the foregoing discussion it can be concluded that endurance changes could result from changes in $\dot{V}o_2$max, muscle glycolytic metabolism, or both. For example, acute alterations in Cao_2 (such as experienced by unacclimatized lowlanders on arrival at high altitude) would influence endurance by altering $\dot{V}o_2$max, but parameters A and B would not be expected to be affected [39]. On the other hand, as will be discussed, endurance changes during the first weeks of altitude acclimatization probably reflect changes in muscle glycolytic metabolism with little [55] or no [135, 141] alteration in $\dot{V}o_2$max.

Changes in blood lactate responses to exercise were the first indication that altitude acclimatization affected muscle metabolism. As mentioned, Edwards [25] reported that acclimatized (6 weeks) subjects exercising at 2810 m exhibited the same or smaller increments in blood lactate as during sea-level exercise at the same power output. Edwards [25] noted, however, that in the cases where blood lactate did not rise as high at high altitude as at sea level, the exercise duration that could be sustained was also less. Other more recent investigations [14, 21, 42] have reported that blood lactate concentration achieved by acclimatized persons during maximal exercise at altitude is lower than at sea level. Data from the recent Operation Everest II study indicate that this reduction in lactate accumulation during maximal exercise is not due to an impairment of muscle glycolytic flux following acclimatization [42]; furthermore, 48 hr after returning to sea level, altitude-acclimatized individuals achieve about the same maximal lactate concentrations as before ascent to altitude [42]. Thus, the lower blood lactates achieved by acclimatized persons during maximal exercise at altitude most likely reflect reduced exercise durations and lower power outputs rather than the effects of any metabolic adaptation.

In contrast, metabolic responses to steady-state submaximal exercise do change with acclimatization in a way suggestive of metabolic adaptation to prolonged altitude exposure. Maher et al. [76] observed that plasma lactate concentrations of sea-level residents did not increase as much during 20 min of exercise at 75% $\dot{V}o_2$max on day 12 of residence at 4300 m as on the 2nd day at high altitude, or at sea level. That lactate accumulation during submaximal exercise decreases with altitude acclimation has been confirmed subsequently [135], including two studies that compared blood lactate concentration following exercise at the same absolute exercise intensity at sea level and at high altitude [3, 136].

The effect of altitude acclimatization on blood lactate accumulation during exercise could reflect an increased lactate removal from blood, a decreased lactate release into blood, or both. The effect of altitude acclimatization on blood lactate clearance during exercise has not been studied, but it seems unlikely that an increase sufficient to account for the dramatic reduction in postexercise lactate concentration observed (see Fig. 3.4) would occur. The fall in cardiac output during acclimatization [43] is associated with a decrease in blood flow to the active [3] and presumably also the inactive muscle. Therefore, removal of lactate from blood by muscle probably remains unchanged or decreases with altitude acclimatization. As mentioned previously, hepatic lactate removal during exercise is already increased under acute hypoxic conditions [100]. A further substantial increase with acclimatization is not very likely because hepatic blood flow is only slightly (nonsignificantly) greater after 6–8 days at high altitude as compared to the 1st day [92]. Although changes in lactate clearance cannot be entirely ruled out, it appears that a change in lactate release from the contracting muscles is a more important factor contributing to the lower postexercise blood lactate concentration observed following altitude acclimatization.

Lactate release from contracting muscles during exercise is reduced following altitude acclimatization. Bender et al. [3] measured leg (iliac venous) blood flow and femoral arterial-iliac venous lactate differences during exercise at several submaximal intensities before and after 18 days of acclimatization to 4300 m. Both before and after altitude acclimatization, the measurements were obtained while the subjects breathed normoxic ($P_{IO_2} = 147$ torr) and hypoxic ($P_{IO_2} = 85$ torr) air mixtures [3]. Lactate release (muscle blood flow $\times$ arteriovenous lactate difference) during exercise was reduced following altitude acclimatization [3]. Interestingly, the reduction in lactate release due to altitude acclimatization was apparent during normoxic as well as hypoxic breathing [3]

Muscle lactate accumulation during exercise at altitude also appears to be lower after acclimatization. Young et al. [136] measured muscle pH and blood lactate changes in lowlanders exercising at the same power output at sea level ($\dot{V}o_2 = 3.2$ liters·min^{-1}, 86% $\dot{V}o_2$max) and at 4300 m ($\dot{V}o_2 = 3.1$ liters·min^{-1}, 97% $\dot{V}o_2$max) after 18 days of acclimatization. The subjects exercised 30 min at sea level, but at 4300 m they were capable of only 12 min of exercise [136]. There were no differences in preexercise muscle pH, but the decrease in muscle pH and increase in blood lactate with exercise were less pronounced on day 18 at high altitude than at sea level [136]. Muscle pH changes during exercise are primarily due to lactic acid formation. Thus the attenuated fall in muscle pH suggests that muscle lactate accumulation was reduced concomitant with the lower postexercise blood lactate concentration observed. Whether or not the smaller change in muscle pH reflected the reduced exercise time during the trial at 4300 m or an effect of altitude acclimatization was not clear, but muscle acidosis did not appear to be limiting exercise endurance after altitude acclimatization [136]. More recently, muscle lactate concentrations following 30 min of exercise at 80% $\dot{V}O_2$max were found to be lower on day 20 of acclimatization at 4300 m than after 30 min of exercise at the same relative intensity at sea level (unpublished observations from this laboratory).

Lowlanders sojourning at high altitude experience changes in acid-base balance [19, 140]. The reduction in muscle lactate accumulation and release into the blood may be, at least partially, mediated by these acid-base changes. Lactate efflux from muscle is subject to the effects of extracellular pH and bicarbonate concentration on the muscle cell membrane [77]. The increased ventilation at altitude causes hypocapnia and respiratory alkalosis. Metabolic alkalosis induced by $NaHCO_3$ ingestion increases blood lactate accumulation during exercise, but endurance improves [60, 119]. The improved endurance with metabolic alkalosis may have been due to a facilitation of muscle lactate efflux because muscle to blood lactate concentration difference was smaller than with metabolic acidosis or in control conditions [119]. In contrast to the metabolic alkalosis induced by ingesting $NaHCO_3$, respiratory alkalosis at high altitude is associated with decreased bicarbonate concentration due to an increased pulmonary carbon dioxide output as well as an increased renal bicarbonate excretion during acclimatization [15]. In isolated perfused frog muscle, the pH effect on lactate efflux (increase with alkalosis) was found to be separate from the effect of bicarbonate concentration; lactate efflux from muscle decreased as bicarbonate concentration in the perfusate fell [77]. The net effect on muscle lactate efflux of the opposing alkaline pH and reduced bicarbonate concentration due to respiratory alkalosis and altitude acclimatization remains to be systematically evaluated.

In addition to alterations in muscle lactate efflux, either a decreased lactic acid production during glycolysis or an increased oxidation of pyruvate could contribute to the decreased muscle lactate accumulation during exercise. The effect of acclimatization on pyruvate oxidation in contracting muscle has not been evaluated, but there is experimental evidence indicating that altitude acclimatization results in a decreased muscle glycogenolysis during exercise. Young et al. [135] measured muscle glycogen utilization of sea-level residents during 30 min of exercise at 85% $\dot{V}O_2$max at sea level, again during the first 2 hr of

FIGURE 3.4

Changes in serum concentrations (mean ± SE) of free fatty acids **(A)**, *glycerol* **(B)**, *lactate* **(C)**, *and muscle glycogen concentration* **(D)** *in eight lowland residents with 30 min of exercise (85% maximum oxygen uptake) at sea level and at high altitude, before and after acclimatization. (From Young AJ, Evans WJ, Cymerman A, Pandolf KB, Knapik JJ, Maher JT: Sparing effect of chronic high-altitude exposure on muscle glycogen utilization.* J Appl Physiol *52:857–862, 1982.)*

exposure to a simulated altitude of 4300 m, and again after 18 days of acclimatization at 4300 m. As shown in Figure 3.4, muscle glycogen utilization and blood lactate accumulation during exercise at high altitude before acclimatization were the same as at sea level, but both were reduced after 18 days of altitude acclimatization [135]. Thus, reduced muscle glycogenolysis appears to contribute to the reduced lactate accumulation and improved endurance associated with altitude acclimatization.

In sea-level investigations of both animals and humans, an increase in plasma free fatty acid concentration induced before exercise by dietary manipulation and heparin administration has been shown to reduce breakdown of muscle glycogen during exercise, suggesting that high plasma free fatty acid levels inhibit muscle glycogenolysis [16]. The decreased muscle glycogenolysis during exercise at high altitude following acclimatization may also be due to increased mobilization and oxidation of plasma free fatty acids. Respiratory exchange ratio during exercise may be [135], but is not always [55, 141], reduced with altitude acclimatization. However, the ventilatory changes occurring with acclimatization may lessen the validity of the respiratory exchange ratio as an indicator of muscle substrate utilization. On the other hand, changes in blood free fatty acid and glycerol concentration during exercise are more reliable indicators of fat metabolism. As shown in Figure 3.4, resting free fatty acid concentrations of lowlanders acutely exposed to a simulated altitude of 4300 m were increased as compared to concentrations at sea level, and there was a further increase apparent after 18 days at high altitude [135]. Glycerol remained unchanged from resting levels during exercise at sea level or during acute high-altitude exposure, but increased substantially on day 18 at altitude [135]. During lipolysis, free fatty acids and glycerol are released from adipose tissue into the blood in a 3 : 1 molar ratio. The large increase in blood glycerol concentration with no change in free fatty acid concentration during exercise on day 18 at 4300 m suggests that, following altitude acclimatization, increased lipolysis and free fatty acid mobilization were balanced by fatty acid removal and oxidation. The effects of altitude acclimatization on blood free fatty acid and glycerol concentrations that were reported by Young et al. [135] are

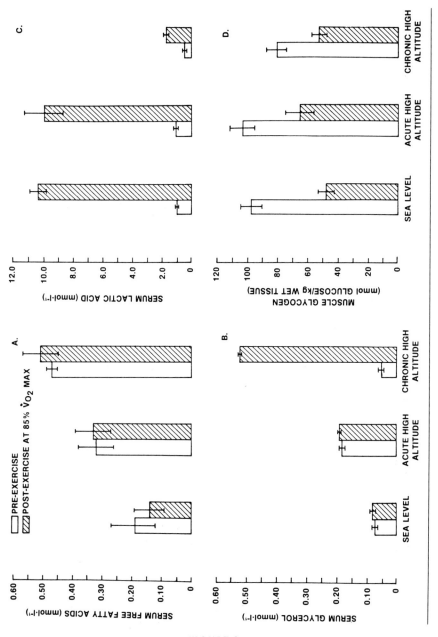

FIGURE 3.4

consistent with observations from other studies [66, 141], but whether or not fat oxidation by contracting muscle is truly increased remains to be confirmed in more detailed studies using quantitatively precise techniques.

During the same time frame that the aforementioned metabolic adaptations to high altitude take place, there is also an increase in sympathetic nervous system activity. This is evidenced by a progressive increase in resting plasma norepinephrine levels with unchanged epinephrine levels [18]. At sea level, increased sympathetic activity stimulates adipose tissue lipolysis [46], and Klain and Hannon [66] suggested that the increased lipolysis during prolonged altitude exposure was mediated by the increased sympathetic nervous activity. Young et al. [135] speculated further that a norepinephrine-mediated increase in lipolysis enabled an increase in fatty acid mobilization and subsequent oxidation by muscle, thereby allowing the glycogen "sparing" effect of altitude acclimatization. Recently, however, administration of the β-adrenergic blocking agent propranolol to subjects during the first 15 days of altitude acclimatization failed to prevent the glycogen sparing adaptation (unpublished observations from this laboratory). This suggests that chronic β-adrenergic stimulation during altitude acclimatization may not account for the reduction in glycogen utilization during exercise.

Several alternative mechanisms might account for the reduction in glycogen utilization due to altitude acclimatization. Although the exaggerated growth hormone response to exercise may persist for up to 5 days at altitude [93], hormonal responses of acclimatized persons exercising at altitude are, with the exception of circulating norepinephrine as discussed above, generally reported to be the same as at sea level [117, 140]. Changes in oxidative and glycolytic enzyme activity in skeletal muscle are related to metabolic adaptations to physical training at sea level and might play a role in altitude adaptation. Animal experiments suggest that altitude acclimatization might increase muscle oxidative enzyme activity [120]. Also, activity of pyridine-linked dehydrogenase enzymes of the mitochondrial electron transport chain are higher in the muscles of lifelong high-altitude residents than in sea-level residents [94]. However, humans residing for 3 weeks at 4300 m exhibited no change in hexokinase, glycogen phosphorylase, lactate dehydrogenase, malate dehydrogenase [136], or citrate synthetase (unpublished observations from this laboratory) activities in the vastus lateralis. Similarly, during a 40-day altitude exposure simulating a progressive ascent to the summit of Mount Everest (282 torr), eight male subjects experienced no changes in the vastus lateralis enzyme activities of succinic dehydrogenase, citrate synthetase, 3-hydroxyacyl-CoA dehydrogenase, pyruvate kinase, or α-glycerophosphate dehydrogenase [41]. Thus, the changes in metabolic responses to exercise observed after 2–3 weeks of altitude acclimatization do not appear to be due to changes in muscle glycolytic or oxidative enzyme activities. However, changes in muscle glycolytic and oxidative enzyme activities in response to increased physical training appear to require about 5–6 weeks to fully develop [121]; therefore, individuals acclimatized to high altitude for long (>2 months) periods may be found to experience adaptations in skeletal muscle enzyme activity.

As shown in Figure 3.3, plasma (and presumably muscle) ammonia accumulation during submaximal exercise at high altitude is reduced following acclimatization as compared to exercise of the same relative intensity at sea level or initially upon arrival at altitude [141]. Therefore, any stimulation of phosphofructokinase during acute hypoxia due to the increased muscle ammonia would be alleviated after altitude acclimatization. Additionally, the reduction in ammonia accumulation may indicate that fewer fast-twitch glycolytic fibers were recruited as compared to exercise at the same power output and relative intensity upon initial arrival at high altitude. Both of these mechanisms could contribute to an acclimatization-induced reduction in muscle glycolysis and lower muscle and blood lactate accumulation during exercise at altitude.

Acclimatized persons exercising at altitude not only accumulate less blood ammonia, but also less muscle IMP [42] compared to persons exercising at sea level. These observations suggest that the energy charge of the muscle adenosine nucleotide pool is maintained during exercise with less reliance on the adenylate kinase reaction after altitude acclimatization. If the capacity for mitochondrial oxidative phosphorylation of ADP to ATP is increased by altitude acclimatization, less ADP would be available for the adenylate kinase reaction; in this way AMP formation and subsequent deamination to IMP and ammonia would be reduced. Although consistent with the experimental observations, this explanation remains speculative.

If the accelerated glycogenolysis and increased lactate accumulation experienced by unacclimatized lowlanders exercising during acute exposure to respiratory hypoxia is indeed due to the development of muscle tissue hypoxia as suggested by Katz and Sahlin [62], then the reduction in lactate accumulation and glycolysis with altitude acclimatization could reflect improved tissue oxygenation. Although temptingly simple, this explanation remains unfounded. First, as mentioned earlier, whether or not acute respiratory hypoxia leads to the development of muscle hypoxia remains controversial. Second, $\dot{V}o_2$ and muscle oxygen delivery during steady-state exercise at high altitude are unchanged by acclimatization and are the same as at sea level. Third, while subjects participating in a 40-day hypobaric chamber simulation of the ascent of Mount Everest exhibited an increased number of capillaries per cross-sectional area of muscle fibers (which could improve muscle tissue oxygenation), the increased capillarization was not due to an increased number of capillaries per fiber, but instead resulted from a decrease in muscle fiber area.

Acclimatization to more moderate altitudes (20 days at 4300 m) does not result in reduced muscle fiber area [137]. Thus, available evidence does not support an improvement in tissue oxygenation as the mechanism underlying the reduction in glycogenolysis and diminished lactate accumulation observed during exercise after altitude acclimatization.

In summary, unacclimatized lowlanders sojourning at high altitude, accumulate more blood and muscle lactate during exercise than at sea level. Lactic acid formation by the contracting muscle is probably increased due to accelerated glycogenolysis, but lactate oxidation in contracting muscles may also be reduced at high altitude. The exact mechanism for the increase in glycolysis and lactate formation remains unresolved, but the development of muscle tissue hypoxia, hormonal effects, and alterations of neuromuscular recruitment during exercise are plausible mechanisms that merit further research. Acclimatization to high altitude is associated with improved endurance for submaximal exercise, which may, at least to some extent, reflect a metabolic adaptation to prolonged high altitude residence. After acclimatization to high altitude, there is less accumulation of blood and muscle lactate and reduced breakdown of muscle glycogen stores during exercise. Whether or not these effects of acclimatization are due to increased mobilization and oxidation of free fatty acids, adaptations in neuromuscular recruitment or improved tissue oxygenation during exercise remains to be demonstrated.

EXERCISE IN HOT ENVIRONMENTS

Cardiovascular and Thermoregulatory Responses

Humans maintain temperature homeostasis via a number of mechanisms that enable heat dissipation to match heat production. The metabolic conversion of biochemical energy into mechanical work also results in the liberation of heat into the muscle. The amount of heat liberated is proportional to the metabolic rate. Heat is conducted from the muscle along thermal gradients through surrounding tissue. Some heat is conducted directly through overlying tissue to the body surface where it can be dissipated into the environment; the remainder is conducted into the blood perfusing the muscle, enabling the circulatory system to transfer the heat by convection to the body core and skin surface. Although some heat is lost via the respiratory system, most heat dissipation occurs at the skin surface by sweat evaporation (insensible heat loss) and radiative convective (sensible heat loss) heat transfer to the ambient environment.

Metabolic heat production in skeletal muscle rapidly increases with the transition from rest to exercise, but heat dissipation mechanisms achieve the new steady state more slowly. The muscle stores heat while heat production exceeds heat dissipation, and muscle temperature (T_m) rises above resting levels. The increase in blood flow to contracting muscle enables a major increase in convective heat transfer away from the muscle. The circulation carries the heat to the body core, resulting in an increase in core temperature. Increasing core (T_c) and skin (T_s) temperatures provide the afferent signal for reflex increases in skin blood flow and sweating, thereby facilitating heat transfer to the skin surface where it can be dissipated to the environment.

The effectiveness of sensible and insensible heat loss mechanisms is influenced by ambient temperature and humidity [105]. As ambient temperature rises, the thermal gradient for heat transfer between the skin and the external environment is diminished, and sensible heat loss is impaired. When ambient temperature exceeds T_s, the gradient for heat transfer is reversed and the body gains heat from the external environment. If humidity is low, a decrease in sensible heat loss can be offset by an increase in evaporative heat loss [89]. As humidity rises, the gradient between skin and ambient dew point is reduced and evaporative heat loss is impaired. There is a fairly broad range of ambient temperature and humidity conditions (the prescriptive zone) over which the rise in T_c during exercise is constant [71]. The upper limit for this temperature range decreases as exercise intensity and metabolic rate increase. At ambient temperatures above this range, heat storage during exercise is increased and the rise in steady-state T_c and, presumably, contracting T_m are more pronounced than that observed within the prescriptive zone. As will be discussed, an increased T_m is probably one of the factors contributing to the changes in metabolic responses to exercise observed during acute heat stress.

A redistribution of regional blood flow is another factor that could influence metabolic responses to exercise in the heat. The increased thermoregulatory demand for skin blood flow during exercise in hot weather is achieved by a reapportionment of the regional distribution of cardiac output [98]. The effect of acute heat stress on cardiac output during exercise depends on the duration and intensity of exercise and degree of heat stress [98]. A reduction in maximal cardiac output and/or a redistribution of blood flow away from active muscle [98] could account for the reduction in $\dot{V}o_2max$ usually observed with acute exposure to hot environments [106]. Cardiac output during high-intensity submaximal exercise is the same or somewhat lower in hot than temperate environmental conditions, whereas cardiac output during prolonged mild exercise may be increased in the heat [98]. Compared to cool conditions, heat stress results in more pronounced sweating, often resulting in dehydration, which reduces blood volume and further compromises the ability of the heart to sustain cardiac output [105].

Acute heat stress and heat acclimation have profound effects on responses of fluid-regulatory hormones to exercise [32]. For the most part, however, hormones that modulate metabolism are unaffected or show a variable response to heat stress [32]. It is possible that effects on metabolic hormones attributed to heat stress may, in fact, be due to the influence of other factors such as hypohydration or psychological factors [32] rather than alterations in body temperature. Thus, changes in energy metabolism during exercise in the heat are probably primarily the result of nonendocrine factors.

As with high altitude, a reduction in $\dot{V}o_2max$ due to heat stress would change the relative exercise intensity elicited by a given power output as compared to temperate conditions. Also, differences in relative intensity between hot and cool environments will result if steady-state $\dot{V}o_2$ during submaximal exercise is different. Oxygen uptake during submaximal exercise in the heat has been reported to be higher, lower, or the same as in temperate environments [98]. In reality, however, the magnitude of the changes in $\dot{V}o_2$ during maximal [106] and submaximal [138] exercise are small and tend to offset each other [138]. Thus, in contrast to the situation at high altitude, differences in relative exercise intensity at a given power output are probably not a major factor in explaining differences in metabolic responses during exercise in hot compared to temperate environmental conditions.

Heat acclimatization/acclimation produced by repeated exercise-heat stress exposure is characterized by adaptations that relieve some of the physiological strain described above. Among the adaptations to chronic exercise-heat stress are reduced body temperature and heart rate responses to exercise, an increased capacity for sweating, and a lower threshold for the onset of cutaneous vasodilation [128]. Other adaptations include changes in vascular fluid regulation and the regional distribution of cardiac output during exercise in the heat [128]. Thus, lower body temperatures and improved perfusion of muscle and other regions may enable changes in exercise metabolism with heat acclimation.

Metabolic Responses

ACUTE EXPOSURE TO HEAT STRESS. As mentioned, the effect of acute heat stress on the $\dot{V}o_2$ elicited during submaximal exercise is controversial. Acute heat stress has been reported to increase [17, 31, 75, 116], decrease [12, 20, 111, 130,, 138], and have no significant effect on [27, 67, 99, 115] $\dot{V}o_2$ during submaximal exercise. Although there are differences among the studies with regard to the mode, duration, and intensity of exercise employed, experience, aerobic fitness and acclimation status of the participating subjects, and environmental conditions during the experiments, the explanation for the disparate observations is not apparent. On the one hand, $\dot{V}o_2$ might increase in the heat due to the additional energy required for tachycardia, sweating and increased ventilation, as well as the generalized increase in tissue metabolism due to increased tissue temperature (Q_{10} effect). On the other hand, $\dot{V}o_2$ might decrease due to an increased muscular efficiency or a reduced oxygen delivery and uptake at the muscle resulting from redistributed cardiac output to the cutaneous circulation. In any event, the magnitude of the difference in $\dot{V}o_2$ measured during exercise in the heat compared to temperate conditions is usually reported to be fairly small, on the order of 80–130 ml·min^{-1}, although a difference of about 200 ml·min^{-1} was reported in one study [130].

The $\dot{V}o_2$ during steady-state exercise reflects only the aerobic (oxidative) metabolic rate during exercise. Total metabolic rate is comprised of an anaerobic (glycolytic) component as well. Therefore, regardless of whether the $\dot{V}o_2$ during exercise is increased, decreased, or unchanged in hot compared to cool conditions, total metabolic rate could be greater in the heat if the anaerobic component increased sufficiently.

Experimental support for this concept is provided in the report of Dimri et al. [20], whose data were recently reviewed and redepicted graphically by Sawka and Wenger [105] as shown in Figure 3.5. Dimri et al. [20] quantified the aerobic component of total metabolic rate by measuring the $\dot{V}o_2$ during three intensities of submaximal exercise in three different ambient environments. The anaerobic component was quantified by measuring the $\dot{V}o_2$ that was in excess of the preexercise resting level during a 30-min recovery period after each exercise. The total oxygen cost (from which the metabolic rate can be calculated) of the exercise bouts was determined by summing the aerobic and anaerobic components. According to the analysis by Dimri et al. [20], total metabolic rate during exercise increased with acute exposure to hot environments due to the progressively greater contribution of the anaerobic component while the aerobic component, reflected by the $\dot{V}o_2$ during exercise, decreased.

The use of the excess $\dot{V}o_2$ measured during the postexercise recovery period to quantify anaerobic metabolism during the preceding exercise period may be quantitatively inaccurate, particularly in hot environmental conditions when body temperatures have increased. Brooks et al. [10] have shown that when the incubation temperature of isolated skeletal muscle mitochondria is raised from 25 to 37°C, both state 3 (maximally stimulated) and state 4 (unstimulated or resting) respiratory rate increase, but above 37°C, the increase in respiration rate with increasing temperature is much more pronounced. Phosphorylation efficiency (reflected by the ADP:O ratio) was constant between 25 and 40°C [10]. As incubation temperature was increased from 40 to 45°C [10], phosphorylation efficiency decreased, but it is unlikely that T_m would rise this high in exercising humans, even with environmental heat stress [10]. One factor contributing to the increased respiration rate and the decreased phosphorylation efficiency appeared to be that mitochondrial ATPase

FIGURE 3.5

Effect of increasing ambient temperature on total metabolic rate (bottom panel) *and relative contribution of aerobic and anaerobic metabolism* (top panel) *in six men during exercise at three different power outputs (subjects had not been heat acclimated but were tropical residents). (Drawn in Sawka MN, Wenger CB: Physiological responses to acute exercise-heat stress. In Pandolf KB, Sawka MN, Gonzalez RR (eds):* Human Performance Physiology and Environmental Medicine at Terrestrial Extremes. *Indianapolis, Benchmark, 1988, pp 97– 151, from data of Dimri GP, Malhotra MS, Gupta JS, Kumar TS, Arora BS: Alterations in aerobic-anaerobic proportions of metabolism during work in heat.* Eur J Appl Physiol *45:43–50, 1980.)*

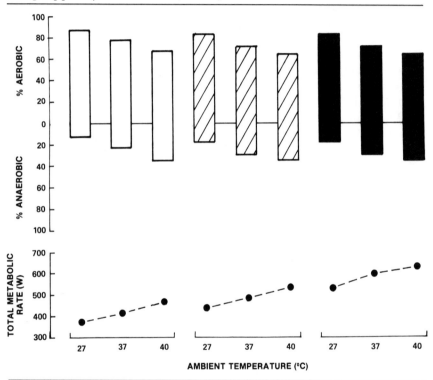

activity was more stimulated, as evidenced by a more pronounced sensitivity to oligomycin inhibition of respiration rate at the higher incubation temperatures [10].

Brooks et al. [11] also showed that the time course for the declines in whole-body $\dot{V}o_2$ and core and muscle temperatures during the postexercise recovery period were very similar. Thus, the $\dot{V}o_2$ measured by Dimri et al. [20] following exercise in the heat may to some degree reflect the Q_{10} effect of elevated body temperatures on the biochemical reactions involved in metabolism during the recovery period. However, there is other evidence indicating that anaerobic (or perhaps more precisely, glycolytic) metabolism in skeletal muscle is more pronounced during exercise in the heat than in temperate conditions. Although blood lactate concentrations during [111] or following [67, 111] progressive incremental exercise to exhaustion have been reported to be the same in hot and temperate environments, indicating no impairment of maximal glycolytic capacity, during steady-state submaximal exercise, blood lactate accumulation is usually observed to be greater under heat-stress conditions [20, 23, 75, 99, 130, 138].

As described earlier, blood lactate concentration during exercise is determined both by lactate release from active muscle into the blood as well as lactate uptake from the blood by the heart, liver, and skeletal muscles. Of these, only hepatic lactate removal has been evaluated for the effect of acute heat stress. Rowell et al. [99] have shown that splanchnic blood flow decreases during exercise, and the decrement is more pronounced during exercise in heat-stress conditions than in the cool. In addition, when hyperthermia develops due to acute heat stress, fractional extraction of arterial lactate by the liver during exercise is decreased compared to temperate conditions [99]. Rowell et al. [99] calculated, however, that the decrease in hepatic lactate extraction could not account for all of the increment in arterial lactate concentration observed during exercise in hot compared to temperate conditions. Therefore, increased lactate efflux from active skeletal muscle, decreased lactate uptake by heart and inactive skeletal muscle, or both must contribute to the increased blood lactate concentrations observed during prolonged exercise in the heat. The effect of heat stress on these vectors of lactate exchange between blood and other body tissues has not been measured.

Lactate exchange between blood and skeletal muscle during exercise would be influenced if heat stress results in a blood flow redistribution away from the muscles. A reduction in inactive muscle blood flow could provide for some of the increase in skin blood flow and cutaneous vascular volume during exercise in the heat, but lactate removal from the blood would be compromised. The effect of heat stress on blood flow to inactive muscle has not been demonstrated. The potential contribution of a redistribution of cardiac output from active muscle to skin during exercise in the heat is large. The studies in which a reduction in $\dot{V}o_2$ during steady-state exercise was observed suggest that muscle oxygen delivery may have been limited by a reduction in muscle blood flow but, as mentioned above, this is not always observed. Until fairly recently, direct measurements of the effect of heat stress on active muscle blood flow during exercise were not available.

Savard et al. [103] reported that acute heat stress did not affect active muscle blood flow in exercising humans. However, there was also no heat-stress effect on blood lactate observed in those experiments [103]. The experimental design used by Savard et al. [103] precludes comparison of physiological and metabolic responses after similar durations of exercise with and without heat stress. In that study [103], subjects wearing a water-perfused suit under a water-impermeable coverall performed two-legged upright cycling (50–60% $\dot{V}o_2max$) for a 25-min control period with no water circulating, and then the suit was perfused with 45–47°C water as exercise was continued for another 25 min. Esophageal temperatures increased about 0.75°C during the control period [103]; thus, the physiological measurements during this period may already reflect the effects of thermal strain. The additional heat stress imposed during the experimental period may have been insufficient to produce a difference in muscle blood flow and blood lactate responses. Studies showing a pronounced increment in blood lactate due to heat stress have employed more severe environmental stress [99, 138] and/or higher intensity exercise [31, 75, 138] as compared to Savard et al. [103]. Acute heat stress has been reported to result in a reduction in active muscle blood flow in exercising sheep [2]. Unfortunately, blood lactate data from that study were not reported. Therefore, a redistribution in blood flow away from skeletal muscle remains as a potential factor to explain the higher blood lactate accumulation observed during exercise in hot environments.

Lactate accumulation within active skeletal muscle is also accelerated by acute heat stress. Edwards et al. [26] observed that lactate and pyruvate concentrations in human muscle increased more following an isometric contraction preceded by heating the leg to a T_m of about 39°C as compared to when T_m was 22 or 33°C. These findings were interpreted as indicating that muscle glycolysis had been accelerated at the higher T_m [26]. Acute heat stress also results in a greater muscle lactate accumulation during continuous dynamic exercise. Young et al. [138] observed that postexercise muscle lactate concentrations were higher when men cycled (30 min, 70% $\dot{V}o_2max$) in the heat (49°C, 20% relative humidity) compared to cool conditions (21°C, 30% relative humidity). Kozlowski et al. [70] used a somewhat different approach but demonstrated a similar effect. As shown in Figure 3.6, dogs running to exhaustion on a treadmill exhibited less muscle lactate accumulation when the increase in T_m during exercise was attenuated by the use of external cooling pads as compared to control experiments without cooling pads [70]. Muscle pyruvate accumulation (not shown) was also blunted when the cooling pads were used [70].

A decrease in lactate efflux from active muscle may be one factor contributing to the increased muscle lactate concentrations observed during exercise in hot environmental conditions. Kozlowski et al. [70] observed higher ratios of muscle-to-blood lactate concentration when exercising dogs were not provided with external cooling as compared to

FIGURE 3.6

Muscle lactate concentrations as a function of muscle temperature measured in dogs running to exhaustion with (closed circles) and without (open circles) external cooling pads applied to the skin surface of the torso. (From Kozlowski S, Brzezinska Z, Kruk B, Kaciuba-Uscilko H, Greenleaf JE, Nazar K: Exercise hyperthermia as a factor limiting physical performance: temperature effect on muscle metabolism. J Appl Physiol *59:766–773, 1985.)*

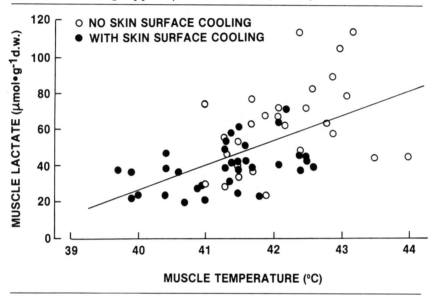

ratios observed when cooling was provided. This suggests that muscle lactate efflux was limited during hyperthermia. However, more pronounced panting in the dogs without cooling may have reduced arterial carbon dioxide and bicarbonate levels. Thus, lactate efflux may have been impaired by reduced bicarbonate levels [77] rather than by hyperthermia, per se. This remains to be clarified. Other data, however, indicate that increased muscle glycolysis contributes to the greater muscle lactate and pyruvate accumulation during exercise in hot as compared to cool environmental conditions.

Fink et al. [31], whose data are shown in Figure 3.7, reported that muscle glycogen depletion during cycling exercise (average power output = 138 W, $\dot{V}O_2$ = 2.1–2.4 liters·min^{-1}) was more rapid in a hot as compared to cold environment. Similarly, Kozlowski et al. [70] showed that, when exercise hyperthermia was limited by the use of external cooling pads, dogs exhibited a slower rate of muscle glycogen breakdown during running. Young et al. [138] observed no difference in muscle glycogen utilization during cycling exercise in hot as compared to

FIGURE 3.7

Changes in muscle glycogen (mean ± SE) in six non-heat acclimated men during three successive bouts of exercise (70–85% maximum oxygen uptake) in hot (41°C) and cold (9°C) ambient conditions. (From Fink WJ, Costill DL, Van Handel PJ: Leg muscle metabolism during exercise in the heat and cold. Eur J Appl Physiol 34:183–190, 1975.)

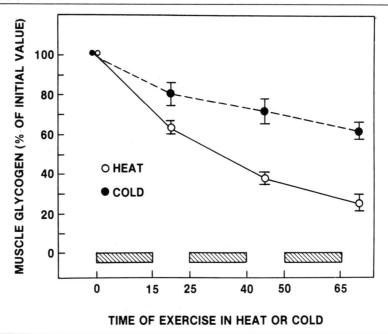

cool environments. However, the respiratory exchange ratio during exercise was slightly (but statistically significantly) higher in the hot as compared to cool conditions, suggesting that oxidation of a carbohydrate substrate other than muscle glycogen may have been increased during exercise in the heat.

Blood glucose might become more important as a substrate for muscle during exercise in heat-stress conditions. Hepatic glucose release is greatly increased during prolonged exercise (50% $\dot{V}o_2$max) in very hot (49°C) as compared to temperate conditions [99]. During severe exercise-heat stress, the reduced splanchnic blood flow combined with increased hepatic metabolism (Q_{10} effect) may result in a relative hepatic hypoxia, which in turn increases hepatic glycogenolysis and glucose release [99]. The increased hepatic glucose release may be an emergency mechanism ensuring adequate blood glucose delivery to the central nervous system and skeletal muscles [99]. Differences in blood glucose availability may explain the discrepancy between the findings of Fink et al. [31] and Young et al. [138] concerning the effect of heat stress on muscle glycogen utilization during exercise. Although exercise intensities were similar, Young et al. [138] had subjects exercise uninterrupted for 30 min, whereas Fink et al. [31] had subjects perform three 15-min exercise bouts, each separated by a 10-min rest period. Furthermore, Young et al. [138] used a more severe heat stress than Fink et al. [31] . Thus, the subjects of Young et al. [138] were probably exposed to greater thermal stress and may have experienced a more pronounced hepatic glucose release during exercise due to a greater reduction in splanchnic blood flow. It is known that blood glucose can be taken up and utilized by active muscle during exercise [57].

There are several mechanisms that could account for an increase in muscle glycolysis during exercise in the heat. More metabolic energy may be required to sustain muscular contractions when T_m are elevated above normal. Edwards et al. [26] observed that when T_m was increased by preheating, the decline in muscle ATP concentration during the first of a series of seven isometric contractions was greater than when the T_m was normal or reduced by precooling. These isometric contractions were 42–65 s in duration; therefore, aerobic ATP formation was assumed to be negligible, due to the almost complete restriction of muscle blood flow and oxygen delivery [26]. Glycolytic ATP formation was accelerated in heated as compared to cooled muscle, thus the rate of ATP utilization for a given amount of tension development must have been accelerated in the heated muscle or else the ATP concentration would not have declined more than in cooled muscle [26]. In agreement with this concept are the data of Asmussen et al. [1], which strongly suggest that the ability of muscle to store elastic energy is less at high than at low muscle temperatures. A reduction in the contribution of stored energy during tension development would have to be offset by an increased release of energy from metabolic sources.

It has been suggested that redistribution of blood flow from active muscle to the skin with exercise in hot conditions could serve to limit aerobic metabolism via various mechanisms associated with tissue hypoxia [31, 64]. As mentioned, whether or not human blood flow during exercise is compromised in the heat is not clear. However, even if muscle blood flow during exercise is reduced by heat stress, the development of any significant muscle hypoxia is unlikely to account for changes in muscle metabolism. Schumacker et al. [109] have presented data from animal experiments indicating that hyperthermia is associated with an increase in the muscle's ability to extract oxygen from the blood, thus allowing $\dot{V}o_2$ to be maintained unchanged despite a reduced oxygen delivery.

The mechanism regulating the increased glycolysis may simply be a Q_{10} effect on muscle glycolytic enzymes due to higher muscle temperatures during exercise in hot compared to cool environments. Alternatively, there is some evidence that during exercise-heat stress either a greater proportion of fast-twitch fibers are recruited or that fast-twitch fibers are more sensitive to the effects of increased muscle temperature and/or decreased muscle blood flow than slow-twitch fibers. As shown in Figure 3.8, individuals having the highest proportion of fast-twitch fibers exhibited the largest heat-stress-induced increments in postexercise muscle lactate concentrations [138]. More definitive studies are needed concerning neuromuscular recruitment during exercise in heat-stress conditions.

FIGURE 3.8

The difference in post exercise muscle lactate concentration in a hot (49°C) as compared to cool (21°C) environment plotted as a function ($p < 0.01$) of the individual percent fast-twitch fibers, before ($r = 0.60$) and after ($r = 0.71$) heat acclimation. (From Young AJ, Sawka MN, Levine L, Cadarette BS, Pandolf KB: Skeletal muscle metabolism during exercise is influenced by heat acclimation. J Appl Physiol *59:1929–1935, 1985.)*

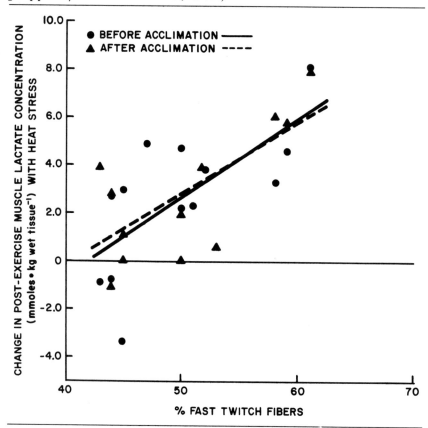

ADAPTATIONS WITH CHRONIC EXPOSURES TO EXERCISE-HEAT STRESS. Adaptations resulting from chronic exposure to environmental stress are termed as acclimatization or acclimation depending on whether they result from changes in the natural environment or controlled laboratory procedures, respectively. Whereas the distinction may be only semantic when considering adaptations to chronic hypoxic exposure, the differences are significant when considering adaptations to chronic heat stress. In general, the effects of heat acclimation programs take place more rapidly and are more pronounced than changes due to natural heat acclimatization, probably because acclimation programs usually involve more severely hot conditions and more intense exercise stress. All of the metabolic adaptations that will be discussed in this section have been observed in laboratory investigations, hence the term acclimation will be used.

A number of investigations have reported an effect of heat acclimation on $\dot{V}o_2$ during maximal and submaximal exercise. Sawka et al. [106] reported that there was a 7–8% decrement in $\dot{V}o_2$max in the heat compared to temperate conditions both before and after acclimation. In that study [106], Sawka and coworkers observed that $\dot{V}o_2$max in both environmental conditions was about 4% higher after acclimation than before, which was attributed to a small training effect due to the acclimation procedure. The occurrence of a small training effect during acclimation may explain why Williams et al. [130] reported that heat-acclimated individuals did not experience a decrement in $\dot{V}o_2$max during exposure to hot as compared to cool conditions. Williams et al. [130] measured $\dot{V}o_2$max in the cool environment first, after which the subjects were heat acclimated and then $\dot{V}o_2$max was determined in the hot environment. Thus, heat acclimation per se does not appear to alleviate the reduction in $\dot{V}o_2$max, which is measured in hot compared to temperate environmental conditions.

In contrast to maximal exercise, $\dot{V}o_2$ during submaximal exercise does appear to be affected by heat acclimation. Most reports indicate that $\dot{V}o_2$ and aerobic metabolic rate during submaximal exercise is reduced by heat acclimation [e.g., see Refs. 27, 104, 110, 116, and 138] although a significant effect is not always observed [64, 65, 115]. Large effects (14–17% reductions) have been reported for stair-stepping [110, 116], but some of the reduction in $\dot{V}o_2$ during stair-stepping can be attributed to increased skill and improved efficiency in performing the task acquired during the acclimation program. In two more recently reported studies, although the acclimation-induced reduction was statistically significant, the magnitude of the effect was reported to be relatively small for treadmill [104] and cycle-ergometer [138] exercise. Although interesting to physiologists, the reduction in aerobic metabolic rate resulting from heat acclimation is probably too small to have major importance for the heat balance equation.

Lactate accumulation in blood and muscle during submaximal exercise is generally found to be reduced following heat acclimation. Although Senay and Kok [110] reported that heat acclimation had no effect on blood lactate turn point, the lactate turn point discerned by their procedure would not necessarily have been changed by a reduction in blood lactate concentrations at the higher intensities. Young et al. [138] had subjects exercise 30 min at 70% $\dot{V}o_2$max in both a very hot (49°C) and a cool (21°C) environment before, and again after, they completed a 9-day heat (49°C) acclimation program. As Figure 3.9 shows, heat acclimation resulted in lower postexercise muscle lactate concentrations, although concentrations were still higher in the heat than in the cool; changes in blood lactate concentrations followed exactly the same pattern [138]. King et al. [64] observed that subjects exercising at 50% $\dot{V}o_2$max intermittently (30-min exercise/30-min rest) for 6 hr in the heat (40°C) exhibited lower blood lactates after the first 30-min bout following 8 days of acclimation (40°C) compared to before, with no apparent differences thereafter. Kirwan et al. [65] observed lower blood lactate concentrations only at the 15th min of exercise at 50% $\dot{V}o_2$max in a hot environment after acclimation (8 days, 40°C) than before, but concentrations after 30–60 min were unaffected. The less pronounced acclimation effect on blood lactate responses observed by King et al. [64] and Kirwan et al. [65] as compared to Young et al. [138] may reflect the less severe environmental conditions for heat acclimation or the lower exercise intensities used in their tests.

There is very little information available on the effects of heat acclimation on lactate efflux into and removal from blood. Kirwan et al. [65] observed that lactate release (product of arteriovenous difference and muscle blood flow) from skeletal muscle during exercise in the heat was the same before and after acclimation. If lactate efflux from active muscle is unaffected by heat acclimation, then lactate removal from the blood by the liver and inactive skeletal muscles must be increased following heat acclimation to account for the reduction in blood lactate accumulation during exercise. This could occur if heat acclimation alleviated the reduction in splanchnic and inactive muscle blood flow during exercise resulting from acute heat stress. There are no data that directly address this issue. However, the reduction in blood (and muscle) lactate accumulation due to heat acclimation is apparent during exercise tests performed in cool as well as hot conditions [138]. Body temperatures, sweating and, therefore probably regional blood flow during exercise in the cool environment were unaffected by acclimation [138]. Thus, while heat acclimation may result in an increase in lactate removal from the blood by the liver and inactive skeletal muscle, the mechanism is probably not an effect on regional blood flow distribution.

Assuming that lactate efflux from active muscle during exercise is unaffected by heat acclimation, then the lower postexercise muscle lac-

FIGURE 3.9

Effects of heat acclimation on changes in muscle lactate concentrations (mean ± SE) in 13 men exercising (70% maximum oxygen uptake) for 30 min in cool (21°C) and hot (49°C) ambient environments. (From Young AJ, Sawka MN, Levine L, Cadarette BS, Pandolf KB: Skeletal muscle metabolism during exercise is influenced by heat acclimation. J Appl Physiol *59:1929–1935, 1985.)*

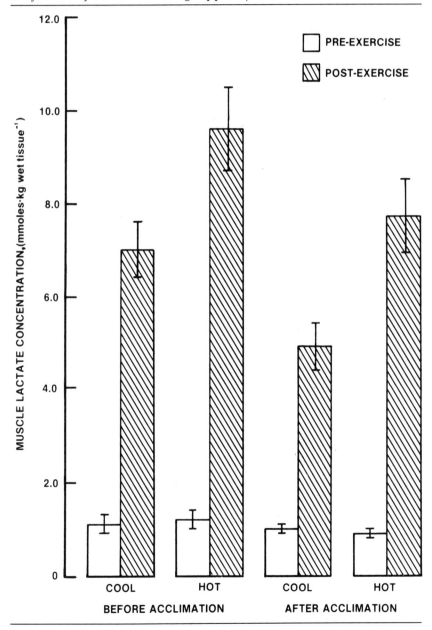

tate concentrations following heat acclimation result from a decreased rate of lactate production, an increased rate of oxidation, or both. King et al. [64] and Kirwan et al. [65] both observed that heat acclimation reduced muscle glycogen utilization during exercise in the heat by 40–50% compared to before acclimation. Young et al. [138] also observed a statistically significant glycogen sparing effect due to heat acclimation, but in that study the reduction in glycogen utilization was small and apparent only during exercise in the cool conditions; glycogen use during exercise in the heat was negligibly affected. As mentioned above, Young et al. [138] used a more severe heat stress and a higher intensity of exercise than used by the other investigators, which may explain the smaller glycogen sparing effect observed in the hot conditions. Thus, a reduction in muscle glycolysis during exercise appears to contribute to the reduction in muscle lactate accumulation resulting from heat acclimation.

The mechanism for the reduction in muscle glycogen use and lactate accumulation associated with heat acclimation remains unidentified. Respiratory exchange ratio is lower [65, 138] and free fatty acid uptake (product of muscle blood flow and arterio venous difference) greater [65] during exercise after than before acclimation. However, the changes reported are very small and it is unlikely that there is a substantial increase in fatty acid oxidation during exercise due to heat acclimation. There is no evidence that heat acclimation alters neuromuscular recruitment pattern or that fast-twitch fibers become any less sensitive to the effects of increased muscle temperature (see Fig. 3.8). Nevertheless, the lower muscle glycogen use and lactate accumulation following heat acclimation regardless of ambient environment, suggests that chronic heat stress may stimulate a metabolic adaptation independent of other physiological responses. One possibility deserving research attention is that a mitochondrial adaptation to chronic heat stress enables mitochondrial phosphorylation efficiency to be better maintained as muscle temperature rises.

In summary, increased body-heat storage and associated thermoregulatory adjustments due to acute heat stress result in alteration in metabolism during exercise as compared to cool conditions. Total metabolic rate during exercise at a given power output is higher in hot than cool environments, possibly because the rate of ATP utilization to develop a given muscle tension is increased as muscle temperature rises. Aerobic metabolism may decrease while oxygen debt, blood and muscle lactate accumulation, and skeletal muscle glycolytic rate are all increased during exercise in the heat as compared to cool conditions. In addition, lactate uptake and oxidation by liver (and probably nonexercising muscle) are impaired in heat-stress conditions. The mechanism for these effects is not clear, but reduced muscle and splanchnic blood flow, altered neuromuscular recruitment pattern, Q_{10} effects on glycolysis, and decreased mitochondrial phosphorylation efficiency may all be contributing factors. Besides thermoregulatory and cardiovascular adjustments, heat acclimation also produces adaptations in metabolic responses to exercise. Heat acclimation may lower total metabolic rate during exercise due to reductions in both aerobic and anaerobic components, but this effect is probably too small to reduce heat storage during exercise. On the other hand, changes in substrate metabolism induced by heat acclimation may contribute to improved endurance. Blood and muscle lactate accumulation and muscle glycogen depletion during exercise are all reduced following heat acclimation. The fact that these metabolic effects of acclimation are observed during exercise in cool as well as hot environments suggests that chronic heat exposure may result in a metabolic adaptation, which is independent of thermoregulatory and cardiovascular alterations.

EXERCISE IN COLD ENVIRONMENTS

Cardiovascular and Thermoregulatory Responses

For the most part, humans protect themselves from the cold by employing various behavioral strategies (e.g., clothing, protective shelter, external heat sources, migration). When these strategies are inadequate to prevent cold stress, humans exhibit two major physiological responses. Peripheral vasoconstriction reduces the thermal gradients along which heat is transferred from the core to the body surface, thus limiting body heat loss to the environment. In addition, metabolic heat production is increased by shivering, thereby tending to offset the increased heat loss. Metabolism during exercise in the cold may be influenced directly by the effects of reduced body temperatures as well as indirectly due to the side effects of shivering and cardiorespiratory and/or neurohumoral responses to cold-induced changes in body temperatures. Both shivering and peripheral vasoconstriction can be elicited during exercise, but the magnitude of these responses appears to vary with the exercise intensity and environmental conditions [56].

The concept of the prescriptive zone, that range of environmental conditions within which T_c responses to exercise were constant [71] was mentioned in the preceding section. Just as the upper temperature limit for this range is reduced as exercise intensity increases, the lower limit for this range is higher as exercise intensity decreases. Above this range, the increment in body temperatures during exercise becomes more pronounced due to the failure of heat dissipation mechanisms to keep pace with heat production [71]. Similarly below this range, T_c and T_m will increase less, remain unchanged, or decrease during exercise, depending on the balance between the rate of heat loss and metabolic heat production. During exercise in the cold, this balance is influenced by many other factors besides exercise intensity (e.g., exercise mode, anthropometry, coefficient for heat transfer), which have been considered in detail elsewhere [123].

Acute exposure to cold air or immersion in cold water elicits a peripheral vasoconstriction, which improves insulation. The body's insulative shell consists of two regions: the superficial shell (skin and subcutaneous fat) and the underlying muscle shell. As T_s declines below about 35°C, blood flow to the superficial shell decreases and insulation increases, achieving maximal values at T_s of about 31°C and lower [127]. In addition, poorly perfused inactive muscle tissue beneath the superficial shell provides as much as 85% of the body's total insulation in resting individuals [127]. During exercise, the insulation provided by muscle tissue decreases as compared to resting conditions due to increased muscle blood flow [127]. This effect, combined with the increased convective heat loss during exercise due to limb movement, results in increased body cooling and lower T_m as compared to temperate environmental conditions. Thus, muscle metabolism may be directly influenced by reduced T_m (Q_{10} effect) during exercise in the cold.

Cold exposure can also elicit a number of hormonal responses that may influence energy metabolism during exercise. For example, decreased body temperatures can result in increased blood norepinephrine and epinephrine concentrations, which may affect muscle metabolism [35]. Furthermore, the metabolic regulatory hormones cortisol and growth hormones appear to be released during exercise in response to a rise in body temperature [35]. Thus, in the cold, the response of these hormones to exercise may be less pronounced due to the attenuation of the increase in body temperature. Insulin and glucogen responses to exercise appear to be somewhat insensitive to the effects of cold [35], although insulin sensitivity of tissues appears increased in cold-exposed humans [124]. The effects of cold exposure on thyroid hormone responses to exercise that have been reported are variable and small [32].

The superficial shell can remain partially or completely vasoconstricted during exercise in the cold if T_s remains less than about 33°C [127], such as when exercise is performed in cold water and/or at low intensity. Active muscle might also remain somewhat vasoconstricted during exercise in the cold, particularly if T_m was low [126]. Blomstrand et al. [8] reported that limb blood flow immediately following exercise was lower when muscle temperatures were reduced by precooling the limb; however, limb blood flow measurements do not discern between skin versus muscle blood flow. Cardiac output during short-term (5 min) exercise in cold air [56] or cold water [80] is the same (heart rate decreases but stroke volume increases) for a given submaximal $\dot{V}O_2$, suggesting that muscle blood flow during exercise is unaffected by cold exposure. The effect of cold exposure on systemic oxygen transport during more prolonged exercise has not been investigated, nor has active muscle blood flow been measured during exercise in the cold. A reduced blood flow to active muscle could influence metabolism during exercise by mechanisms already discussed.

Maximal oxygen uptake can be reduced in the cold. The reduction in $\dot{V}O_2max$ is not due to cold exposure per se, but rather appears to be dependent on the reduction in T_c. For example, no decrease in $\dot{V}O_2max$ is observed when T_c is reduced by about 0.5°C [108]. With more pronounced reduction in T_c [5, 52, 56, 87,91] and/or T_m [5, 52, 91], significant decrements in $\dot{V}O_2max$ were observed. Myocardial contractility may be impaired when body temperatures are low [5], and maximal heart rate is also lower when body temperature is reduced [5, 52, 56, 87]. This suggests that the reduction in $\dot{V}O_2max$ is due to a reduced maximum cardiac output. The decrement in $\dot{V}O_2max$ may be proportional to the reduction in body temperature [5, 52], and decrements as high as 15–18% compared to measurements at normal body temperatures have been reported [5, 52, 87]. Thus, for a given $\dot{V}O_2$, exercise in the cold may require a greater % $\dot{V}O_2max$ than in temperate conditions, and muscle metabolism may be affected similarly to the effect of high-altitude exposure.

The occurrence of shivering may be another factor influencing muscle metabolism during both rest and exercise. At low exercise intensities, $\dot{V}O_2$ is generally observed to be higher in cold environments than in temperate control conditions [52, 53, 56, 80, 87, 114]. The increased $\dot{V}O_2$ is usually attributed to the added oxygen requirements for shivering. The difference in $\dot{V}O_2$ between cold and temperate conditions diminishes and eventually disappears as exercise intensity is increased [52, 53, 108, 114]. The exercise intensity below which $\dot{V}O_2$ is reported to be elevated in cold exposure varies depending on environmental and body-composition factors governing heat transfer to the environment. Peripheral and central afferent stimuli for shivering are provided by reductions in T_s and T_c, respectively [53, 88]. When metabolic heat production during exercise sufficiently offsets body-heat loss, shivering is suppressed [53, 56, 108]. This may occur because T_c and T_s are maintained above the threshold for shivering stimulation [53, 56]. However, even when body temperatures are reduced below values thought to represent the threshold for stimulation of shivering, moderate to high intensity exercise appears to suppress shivering [108].

Humans show several different patterns of adaptation in response to chronic cold stress [134]. Those adaptations have been documented in resting individuals, however, and they are observed more rarely than adaptations to chronic heat or high altitude. Probably for those reasons, the effects of cold acclimatization/acclimation on physiological responses to exercise have not been studied in detail.

Metabolic Responses

Before considering the effects of cold stress on exercise metabolism, the metabolism of shivering will be briefly examined. Horvath [56] has referred to shivering as a "quasi-exercising" state, in that muscles contract, metabolic heat is produced, but no external work is performed. Shivering consists of repeated involuntary contractions of the skeletal muscles. Shivering may begin immediately upon exposure to cold, or not for several minutes [56]. Usually observed in the neck and jaw muscles first, shivering spreads progressively to the torso and then limb muscles [56]. Cold-induced shivering is usually observed to result in a 2–3-fold increase in metabolic rate as compared to rest [78, 139], but as much as a 5-fold increase in metabolism is possible [56].

As with exercise, muscles actively engaged in shivering require an adequate supply of metabolic energy substrates. Shivering induced by cold exposure results in only a small increase [78, 139] or no change [84] in blood lactate concentration. The small changes in blood lactate concentration apparently belie rather large increases in the rate of lactate appearance in the blood during shivering. Minaire et al. [84] used radioactively labeled lactate infusion techniques to demonstrate that while blood lactate concentrations were unchanged by cold-induced shivering, the overall rates of lactate turnover were more than double the turnover rates measured in thermoneutral conditions. Thus, both lactate release from the muscles into the blood and removal of lactate from the blood were increased during shivering. In addition, lactate oxidation rate is about 40% of the rate of lactate removal from blood in dogs resting in thermoneutral conditions, but in cold-exposed shivering dogs, oxidation rate is about 70% of the rate of removal, which is comparable to lactate oxidation in exercising dogs [84]. These findings indicate that both glycolytic and oxidative muscle metabolism are increased during shivering.

Carbohydrate utilization, estimated from indirect calorimetry and respiratory exchange ratios, is markedly increased in shivering cold-exposed humans [124, 125]. For example, in seven men resting nude for 2 hr in air at 29°C, metabolic heat production due to carbohydrate oxidation was reported to average 140 kJ, but was about 750 kJ during a 2-hr exposure to 10°C air [125]. Although the cold-induced increment in metabolic heat production due to fat oxidation was, when expressed as a percent of the value measured in warm conditions, not as pronounced, fat oxidation does contribute very substantially to total metabolic heat production during shivering in the cold. In the aforementioned experiments, fat oxidation accounted for production of about 350 kJ of metabolic heat in men resting 2 hr at 29°C, but over 625 kJ during 2-hr of exposure at 10°C [125]. The greater increment in carbohydrate versus fat oxidation, relative to basal levels in warm conditions, may be hormonally mediated. Cold exposure appears to increase the insulin sensitivity of peripheral tissues, thereby enhancing glucose uptake [124].

Hypoglycemia impairs shivering during cold exposure. Haight and Keatinge [44] employed a combination of heavy exercise followed by alcohol ingestion to produce hypoglycemia in subjects before they were exposed to cold air. These subjects exhibited less shivering, lower metabolic rates, and larger decrements in body temperature compared to control trials when hypoglycemia was prevented by glucose ingestion [44]. Gale et al. [37] observed that subjects exposed to cold air stopped shivering and their metabolic rate and T_c fell when plasma glucose concentration fell below 2.5 mmol·liter^{-1} due to insulin infusion. Interestingly, intravenous glucose administration restored shivering in both an arterially occluded leg as well as a nonoccluded leg, suggesting that blood glucose may have been acting centrally rather than at the active muscle [37].

Whether or not muscle glycogen is a substrate for and can limit shivering, thermogenesis remains controversial. Young et al. [139] measured vastus lateralis muscle glycogen concentrations in eight subjects, before and after 2–3 hr of immersion in 18°C water repeated on two occasions. In one trial, preimmersion muscle glycogen levels had been substantially reduced by a 3-day exercise/low carbohydrate diet regimen preceding the test, and in the other trial, high preimmersion muscle glycogen levels were maintained by a 3-day rest/high carbohydrate diet regimen [139]. Shivering was visible in both trials, with no significant difference in metabolic rate or body cooling between the trials, and no significant change in muscle glycogen concentration during either trial [139]. Plasma glycerol and free fatty acid concentrations increased during immersion more in the low than high glycogen trial, and plasma glucose levels remained in the euglycemic range during both immersions [139]. These findings were interpreted as indicating that either muscle glycogen was not depleted in shivering muscle due to the availability of alternative metabolic substrates, or the vastus lateralis was not participating in the whole-body shivering response [139].

Martineau and Jacobs [78] also used 3-day diet/exercise manipulations in order to achieve high, low, and normal muscle glycogen levels in their eight subjects prior to immersing them for about 1 hr in 18°C water. In contrast to results of Young et al. [139], Martineau and Jacobs [78] observed a statistically significant reduction in vastus lateralis glycogen concentration during the trials in which the subjects had high or normal preimmersion glycogen levels, and no significant change when preimmersion glycogen levels had been reduced. Metabolic rate was slightly but significantly lower during the first 30 min of the low compared to the high and normal glycogen trials, with no differences between trials for the remainder of the immersion duration [78]. Body cooling rate was also greater during the low glycogen trial as compared to the others [78]. More pronounced increases in plasma glycerol and free fatty acid concentrations were observed during the low than high glycogen immersions [78]. The authors concluded that muscle glycogen was depleted during shivering, and that shivering thermogenesis was limited when muscle glycogen levels were reduced, resulting in more rapid body cooling during cold water immersion [78].

Figure 3.10 shows the individual pre- and postimmersion muscle glycogen concentrations of the subjects of Young et al. [139] during the high and low glycogen immersion trials, along with the pre- and postimmersion glycogen concentrations (mean ± SE) for the three trials reported by Martineau and Jacobs [71]. Although these investigations were conducted using nearly identical experimental designs and procedures, one important difference may explain the discrepancy between the two studies. Martineau and Jacobs studied extremely lean subjects; in fact, the leanest subject studied by Young et al. was fatter than the fattest of Martineau and Jacobs [78, 139]. The importance of body fat in providing resistance to body heat loss during cold exposure is well known [123, 127, 134] Based on their hydrostatically determined body fat content (9%), it can be estimated that the subjects studied by Martineau and Jacobs [78] had an average subcutaneous fat thickness of 0.9 mm, whereas the subcutaneous fat thickness of the subjects studied by Young et al. [139] ranged from 1.8 to 8 mm. Therefore, estimated [127] maximal superficial shell insulation of the subjects of Young et al. [139] was two to four times that of the subjects of Martineau and Jacobs [78]. Obviously, leaner subjects would be expected to experience a more rapid body cooling rate, which the data do show. Tikuisis et al. [122] have observed that there is an inverse relationship between adiposity and the metabolic response to a given reduction in body temperatures, thus metabolic heat production is stimulated more in lean than in fat individuals, even if they experience a similar reduction in core temperature.

Although the subjects studied by Martineau and Jacobs [78] were leaner and lost body heat more rapidly than those studied by Young et al. [139], the significant reduction in muscle glycogen levels during cold water immersion cannot necessarily be attributed to more pronounced shivering in the former. In both studies, metabolic rate after 60 min of cold water immersion was about 160 W/m^2, which corresponded to 25–30% of $\dot{V}o_2$max [78, 139]. Assuming that metabolic control during shivering and exercise are similar, relatively little glycogen depletion would have been expected at this low (compared to moderate intensity exercise) metabolic rate. Furthermore, the subjects of Young et al. [139] remained immersed and shivering for a longer period (2–3 versus 1 hr) than those of Martineau and Jacobs [78]. Therefore, shivering per se does not necessarily result in vastus lateralis glycogen depletion, and

FIGURE 3.10

Comparison of muscle glycogen concentrations before and after 1–3 hr of immersion in cold (18°C) water. Individual data points from Young et al. [139] show concentrations measured in four fat (>17%, closed symbols) and four lean (<12%, open symbols) subjects immersed once with high preimmersion glycogen levels (triangles) and again with low preimmersion glycogen levels (circles). In addition, data (mean ± SE, N = 8) reported by Martineau and Jacobs [78] from similar experiments are shown with points marked H, N, and L representing high, normal, and low preimmersion glycogen trials, respectively.

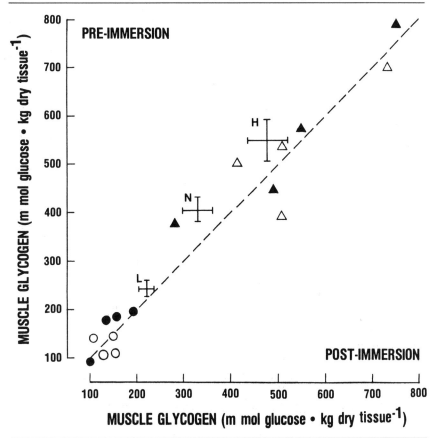

other mechanisms to account for the reduction in glycogen concentrations observed by Martineau and Jacobs [78] should be researched. Perhaps cooling increases glycolytic rate even in resting muscle, thereby satisfying ATP requirements with less efficient metabolic processes, but with a greater heat production (nonshivering thermogenesis?).

Despite the paucity of research on the effect of cold on human muscle metabolism during exercise, there is evidence that the rate of muscle glycolysis is increased during exercise in the cold. Blood lactate accumulation during sustained (i.e., >20 min) submaximal exercise has been reported to be increased by cold stress as compared to temperate conditions [35, 52, 87], although others have reported no change [48, 58]. The discrepancy probably relates to the degree of cold stress. The studies in which lactate responses to exercise were not altered were performed in an air environment and subjects experienced little or no reduction in T_c and no significant elevation in $\dot{V}o_2$ during exercise compared to control conditions [48, 58]. In contrast, studies reporting increased lactate accumulation in the cold involved cold water immersion and observed pronounced reductions in T_c and marked increases in $\dot{V}o_2$ during exercise compared to control conditions [35, 52, 87]. Furthermore, as mentioned above, shivering results in an increased rate of lactate turnover often with no change in blood lactate concentrations [84]. Therefore, changes in blood lactate concentration may be an especially poor indicator of muscle metabolism during exercise in the cold.

Muscle glycogen utilization during sustained submaximal exercise can be greater in cold than in temperate environments. Jacobs et al. [58] measured vastus lateralis glycogen concentration changes experienced by subjects cycling 30 min in 9 versus 21°C air. Each subject exercised at the same power output in both environments; half of the subjects exercised at a low (55 W) power output, while the others exercised at a moderate (103 W) power output [58]. The subjects exercising at the low power output experienced a greater depletion of muscle glycogen in the cold than in the temperate environment [58]. Figure 3.11 shows the difference between the two environments in glycogen utilization during low-intensity exercise. Those subjects who exercised at the higher power output experienced similar amounts of glycogen depletion in both environments [58]. The authors credited the increased glycogen breakdown during the low-intensity exercise to the additional energy required for shivering, whereas heat production during the higher intensity exercise was presumed adequate to obviate the need for shivering [58]. However, neither $\dot{V}o_2$ nor respiratory exchange ratio during exercise differed between the two trials indicating that metabolic rate was no greater in the cold than in the temperate environment [55]. Therefore, it seems tenuous to attribute the greater muscle glycogen utilization to the occurrence of shivering. Whether or not muscles actively contracting during exercise can also shiver has not been demonstrated. There are other mechanisms by which muscle glycogenolysis/glycolysis during exercise might be accelerated in cold conditions.

Blomstrand et al. [6–8] have studied the effects of reduced T_m on muscle metabolism during exercise to exhaustion (1–3 min) at very high power outputs (350–370 W). In these investigations, subjects completed one trial when preexercise T_m had been reduced by about 6°C by immersing the legs for 30 min in 12°C water, and an additional trial was

FIGURE 3.11

Change in muscle glycogen in six men exercising at low intensity (55 W) in temperate and cold environments. NS, not significant. (Drawn from data of Jacobs I, Romet TT, Kerrigan-Brown D: Muscle glycogen depletion during exercise at 9°C and 21°C. Eur J Appl Physiol 54:35–39, 1985.)

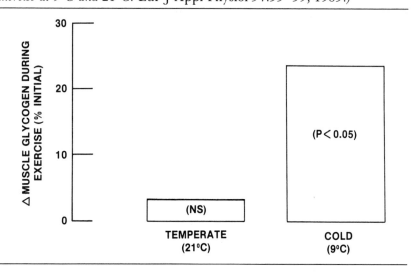

completed without the precooling of the legs [6–8]. T_m increased with exercise in both trials, but postexercise T_m was still about 3°C lower when the legs had been precooled than in the control experiments [6–8]. The decrease in muscle glycogen [7] and the increase in muscle glucose 6-phosphate and lactate [6–8] concentrations were all more pronounced during exercise when T_m were reduced. However, the increments were smaller in subjects whose T_m was reduced below 28°C, which might reflect the point at which muscle glycolysis is impaired due to the Q_{10} effect of profound reductions in T_m. The $\dot{V}o_2$ during these exercise bouts was the same when T_m was reduced as when it was normal, indicating that shivering was not a factor [6, 8]. Calf blood flow measurements made following exercise using venous occlusion plethysmography were lower in the trials with reduced T_m, leading the authors to suggest that reduced muscle blood flow during exercise impaired oxygen delivery, increased glycolysis, and reduced muscle lactate release [8]. That conclusion may be unwarranted because the blood flow measurements were not made during the exercise, and venous occlusion plethysmography cannot discern between muscle and skin blood flow. Although data from animal experiments suggest that muscle fiber recruitment might be influenced by cold stress [96], Blomstrand et al. [7] observed no evidence that muscle cooling had a selective effect on the glycogen utilization of fast- or slow-twitch muscle fibers in exercising humans.

There are two additional factors that might contribute to an increased muscle glycolysis and lactate accumulation during exercise in the cold. Mechanical efficiency of the muscle may be diminished as T_m decreases. Muscle force generation at a given contraction velocity is reduced by muscle cooling [4]; therefore, it has been suggested [8] that, to generate the force required for a given power output, a greater amount of muscle mass may need to be recruited. Alternatively, the increased glycolysis in cold versus temperate conditions may reflect the effects of elevated catecholamine concentrations. The increase in plasma epinephrine and norepinephrine during short-duration high-intensity exercise is more pronounced when muscle temperatures are reduced by cooling the muscle before exercise [8]. Similarly, plasma epinephrine and norepinephrine concentrations rise higher during prolonged [60-min) submaximal exercise in cold (21°C) than in comfortable (27°C) water [35]. Catecholamine responses to exercise are determined to some extent by the % $\dot{V}o_2$max [90, 133] and, as described previously, $\dot{V}o_2$max may be decreased when body temperature is lowered by cold stress. Therefore, the more pronounced catecholamine increase during exercise in the cold may reflect an increased relative exercise intensity, or may be a direct effect of cold stimulation of thermoreceptors. In any event, the increased catecholamine concentrations during exercise in the cold may result in increased stimulation of glycogen phosphorylase and accelerated muscle glycolysis [95].

In summary, the increased metabolic heat production elicited in humans exposed to cold stress results from increased oxidation of both carbohydrate and fat. The increment in the former is, relative to resting levels in warm conditions, more pronounced than the latter, although both are substantially increased. Increased oxidation of carbohydrate in resting humans may result in a decrease in muscle glycogen concentration during cold exposures of an hour or more, if the individuals are fairly lean. This may reflect the utilization of muscle glycogen stores by shivering activity, or an increased rate of glycolysis in the resting muscle stimulated by whole-body and muscle cooling. Individuals having moderate or substantial amounts of subcutaneous fat do not experience a measurable decrease in muscle glycogen during up to 3 hr of rest in the cold either because metabolic heat production is not stimulated as intensely as in leaner persons or because there are ample alternatives to muscle glycogen available to sustain shivering thermogenesis.

Whether or not muscle metabolism during exercise is affected by cold exposure appears to depend on the exercise intensity and magnitude of reduction in core and muscle temperature. With low-intensity exercise, and/or reduced muscle temperatures, muscle glycogen breakdown and glycolytic flux are accelerated; this effect may be attenuated or eliminated with profound lowering of muscle temperature. With muscle cooling, muscle lactate production is accelerated due to accelerated glycolysis during exercise; however, blood lactate concentration may be the same or only slightly greater than during exercise in temperate conditions due to an increase in the rate that lactate is removed from the blood and oxidized. A more pronounced catecholamine response to exercise during cold stress probably stimulates the increased muscle glycogenolysis but the occurrence of shivering and changes in muscle blood flow may also be a contributing factor. The effects of cold acclimation/acclimatization on human muscle metabolism during exercise have not been studied.

CONCLUSION

Human skeletal muscle metabolism during exercise is altered by exposure to the environmental extremes of high altitude, heat, and cold. An effect common to all three of the extreme environments is that unacclimatized individuals exhibit greater muscle glycogen breakdown, glycolytic flux, and lactate accumulation during exercise as compared to individuals exercising in temperate conditions at sea level.

The amount of force required to sustain a given power output is unaffected by the environmental conditions. However, the muscle's ability to develop tension at a given velocity may be altered by increased or decreased muscle temperature; thus, neuromuscular recruitment pattern and ultimately muscle metabolism would have to change to sustain exercise performance. Neuromuscular recruitment pattern during exercise may itself be altered by centrally mediated effects of hypoxemia, hyperthermia, and/or hypothermia.

The effect of extreme environments on muscle metabolism may also reflect the general inaccuracy of human energy metabolism during exercise. Galbo et al. [36] have observed that fuel mobilization and utilization during exercise is rarely precisely adjusted to energy needs of the active muscles because these processes respond to a feed-forward type of control. Among the factors involved in this feed-forward control system are the hormonal responses to exercise and blood flow to the active muscle, both of which influence the delivery of oxygen and exogenous fuels to the muscle. Hormonal and blood flow responses to exercise are themselves subject to the effects of heat, cold, and hypoxia. Therefore, environmental stress may provide nonmetabolic error signals influencing muscle metabolism [36]. Furthermore, the enzymes catalyzing the biochemical reactions making up the metabolic pathways are stimulated and inhibited by a variety of local factors in the intracellular regions where these reactions take place. These local factors include temperature, pH, and oxygen tension as well as substrate and cofactor availability, all of which may be affected by exposure to extreme environments.

Overall, acclimatization to extreme environments tends to limit performance decrements, while reducing the physiological strain imposed by the environments. Therefore, it is not surprising that the accelerated glycogen breakdown and lactate accumulation during exercise under acute heat stress or hypoxia abate with acclimatization to the environment. Whether or not cold adaptations include changes in muscle metabolism during exercise has yet to be determined, but in general, humans demonstrate less significant adaptations to chronic cold stress than to heat or high altitude. The metabolic adaptations to chronic heat stress or prolonged high-altitude exposure are probably secondary to adapted hormonal, cardiovascular, and thermoregulatory responses to environmental stress. However, the fact that metabolic adaptations are still evident with the restoration of normoxia/normothermia suggests that they may be independent of the other acclimatization effects and may involve a cellular level of adaptation to environmental stress.

DISCLAIMER AND DISTRIBUTION STATEMENTS

The views, opinions, and/or findings contained in this chapter are those of the author and should not be construed as an official Department of the Army position, policy, or decision, unless so designated by other official documentation.

Approved for public release; distribution is unlimited.

REFERENCES

1. Asmussen E, Bonde-Petersen F, Jorgensen K: Mechano-elastic properties of human muscles at different temperatures. *Acta Physiol Scand* 96:83–93, 1976.
2. Bell AW, Hales JRS, King RB, Fawcett AA: Influence of heat stress on exercise-induced changes in regional blood flow in sheep. *J Appl Physiol* 55:1916–1923, 1983.
3. Bender PR, Groves BM, McCullough RE, McCullough RG, Trad L, Young AJ, Cymerman A, Reeves JT: Decreased exercise muscle lactate release following high altitude acclimatization. *J Appl Physiol* 67:1456–1462, 1989.
4. Bergh U, Ekblom B: Influence of muscle temperature on maximal muscle strength and power output of human skeletal muscles. *Acta Physiol Scand* 107:33–37, 1979.
5. Bergh U, Ekblom B: Physical performance and peak aerobic power at different body temperatures. *J Appl Physiol* 46:885–889, 1979.
6. Blomstrand E, Bergh U, Essen-Gustavsson B, Ekblom B: Influence of low muscle temperature on muscle metabolism during intense dynamic exercise. *Acta Physiol Scand* 120:229–236, 1984.
7. Blomstrand E, Essen-Gustavsson B: Influence of reduced muscle temperature on metabolism in type I and type II human muscle fibres during intensive exercise. *Acta Physiol Scand* 131:569–574, 1987.
8. Blomstrand E, Kaijser L, Martinsson A, Bergh U, Ekblom B: Temperature- induced changes in metabolic and hormonal responses to intensive dynamic exercise. *Acta Physiol Scand* 127:477–484, 1986.

9. Bouissou P, Peronnet F, Brisson G, Helie R, Ledoux M: Metabolic and endocrine responses to graded exercise under acute hypoxia. *Eur J Appl Physiol* 55:290–294, 1986.

10. Brooks GA, Hittelman KJ, Faulkner JA, Beyer RE: Temperature, skeletal muscle mitochondrial functions, and oxygen debt. *Am J Physiol* 220:1053–1059, 1971.

11. Brooks GA, Hittelman KJ, Faulkner JA, Beyer RE: Tissue temperatures and whole-animal oxygen consumption after exercise. *Am J Physiol* 221:427–431, 1971.

12. Brouha L, Smith PE, De Lanne R, Maxfield ME: Physiological reactions of men and women during muscular activity and recovery in various environments. *J Appl Physiol* 16:133–140, 1960.

13. Buskirk ER, Kollias J, Akers RF, Prokop EK, Reategui ER: Maximal performance at altitude and on return from altitude in conditioned runners. *J Appl Physiol* 23:259–266, 1967.

14. Cerretelli PJ, di Prampero PE: Aerobic and anaerobic metabolism during exercise at altitude. *Med Sport Sci* 19:1–19, 1985.

15. Chiodi H: Respiratory adaptations to chronic high altitude hypoxia. *J Appl Physiol* 10:81–87 1957.

16. Conlee RK: Muscle glycogen and exercise endurance: a twenty-year perspective. In Pandolf KB (ed): *Exercise and Sport Sciences Reviews*. New York, MacMillan, 1987, pp 1–28.

17. Consolazio CF, Matoush LRO, Nelson RA, Torres JB, Isaac G: Environmental temperature and energy expenditures. *J Appl Physiol* 18:65–68, 1963.

18. Cunningham WL, Becker EJ, Kreuzer F: Catecholamines in plasma and urine at high altitude. *J Appl Physiol* 20:607–610, 1965.

19. Dempsey JA, Forster HV: Mediation of ventilatory adaptations. *Physiol Rev* 62:262–346, 1982.

20. Dimri GP, Malhotra MS, Gupta JS, Kumar TS, Arora BS: Alterations in aerobic-anaerobic proportions of metabolism during work in heat. *Eur J Appl Physiol* 45:43–50, 1980.

21. Dill DB, Myhre LG, Brown DK, Burrus K, Gehlsen G: Work capacity in chronic exposures to altitude. *J Appl Physiol* 23:555–560, 1967.

22. Dudley GA, Staron RS, Murray TF, Hagerman FC, Luginbuhl A: Muscle fiber composition and blood ammonia levels after intense exercise in humans. *J Appl Physiol* 54:582–586, 1983.

23. Eccles RM, Loyning Y, Oshima T: Effects of hypoxia on the monosynaptic reflex pathway in the cat spinal cord. *J Neurophysiol* 29:315–332, 1966.

24. Edgerton VR, Roy RR, Gregor RJ, Hager CL, Wickiewicz T: Muscle fiber activation and recruitment. In Knuttgen HG, Vogel JA, Poortmans J (eds): *Biochemistry of Exercise*. Champaign, IL, Human Kinetics, 1983 pp 31–49.

25. Edwards HT: Lactic acid in rest and work at high altitude. *Am J Physiol* 116:367–375, 1936.

26. Edwards RHT, Harris RC, Hultman E, Kaijser L, Koh D, Nordesjo LO: Effect of temperature on muscle energy metabolism and endurance during successive isometric contractions, sustained to fatigue, of the quadriceps muscle in man. *J Physiol* 220:335–352, 1972.

27. Eichna LW, Park CR, Nelson N, Horvath SM, Palmes ED. Thermal regulation during acclimatization in a hot dry desert type environment. *Am J Physiol* 163:585–597, 1950.

28. Escourrou P, Johnson DG, Rowell LB: Hypoxemia increases plasma catecholamine concentrations in exercising humans. *J Appl Physiol* 57:1507–1511, 1984.

29. Eyzaguirre C, Fidone SJ: *Physiology of the Nervous System*. ed 2. Chicago, Year Book, 1975, pp 202–204.

30. Fagraeus L, Karlsson J, Linnarsson D, Saltin B: Oxygen uptake during maximal work at lowered and raised ambient air pressures. *Acta Physiol Scand* 87:411–421, 1973.

31. Fink WJ, Costill DL, Van Handel PJ: Leg muscle metabolism during exercise in the heat and cold. *Eur J Appl Physiol* 34:183–190, 1975.
32. Francesconi, BP: Endocrinological responses to exercise in stressful environments. In Pandolf KB (ed): *Exercise and Sport Sciences Reviews*. New York, MacMillan, 1988, pp 255–284.
33. Friedemann TE, Haugen GE, Kmieciak TC: The level of pyruvic and lactic acids and lactic pyruvic ratio in the blood of human subjects. The effect of food, light, muscular activity, and anoxia at high altitude. *J Biol Chem* 157:673–689, 1945.
34. Fulco, CS, Cymerman A: Human performance and acute hypoxia. In Pandolf KB, Sawka MN, Gonzalez RR (eds): *Human Performance Physiology and Environmental Medicine at Terrestrial Extremes*. Indianapolis, Benchmark, 1988, pp 467–495.
35. Galbo H, Houston ME, Christensen NJ, Holst JJ, Nielsen B, Nygaard E, Suzuki J: The effect of water temperature on the hormonal response to prolonged swimming. *Acta Physiol Scand* 105:326–337 1979.
36. Galbo H, Richter EA, Sonne B: On the accuracy of fuel mobilization in exercise. In Saltin B (ed): *Biochemistry of Exercise VI*. Champaign, IL, Human Kinetics, 1986, pp 223–226.
37. Gale EAM, Bennett T, Green Hilary J, MacDonald IA: Hypoglycemia, hypothermia, and shivering in man. *Clin Sci Lond* 61:463–469, 1981.
38. Glesser MA, Vogel JA: Endurance capacity for prolonged exercise on the bicycle ergometer. *J Appl Physiol* 34:438–442, 1973.
39. Glesser MA, Vogel JA: Effects of acute alteration of $\dot{V}o_2$max on endurance capacity of men. *J. Appl Physiol* 34:443–447, 1973.
40. Gollnick PD, Hermansen L: Biochemical adaptations to exercise: anaerobic metabolism. In Wilmore JH (ed): *Exercise and Sport Sciences Reviews*. New York, Academic Press, 1973, pp 1–43.
41. Green HJ, Sutton JR, Cymerman A, Young PM, Houston CS: Operation Everest II: adaptations in human skeletal muscle. *J Appl Physiol* 66: 2454–2461, 1989.
42. Green HJ, Sutton J, Young PM, Cymerman A, Houston CS: Operation Everest II: muscle energetics during maximal exhaustive exercise. *J Appl Physiol* 66:142–150, 1989.
43. Grover RF, Weil JV, Reeves JT: Cardiovascular adaptation to exercise at high altitude. In Pandolf KB (ed): *Exercise and Sport Sciences Reviews*. New York, MacMillan, 1986, pp 269–302.
44. Haight JSL, Keatinge WR: Failure of thermoregulation induced by exercise and alcohol in man. *J Physiol Lond* 229:87–97, 1973.
45. Harboe M: Lactic acid content in human venous blood during hypoxia at high altitude. *Acta Physiol Scand* 40:248–253, 1957.
46. Havel RJ: Autonomic nervous system and adipose tissue. In *Handbook of Physiology, Adipose Tissue*. Washington, D.C., American Physiological Society, 1965, pp 575–582.
47. Hermansen L, Saltin B: Blood lactate concentration during exercise at acute exposure to altitude. In Margaria R (ed): *Exercise at Altitude*. New York, Excerpta Medica Foundation, 1967, pp 48–53.
48. Hessemer V, Langusch D, Bruck K, Bodeker RH, Breidenbach T: Effect of slightly lowered body temperatures on endurance performance in humans. *J Appl Physiol* 57:1731–1737, 1984.
49. Hill AV, Lupton H: Muscular exercise, lactic acid and the supply and utilization of oxygen. *O J Med* 16:135–171, 1923.
50. Hogan MC, Cox RH, Welch HG: Lactate accumulation during incremental exercise with varied inspired oxygen fractions. *J Appl Physiol* 55:1134–1140, 1983.
51. Holloszy JO: Biochemical adaptations to exercise: aerobic metabolism. In Wilmore JH (ed): *Exercise and Sport Sciences Reviews*. New York, Academic Press, 1973, pp 45–71.

52. Holmer I, Bergh U: Metabolic and thermal response to swimming in water at varying temperatures. *J Appl Physiol* 37:702–705, 1974.
53. Hong SI, Nadel ER: Thermogenic control during exercise in a cold environment. *J Appl Physiol* 47:1084–1089, 1979.
54. Horstman DH, Gleser M, Delahunt J: Effects of altering O_2 delivery on $\dot{V}o_2$ of isolated, working muscle. *Am J Physiol* 230:327–334, 1976.
55. Horstman DH, Weiskopf R, Jackson RE: Work capacity during 3-week sojourn at 4300 m; effects of relative polycythemia. *J Appl Physiol* 49:311–318, 1980.
56. Horvath SM: Exercise in a cold environment. In Miller DI (ed): *Exercise and Sport Sciences Reviews*. Philadelphia, Franklin Institute Press, 1981, pp 221–263.
57. Ivy JL: The insulin-like effect of muscle contraction. In Pandolf KB (ed): *Exercise and Sport Sciences Reviews*. New York, MacMillan, 1987, pp 29–51.
58. Jacobs I, Romet TT, Kerrigan-Brown D: Muscle glycogen depletion during exercise at 9°C and 21°C. *Eur J Appl Physiol* 54:35–39, 1985.
59. Jones NL, Robertson DG, Kane JW, Hart RA: Effect of hypoxia on free fatty acid metabolism during exercise. *J Appl Physiol* 33:733–738, 1972.
60. Jones NL, Sutton JR, Taylor R, Toews CJ: Effect of pH on cardiorespiratory and metabolic responses to exercise. *J Appl Physiol* 43:959–964, 1977.
61. Jorfeldt L: Metabolism of L(+)-lactate in human skeletal muscle during exercise. *Acta Physiol Scand Suppl* 338:1–67, 1970.
62. Katz A, Sahlin K: Effect of decreased oxygen availability on NADH and lactate contents in human skeletal muscle during exercise. *Acta Physiol Scand* 131:119–127, 1987.
63. King CE, Dodd SL, Cain SM: O_2 delivery to contracting muscle during hypoxia or CO hypoxia. *J Appl Physiol* 63:726–732, 1987.
64. King DS, Costill DL, Fink WJ, Hargreaves M, Fielding RA: Muscle metabolism during exercise in the heat in unacclimatized and acclimatized humans. *J Appl Physiol* 59:1350–1354, 1985.
65. Kirwan JP, Costill DL, Kuipers H, Burrell MJ, Fink WJ, Kovaleski JE, Fielding RA: Substrate utilization in leg muscle of men after heat acclimation. *J Appl Physiol* 63:31–35, 1987.
66. Klain GJ, Hannon JP: Effects of high altitude on lipid components of human serum. *Proc Soc Exp Biol Med* 129:646–649, 1969.
67. Klausen K, Dill DB, Phillips EE, McGregor D: Metabolic reactions to work in the desert. *J Appl Physiol* 22:292–296, 1967.
68. Knuttgen HG, Saltin B: Oxygen uptake, muscle high-energy phosphates, and lactate in exercise under acute hypoxic conditions in man. *Acta Physiol Scand* 87:368–376, 1973.
69. Knuttgen HG, Saltin B: Muscle metabolites and oxygen uptake in short-term submaximal exercise in man. *J Appl Physiol* 32:690–694, 1972.
70. Kozlowski S, Brzezinska Z, Kruk B, Kaciuba-Uscilko H, Greenleaf JE, Nazar K: Exercise hyperthermia as a factor limiting physical performance: temperature effect on muscle metabolism. *J Appl Physiol* 59:766–773, 1985.
71. Lind AR: A physiological criterion for setting thermal environmental limits for everyday work. *J Appl Physiol* 18:51–56, 1963.
72. Linnarsson D, Karlsson J, Fagraeus L, Saltin B: Muscle metabolites and oxygen deficit with exercise in hypoxia and hyperoxia. *J Appl Physiol* 36:399–402, 1974.
73. Lorentzen FV: Lactic acid in blood after various combinations of exercise and hypoxia. *J Appl Physiol* 17:661–664, 1962.
74. Lowenstein JM: Ammonia production in muscle and other tissues: the purine nucleotide cycle. *Physiol Rev* 52:82–414, 1972.
75. MacDougall JD, Reddan WG, Layton CR, Dempsey JA:. Effects of metabolic hyperthermia on performance during heavy prolonged exercise. *J Appl Physiol* 36:538–544, 1974.

76. Maher JT, Jones LG, Hartley LH: Effects of high-altitude exposure on submaximal endurance capacity of men. *J Appl Physiol* 37:895–898, 1974.

77. Mainwood BW, Worsley-Brown P: The effects of extracellular pH and buffer concentiation on the efflux of lactate from frog sartorius muscle. *J Physiol* 250:1–22, 1975.

78. Martineau L, Jacobs I: Muscle glycogen availability and temperature regulation in humans. *J Appl Physiol* 66:72–78, 1989.

79. Mazzeo RS, Brooks GA, Sutton J, Butterfield G, Wolfel G, Groves B, Reeves JT: Catecholamine response at rest and during exercise at sea level, acute and chronic exposure to high altitude, (Abstract). *Med Sci Sports Exerc* 21:S61, 1989.

80. McArdle WD, Magel JR, Lesmes GR, Pechar GS: Metabolic and cardiovascular adjustment to work in air and water at 18, 25 and 33°C. *J Appl Physiol* 40:85–90, 1976.

81. McLellan T, Jacobs I, Lewis W: Acute altitude exposure and altered acid-base states, I. effects on the exercise ventilation and blood lactate responses. *Eur J Appl Physiol* 57:435–444, 1988.

82. McLellan T, Jacobs I, Lewis W: Acute altitude exposure and altered acid-base states. II. effects on exercise performance and muscle and blood lactate. *Eur J Appl Physiol* 57:445–451, 1988.

83. McManus BM, Horvath SM, Bolduan N, Miller JC: Metabolic and cardiorespiratory responses to long-term work under hypoxic conditions. *J Appl Physiol* 36:177–182, 1974.

84. Minaire Y, Pernod A, Jomain M-J, Mottaz M: Lactate turnover and oxidation in normal and adrenal-demedullated dogs during cold exposure. *Can J Physiol Pharmacol* 49:1063–1070, 1971.

85. Mutch BJC, Banister EW: Ammonia metabolism in exercise and fatigue: a review. *Med Sci Sports Exerc* 15:41–50, 1983.

86. Naimark A, Jones NL, Lal S: The effect of hypoxia on gas exchange and arterial lactate and pyruvate concentration during moderate exercise in man. *Clin Sci* 28:1–13, 1965.

87. Nadel ER, Holmer I, Bergh U, Astrand P-O, Stolwijk JAJ: Energy exchanges of swimming man. *J Appl Physiol* 36:465–471, 1974.

88. Nielsen B: Metabolic reactions to changes in core and skin temperature in man. *Acta Physiol Scand* 97:129–138, 1976.

89. Nielsen M: Die regulation der korpertemperatur bei muskelarbeit. *Skand Arch Physiol* 79:193–230, 1938.

90. Peronnet F, Cleroux J, Perrault, H, Cousineau D, deChamplain J, Nadeau R: Plasma norepinephrine response to exercise before and after training in humans. *J Appl Physiol* 51:812–815, 1981.

91. Pirnay F, Deroanne R, Petit JM: Influence of water temperature on thermal, circulatory and respiratory responses to muscular work. *Eur J Appl Physiol* 37:129–136, 1977.

92. Ramsoe K, Jarnum S, Preisig R, Tauber J, Tygstrup N, Westergaard H: Liver function and blood flow at high altitude. *J Appl Physiol* 28:725–727, 1970.

93. Raynaud J, Drouet L, Martineaud JP, Bordachar J, Coudart J, Durand J: Time course of plasma growth hormone during exercise in humans at altitude. *J Appl Physiol* 50:229–233, 1981.

94. Reynafarje B: Myoglobin content and enzymatic activity of muscle and altitude adaptation. *J Appl Physiol* 17:301–305, 1962.

95. Richter EA, Ruderman NB, Gavras H, Belur ER, Galbo H: Muscle glycogenolysis during exercise: dual control by epinephrine and contractions. *Am J Physiol* 242:E25–E32, 1982.

96. Rome LC, Loughna PT, Goldspink G: Muscle fiber activity in carp as a function of swimming speed and muscle temperature. *Am J Physiol* 247:R272–R279, 1984.

97. Rose MS, Houston CS, Fulco CS, Coates G, Sutton JR, Cymerman A: Operation Everest II: nutrition and body composition. *J Appl Physiol* 65:2545–2552, 1988.
98. Rowell LB: Human cardiovascular adjustments to exercise and thermal stress. *Physiol Rev* 54:75–159, 1974.
99. Rowell LB, Brengelmann GL, Blackmon JR, Twiss RD, Kusumi F: Splanchnic blood flow and metabolism in heat-stressed man. *J Appl Physiol* 24:475–484, 1969.
100. Rowell LB, Blackmon JR, Kenny MA, Escourrou P: Splanchnic vasomotor and metabolic adjustments to hypoxia and exercise in humans. *Am J Physiol* 247:H251-H258, 1984.
101. Saltin B, Gagge AP, Stolwijk JAJ: Muscle temperature during submaximal exercise in man. *J Appl Physiol* 25:679–688, 1968.
102. Saltin B, Karlsson J: Muscle glycogen utilization during work of different intensities. In Pernow B, Saltin B (eds): *Muscle Metabolism During Exercise.* New York, Plenum Press, 1971, pp 289–299.
103. Savard GK, Nielsen B, Laszczynska J, Larsen BE, Saltin B: Muscle blood flow is not reduced in humans during moderate exercise and heat stress. *J Appl Physiol* 64:649–657, 1988.
104. Sawka MN, Pandolf KB, Avellini BA, Shapiro Y: Does heat acclimation lower the rate of metabolism elicited by muscular exercise? *Aviat Space Environ Med* 54:27–31, 1983.
105. Sawka MN, Wenger CB: Physiological responses to acute exercise-heat stress. In Pandolf KB, Sawka MN, Gonzalez RR (eds): *Human Performance Physiology and Environmental Medicine at Terrestrial Extremes.* Indianapolis, Benchmark, 1988, pp 97–151.
106. Sawka MN, Young AJ, Cadarette BS, Levine L, Pandolf KB: Influence of heat stress and acclimation on maximal aerobic power. *Eur J Appl Physiol* 53:294–298, 1985.
107. Schmeling WT, Forster HV, Hosko MJ: Effect of sojourn at 3200-m altitude on spinal reflexes in young adult males. *Aviat Space Environ Med* 48:1039–1045, 1977.
108. Schmidt V, Bruck K: Effect of a precooling maneuver on body temperature and exercise performance. *J Appl Physiol* 50:772–778, 1981.
109. Schumacker PTJ, Rowland J, Saltz S, Nelson DP, Wood LSH: Effects of hyperthermia and hypothermia on oxygen extraction by tissues during hypovolemia. *J Appl Physiol* 63:1246–1252, 1987.
110. Senay LC, Kok R: Effects of training and heat acclimatization on blood plasma contents of exercising men. *J Appl Physiol* 43:591–599, 1977.
111. Smolander J, Kilar P, Korhonen O, Ilmarinen R: Aerobic and anaerobic responses to incremental exercise in a thermoneutral and a hot dry environment. *Acta Physiol Scand* 128:15–21, 1986.
112. Squires RW, Buskirk ER: Aerobic capacity during acute exposure to simulated altitude, 914 to 2286 m. *Med Sci Sports Exerc* 14:36–40, 1982.
113. Stanley WC, Gertz EW, Wisneski JA, Neese RA, Morris DA, Brooks GA: Lactate extraction during net lactate release in legs of humans during exercise. *J Appl Physiol* 60:1116–1120, 1986.
114. Stromme, S, Andersen KL, Elsner RW: Metabolic and thermal responses to muscular exertion in the cold. *J Appl Physiol* 18:756–763, 1963.
115. Strydom NB, Wyndham CH, Williams CG, Morrison JF, Bredell GAG, Benade AJS, Von Rahden M: Acclimatization to humid heat and the role of physical conditioning. *J Appl Physiol* 21:636–642, 1966.
116. Strydom NB, Wyndham CH, Williams CG, Morrison JF, Bredell GAG, Von Rahden MJ, Peter J: Energy requirements of acclimatized subjects in humid heat. *Fed Proc* 25:1366–1371, 1966.
117. Sutton JR: Scientific and medical aspects of the Australian Expedition. *Med J Aust* 2:355–361, 1971.
118. Sutton JR: Effect of acute hypoxia on the hormonal responses to exercise. *J Appl Physiol* 42:587–592, 1977.

119. Sutton JR, Jones NL, Toews CJ: Effect of pH on muscle glycolysis during exercise. *Clin Sci* 61:331–338, 1981.

120. Tappan DV, Reynafarje B, Potter VR, Hurtado A: Alterations in enzymes and metabolites resulting from adaptation to low oxygen tension. *Am J Physiol* 190:93–98, 1957.

121. Terjung RL, Hood DA: Biochemical adaptations in skeletal muscle induced by exercise training. In Layman DA (ed): *Nutrition and Aerobic Exercise.* Washington DC, American Chemical Society, 1986, pp 8–27.

122. Tikuisis P, Gonzalez RR, Oster RA, Pandolf KB: Role of body fat in the prediction of the metabolic response for immersion in cold water. *Undersea Biomed Res* 15:123–134, 1988.

123. Toner MN, McArdle WD: Physiological adjustments of man to the cold. In Pandolf KB, Sawka MN, Gonzalez RR (eds): *Human Performance Physiology and Environmental Medicine at Terrestrial Extremes.* Indianapolis, Benchmark, 1988, pp 361–399.

124. Vallerand AL, Frim J, Kavanagh MF: Plasma glucose and insulin responses in cold-exposed humans. *J Appl Physiol* 65:2395–2399, 1988.

125. Vallerand AL, Jacobs I: Rates of energy substrates utilization during human cold exposure. *Eur J Appl Physiol* 58:873–878, 1989.

126. Vanhoutte PM: Physical factors of regulation. *Handbook of Physiology. The Cardiovascular System.* Bethesda, MD, American Physiological Society, 1980, pp 443–474.

127. Viecsteinas A, Ferretti G, Rennie DW: Superficial shell insulation in resting and exercising men in cold water. *J Appl Physiol* 52:1557–1564, 1982.

128. Wenger CB: Human heat acclimatization. In Pandolf KB, Sawka MN, Gonzalez RR (eds): *Human Performance Physiology and Environmental Medicine at Terrestrial Extremes.* Indianapolis, Benchmark, 1988, pp 153–197.

129. Willer JC, Miserocchi G, Gautier H: Hypoxia and monosynaptic reflexes in humans. *J Appl Physiol* 63:639–645, 1987.

130. Williams CG, Bredell GAG, Wyndham CH, Strydom NB, Morrison JF, Peter J, Fleming PW, Ward JS: Circulatory and metabolic reactions to work in heat. *J Appl Physiol* 17:625–638, 1962.

131. Wilson DF, Erecinska M, Drown C, Silver IA: Effect of oxygen tension on cellular energetics. *Am J Physiol* 233:C135–140, 1977.

132. Wilson DF, Erecinska M, Silver IA: Metabolic effects of lowering oxygen tension in vivo. In Bicher HI, Bruley DF (eds): *Oxygen Transport to Tissue—IV.* New York, Plenum Press, 1983, pp 293–301.

133. Winder WW, Hickson RC, Hagberg JM, Ehsani AA, McLane JA: Training-induced changes in hormonal and metabolic responses to submaximal exercise. *J Appl Physiol* 46:766–771, 1979.

134. Young AJ: Human adaptation to cold. In Pandolf KB, Sawka MN, Gonzalez RR (eds): *Human Performance Physiology and Environmental Medicine at Terrestrial Extremes.* Indianapolis, Benchmark, 1988, pp 401–434.

135. Young AJ, Evans WJ, Cymerman A, Pandolf KB, Knapik JJ, Maher JT: Sparing effect of chronic high-altitude exposure on muscle glycogen utilization. *J Appl Physiol* 52:857–862, 1982.

136. Young AJ, Evans WJ, Fisher EC, Sharp RL, Costill DL, Maher JT: Skeletal muscle metabolism of sea-level natives following short-term high-altitude residence. *Eur J Appl Physiol* 52:463–466, 1984.

137. Young AJ, Neufer PD, Hesslink RL, Reeves JT: Muscle fiber size in lowland residents before and after altitude acclimatization (Abstract). *Physiologist* 31:a146, 1988.

138. Young AJ, Sawka MN, Levine L, Cadarette BS, Pandolf KB: Skeletal muscle metabolism during exercise is influenced by heat acclimation. *J Appl Physiol* 59:1929–1935, 1985.

139. Young AJ, Sawka MN, Neufer PD, Muza SR, Askew EW, Pandolf KB: Thermoregulation during cold water immersion is unimpaired by low muscle glycogen levels. *J Appl Physiol* 66:1809–1816, 1989.
140. Young AJ, Young PM: Human acclimatization to high terrestrial altitude. In Pandolf KB, Sawka MN, Gonzalez RR (eds): *Human Performance Physiology and Environmental Medicine at Terrestrial Extremes.* Indianapolis, Benchmark, 1988, pp 497–543.
141. Young PM, Rock PB, Fulco CS, Trad LA, Forte VA, Cymerman A: Altitude acclimatization attenuates plasma ammonia accumulation during submaximal exercise. *J Appl Physiol* 63:758–764, 1987.

4
Physiological Adaptations to Weightlessness: Effects on Exercise and Work Performance

VICTOR A. CONVERTINO, Ph.D.

"The aspiration to travel beyond the atmosphere is like the desire to study the ocean floor, the interior of the Earth's crust, to invent a submarine, to fly through the air, improve life, treat disease, and explore the heavens."

KONSTANTIN TSIOLKOVSKY, 1857–1935
Russian School Teacher

The need of people to explore, live, and work in a world of varying conditions of pressures and temperatures has required their physiological adaptation to these environments. This relationship has led to a wealth of scientific experiments in a field that we know as environmental and exercise physiology. One environmental factor that has received little attention until recently is gravity, probably because it is virtually constant on earth. However, with the emergence of travel to space and visit to planets with lower gravitational forces (e.g., the moon) in order to expand our knowledge about the universe and explore its resources, the reduction in gravity and its effects on a human's ability to work and exercise have become important issues.

The "doors" to the world of microgravity were opened to humans when the Soviets launched Yuri Gagarin into space on April 12, 1961. The early space programs were primarily experimental to determine if humans could go to space and safely return. The early flights were limited to relatively short durations and confined to small spacecrafts that required little physical work. In the 28 years of human spaceflight, over 230 astronauts and cosmonauts (10 of them women) have actually flown in space, over 100 of whom have returned to space for multiple visits. The requirement to perform physical work and ambulation in a microgravity environment was emphasized by the successful U.S. landing of 12 astronauts on the moon during Apollo flights 11 through 17. The commitment to a permanent presence in space has been underscored by three missions of the first U.S. space station Skylab (nine astronauts) of 28, 59, and 84 days and the flights of the Soviet space station Mir, in which 11 cosmonauts have flown over 6 months with the current record being 366 days by Musa Manarov and Vladimir Titov.

119

DEFINITIONS AND DESCRIPTIONS OF SPACE MISSIONS

Throughout this review, reference will be made to data collected during specific spaceflight missions from both U.S. and Soviet programs. Most of the data will be identified with the name of a specific space mission on which the experiment was conducted. To gain some understanding and perspective of what these data mean, the following section is presented to define the names of the various spacecraft used in human spaceflight and briefly to describe the evolution and purpose of each program.

United States Space Program

The U.S. manned space program began with the flight of Alan B. Shepard on May 5, 1961, less than 1 month after the first manned Soviet flight of Yuri Gagarin. The Mercury space capsule was the first craft used in the program. It was very small and could hold only one astronaut. The program consisted of six manned flights (two balistic and four orbital flights) from May 1961 to May 1963 and its objectives included protecting the crew member against the space environment, ensuring reliable operation of spacecraft systems, assuring safe and accurate reentry and landing, and establishing the basic parameters of human response to spaceflight [42].

The second generation of U.S. spacecraft was the Gemini "capsule" that had the capacity for carrying two astronauts. It also was small and restricted movement of astronauts. However, this program provided the United States with experience in rendezvous, docking, extravehicular activities (EVA), and longer exposure to microgravity (up to 14 days) in preparation for the Apollo program. This program consisted of 10 manned missions from March 1965 to November 1966 and provided the first U.S. opportunity to learn about a human's ability to work in space.

The third generation of human spaceflight for the United States was the Apollo program, lasting from October 1968 to July 1975. The Apollo spacecraft could transport three astronauts, but remained small and restricted movement. However, there were three major accomplishments associated with the Apollo program. The first was the successful landing and return of six crews from the moon. The second was the successful use with the first U.S. space station, Skylab, during three missions lasting 28, 59, and 84 days in duration. Finally, the Apollo craft was used in the first successful rendezvous with a Soviet spacecraft, Soyuz-19. Through monitoring and analyzing various lunar, EVA, and exercise activities during these missions, this program provided extensive physiological data on the capability of humans to work and exercise in microgravity environments. The majority of the U.S. data presented in this review were obtained from the Apollo programs.

Nearly 6 years after the last Apollo flight, the United States launched its most recent generation of spacecraft, the Space Shuttle. The shuttle program was designed to provide a reusable space transportation system (STS) in a form that could transport relatively large crews (to date as many as eight in one mission) to space and allow them to return safely by conventional aircraft landing techniques. Although the shuttle flights have been relatively short in duration (2–10 days), some dedicated life sciences missions have provided data on the capability of humans to live and work in space. Current plans are to extend the duration of shuttle flights to 16–28 days and eventually have a permanently orbiting space station to transport crews for long stays in space.

Soviet Space Program

The Soviet space program began with the Vostok spacecraft. Like the U.S. Mercury spacecraft, this capsule was small, carried only one cosmonaut, and was used to test for reliable operation and safety for future program missions.

After six successful Vostok flights from April 1961 to June 1963, the Soviets initiated their Voskhod series of flights. This craft could carry up to three cosmonauts and was used to obtain more comprehensive medical data in flight as well as produced the first EVA in the form of a 12-min "space walk." The Voskhod program consisted of only two missions, but provided the Soviets with information about physiological adaptation and work capability of humans in space.

In April of 1967, the Soviets embarked on their long-running Soyuz program. The Soyuz spacecraft was developed to provide support to space station operations such as supply and crew transport [42]. The most significant accomplishment of the Soyuz program was the development of the first Soviet space station, Salyut. There were seven Salyut space stations launched between 1971 and 1986, although Salyut-2 failed in 1973 and was never occupied. The Soyuz-Salyut missions included physical work tasks such as rendezvous, docking, and EVA. Medical monitoring of cosmonauts continued to focus on the physiological effects of weightlessness and the development of countermeasures that would enable cosmonauts to fly for extended periods of time. Through this program, experience has been gained about the use and efficacy of various countermeasures to physical deconditioning such as "chest expanders," isometric exercises, elastic tension straps, and the "Penguin" suit (a suit that applies constant loading to the muscles of the legs and torso). With the experience of the Salyut space station, the Soviets extended human stay-time in space up to 237 days. The majority of data presented in this review on exercise and work performance in weightlessness was generated from the Soyuz-Salyut spaceflight program.

This Salyut space station program led to the evolution of the next generation space station called Mir (peace). This new station features improved crew facilities for living and separate laboratory modules for scientific work. With this station, the Soviets have completed the longest manned spaceflight to date (366 days). The data and experience gained from living and working for long durations in these space stations will contribute important insight into the limitations of humans to extend missions far beyond Earth, such as a voyage to Mars.

Perspective on Availability of Human Spaceflight Data

Exercise testing has gained wide use for the evaluation of the physiological adaptation to weightlessness. It was first performed in weightlessness on the Soviet Voskhod spacecraft and was later used in the system of medical monitoring of crew members on Gemini 4, Gemini 5, and Gemini 7 spacecrafts. However, the difficulty of interpreting spaceflight data due to limitations in conducting exercise and other physiological experiments in microgravity should be appreciated. Many exercise devices developed for spaceflight have not allowed for accurate calibration or controlled conditions for repeatability. Many tests, experimental conditions, and exercise activities conducted during spaceflight are not standardized and rarely is all activity reported. There has been little control over pretest activities in an attempt to establish repeatable baseline data.

Most of the extensive data on exercise and work in space has been generated from missions involving only two or three crew members. The problems in generalizing to a larger population the results of data from few subjects are apparent. Nevertheless, one-of-a-kind spaceflight data should not be ignored. The ability to accumulate and examine data from multiple crew missions provides an opportunity to begin to analyze trends and consistencies. In this regard, it was necessary to extract the majority of the data presented in this review from translated Soviet literature and U.S. government technical documents, many of which are not readily available to the scientific community. Raw data reported in these documents were statistically analyzed by the author to provide a more concise presentation of spaceflight results.

Within these various limitations, it is the purpose of this review to present and summarize the available data from both U.S. and Soviet space missions regarding human physiological adaptations to exercise and work in weightlessness. The emphasis will be placed on human data collected during and after actual spaceflight, with very limited reference to groundbase or animal studies. Through comparison and integration of common data generated from various spaceflights, an attempt is made to generalize the limitations to work and the role of exercise during and after exposures to weightlessness.

INFLIGHT RESPONSES TO EXERCISE

Cardiovascular Responses

The concept of cardiovascular "deconditioning" as a consequence of weightlessness has been advanced [3, 4], in part due to the reduction of end-diastolic volume and stroke volume after spaceflight and their slow recovery [5]. The investigators interpreted these data to indicate impairment of ventricular performance. Contrary to this hypothesis, there is little evidence to suggest that functional deconditioning of the cardiovascular system occurs during spaceflight. Despite the reduction in resting end-diastolic volume and stroke volume after spaceflight, ejection fraction was unchanged [5], suggesting normal myocardial function. Hemodynamic responses, measured during preflight supine rest and averaged over days 13–21 of flight, in the three cosmonauts who flew the 23-day Salyut-1 space station mission are presented in Table 4.1 [32]. Tragically, this flight ended with loss of the three crew members due to spacecraft depressurization during reentry. However, their data and those of the 63-day Salyut-4 mission provided us with early evidence of little effect on resting heart rate and stroke volume with up to 2 months of exposure to microgravity. In all subjects, a slight elevation in blood pressure was observed, which must have been accounted for by increased systemic peripheral resistance because cardiac output remained constant compared to preflight levels. Degtyarev et al. [32] concluded that cardiac ventricular function was not impaired because all cosmonauts in the Salyut-1 flight demonstrated an increase in pulse wave propagation ve-

TABLE 4.1
Cardiac and Hemodynamic Responses at Rest before and during Spaceflight

Variables	Salyut-1 23-Day Mission		Salyut-4 63-Day Mission	
	Preflight	*Inflight Days 13–21*	*Preflight*	*Inflight Day 56*
Heart rate, bpm	64 ± 5	65 ± 5	65 ± 3	65 ± 3
Stroke volume, ml	94 ± 3	96 ± 9	84 ± 5	90 ± 2
Cardiac output, liters/min	6.0 ± 0.5	6.1 ± 0.1	5.5 ± 0.3	5.9 ± 0.3
Systolic blood pressure, mm Hg	113 ± 7	122 ± 4*	120 ± 5	130 ± 6*
Diastolic blood pressure, mm Hg	73 ± 3	80 ± 2*	86 ± 4	86 ± 1
Mean arterial pressure, mm Hg	86 ± 4	94 ± 2*	97 ± 4	101 ± 2
Aortic pulse wave propagation velocity, m/s	4.4 ± 0.4	4.9 ± 0.1*	6.5 ± 0.6	6.4 ± 0.6
Systemic peripheral resistance, units	15.0 ± 2.7	16.9 ± 2.0*	18.6 ± 1.7	16.9 ± 1.2

Values represent mean ± SE. Asterisk indicates that all cosmonauts changed in the same direction to preflight values. Salyut-1 data (*N* = 3) are derived from Degtyarev et al. [32] and Salyut-4 data (*N* = 2) are derived from Degtyarev et al. [36].

locity, which they interpreted as an index of greater left ventricular contractility. Similar results were reported from the two cosmonauts of the 16-day mission of Soyuz-14/Salyut-3 [48], two cosmonauts of the 18-day Soyuz-24/Salyut-5 flight [81], two cosmonauts who flew on the 49-day orbital mission of Soyuz-21/Salyut-5 [81], and 10 cosmonauts of the Salyut-6 space station [103]. With the exception of an elevated resting systolic blood pressure, all resting hemodynamic parameters returned to preflight levels by day 56 of the 63-day mission of Salyut-4 (Table 4.1) [36, 101]. Consistent in all flights, the data suggest that cardiac function is not compromised in the resting condition and that after a transient change, hemodynamic homeostasis is restored to normal $1g$ levels.

Most of the physical work that is performed during spaceflight involves the arms and upper body while the legs are used primarily for stabilization of the body. There are limited data from spaceflight on cardiovascular responses to standardized work rates using the arms. The two cosmonauts who flew the 18-day Soyuz-9 mission were examined during exercise that consisted of a standardized arm flexion producing 15–18 kg of torque [13]. Each exercise test consisted of 10 repetitions at a rate of one per second, separated by 5 s of rest and repeated four times. The estimated energy expenditure was 160–180 kcal/hr or an oxygen uptake ($\dot{V}o_2$) of about 0.5–0.6 liters/min, representing about 30–35% $\dot{V}o_2$max for two arms [61]. Both heart rate (Fig. 4.1) and respiration were lower or similar during flight compared to preflight conditions. These data suggested that the cardiovascular demand for arm work during flight was not impaired and work performance of the cosmonauts during the entire 18-day orbital flight was reported as "at an adequately high level."

The cardiovascular response to leg exercise has been the center of study during spaceflight. During the 23-day mission of Salyut-1, two cosmonauts were "strapped with bands to an exerciser strip" and performed exercise tests that consisted of 30 squats per minute [35]. The work rate was calculated to about 1100 kgm/min, although this was variable during flight compared to preflight. During the inflight exercise, heart rate, cardiac output, and arterial pressures were slightly higher than those measured preflight. These responses occurred by the 9th day of flight and did not progress with the duration of the mission. Clinical electrocardiographic analysis and dynamics of the ejection phases of the heart determined from ECG analysis were unchanged, suggesting no apparent effect of microgravity in this flight on cardiac function during exercise [43]. Similar observations were reported for the 30-day mission of Salyut-4 [43]. It was concluded that despite small alterations in cardiac and hemodynamic responses to exercise, there was little compromise of the cardiovascular capacity to support moderate work levels during 23–30 days exposure to microgravity.

FIGURE 4.1

Mean heart rate response in two cosmonauts during rest and during arm and leg exercise in spaceflight compared to 1g preflight levels (solid horizontal lines). *(Data were extracted and plotted from Butusov AA, Lyamin VR, Lebedev AA, Polyakova AP, Svistunov IB, Tishler VA, Shulenin AP: Results of routine medical monitoring of cosmonauts during flight on the 'Soyuz-9' ship.* Kosm Biol Med *4(6):35–39, 1970, and Doroshev VG, Batenchuk-Tusko TV, Lapshina NA, Kukushkin YA, Kalmykova ND, Ragozin VN: Changes in hemodynamics and phasic structure of the cardiac cycle in the crew on the second expedition of Salyut-4.* Kosm Biol Aviakosm Med *11(2):26–31, 1977.)*

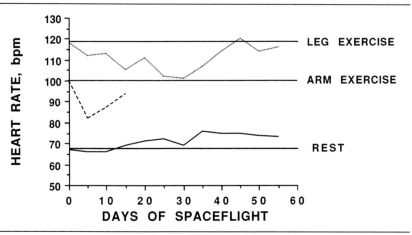

During the 63-day Salyut-4 orbital spaceflight, the heart rate during rest and a 5-min standardized exercise on the cycle ergometer (450 kgm/min, $\dot{V}O_2$ = 1.2 liters/min) was not significantly altered (Fig. 4.1) [101]. These findings were similar to those of the three U.S. Skylab missions (28, 59, and 84 days) in which mean heart rate of 153 bpm and systolic blood pressure of 200 mm Hg was measured both preflight and inflight during a standardized 5-min work rate on the cycle ergometer (75% $\dot{V}O_2max$, $\dot{V}O_2$ = 2.0 liters/min), performed by each of nine astronauts [76]. It can be concluded from these U.S. and Soviet data of hemodynamic reactions to physical work that normal cardiovascular function during spaceflight can be retained for up to 3 months with inflight exercise.

During the 140-day flight of the orbital station Salyut-6, two crew members performed five standardized exercise tests over the course of the mission on a cycle ergometer at a work rate of 750 kgm/min for 5 min [107]. The hemodynamic responses measured during exercise before and during the mission are presented in Table 4.2. In comparison to

TABLE 4.2
Preflight and Inflight Cardiac and Hemodynamic Responses at Standardized Exercise (750 kgm/min for 5 min) for the 140-Day Soviet Salyut-6 Mission

Variables	Preflight	Inflight Days				
		29	41	62	97	119
Heart rate, bpm	113 ± 5	113 ± 4	124 ± 12*	116 ± 8	122 ± 7*	128 ± 13*
Stroke volume, ml	136 ± 19	133 ± 20	134 ± 30	120 ± 26*	131 ± 34*	112 ± 20*
Cardiac output, liters/min	15.3 ± 1.5	15.0 ± 1.7	16.2 ± 2.2*	13.7 ± 2.1*	15.8 ± 3.2	14.1 ± 1.2*
Systolic blood pressure, mm Hg	156 ± 2	157 ± 9	156 ± 1	149 ± 2*	144 ± 4*	146 ± 3*
Diastolic blood pressure, mm Hg	70 ± 4	69 ± 2	70 ± 3	68 ± 5	73 ± 2	69 ± 1
Aortic pulse wave propagation velocity, m/s	7.5 ± 0.6	7.2 ± 0.8	7.5 ± 0.9	7.9 ± 0.9*	7.8 ± 0.7*	8.5 ± 1.5*
Systemic peripheral resistance, units	13.6 ± 2.1	12.8 ± 0.9	10.7 ± 2.0*		12.4 ± 2.9*	

Values represent mean ± SE ($N = 2$). Asterisk indicates that all cosmonauts changed in the same direction compared to preflight values. Data are derived from Yegorov et al. [107].

preflight tests, the cardiovascular responses to exercise during flight were characterized by few alterations during the 1st month of flight but followed by progressive reductions in systolic blood pressure, systemic peripheral resistance, stroke volume, and cardiac output by day 62 of flight despite elevations in heart rate. Similar observations were reported at the end of the 63-day Salyut-4 mission [38], on other Salyut-6 missions lasting from 96 to 184 days [103], and on the later Salyut-7/Soyuz-T 150-day mission [102]. Despite decreased cardiac output during the second half of the mission, Soviet investigators proposed an increase in myocardial contractility as indicated by greater velocity of propagation of the pulse wave over the aorta. Although the mechanism of increased contractility is not clear, a role of elevated myocardial adrenergic stimulation has been suggested [108]. Thus, the reduction in stroke volume and cardiac output during exercise in weightlessness of long duration was attributed to the reduction in circulating blood volume and its effect on venous return rather than an impairment of cardiac function.

From Salyut missions consistent evidence for increased cardiac contraction in the face of reduced stroke volume, cardiac output, and elevated heart rate during exercise in weightlessness of 96–184 days duration suggests the absence of deconditioning with respect to myocardial dysfunction. This concept was most recently supported by the echocardiographic data collected of two cosmonauts from the Salyut-7 237-day mission [1]. During flight, both cosmonauts demonstrated similar hemodynamic changes in response to rest and graded exercise (125 and 175 W) compared to preflight responses. The average data are presented in Figure 4.2. Stroke volume increased very little during inflight exercise, representing a 30% lower level than that at an identical exercise level before the flight. Inflight heart rates were 12 and 17% higher at 125 and 175 W, respectively, compared to preflight, but cardiac output remained lower during inflight exercise. Left ventricular filling volume (end-diastolic volume) was significantly depressed during rest and did not increase with graded exercise in weightlessness. Stroke volume was maintained by greater myocardial contraction as indicated by lesser end-systolic reserve and elevated ejection fraction (Fig. 4.2). These flight data were similar to those of groundbase data [51] and support the notion that blood volume reduction rather than deterioration of myocardial function plays the leading role in the decrease of left ventricular end-diastolic and stroke volumes during rest and exercise in weightlessness.

Although the cardiovascular adaptations to support rest and exercise during spaceflight appear adequate and effective, some isolated cardiac episodes have been reported that could have clinical importance to the health and performance of the astronaut. During the second orbit of a 2-day Soyuz-12 mission, Vasily Lazarev registered one group of five atrial extrasystoles [48]. There were no further episodes reported on this cosmonaut and the short duration of the mission may have prevented fur-

FIGURE 4.2

Cardiac responses of two cosmonauts during rest and at 125 and 175 W of exercise on a cycle ergometer before (open bars) *and during* (hatched bars) *the Salyut-7 237-day mission.* Bars *and* lines *represent mean ± SE, respectively.* Asterisks *indicate that both subjects changed in the same direction. (Modified from Atkov OY, Bednenko VS, Fomina GA: Ultrasound techniques in space medicine.* Aviat Space Environ Med *58 (Suppl 9):A69–A73, 1987.)*

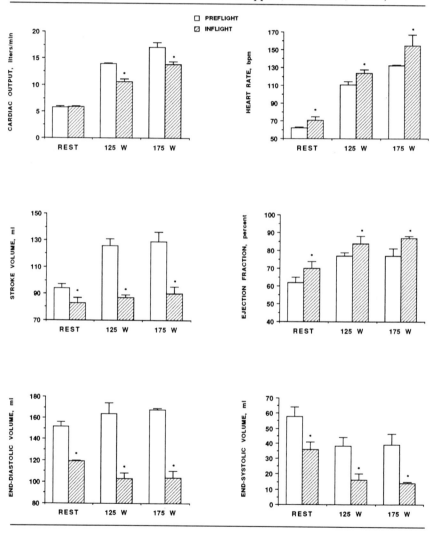

ther symptoms. During an exercise test performed after the 63-day Soyuz-18/Salyut-4 flight, Pyotr Klimuk showed infrequent individual and grouped supraventricular extrasystoles [7]. In the U.S. space program, the most serious finding of aberrations in cardiac electrical activity were noted in the lunar module pilot and the commander of the 12-day Apollo 15 moon mission. The two-person crew had engaged in strenuous activity on the lunar surface, during which time the lunar module pilot experienced premature ventricular contractions (PVCs), 12 bigeminis, and premature atrial contractions (PACs). The mission commander experienced PVCs and PACs that lasted for about 1 hr on the morning of reentry. Postflight examinations of the Apollo 15 crew revealed potassium deficits, which were linked to the irregular heartbeats [10]. Later, a single episode of PVCs during heavy exercise testing (75% $\dot{V}o_2max$) inflight was observed in one astronaut on the 4th inflight day of the 28-day U.S. Skylab 2 mission [90]. However, during the remainder of the flight, no ectopic beats were detected. The clinical importance of these abnormal cardiac electrical activities are currently unclear. However, their occurrence during heavy physical activity may have important implication for limitations to exercise and work during spaceflight and further investigation is warranted.

Metabolic Responses and Mechanical Efficiency

During the U.S. Skylab missions, inflight metabolic measurements were performed during cycle ergometer exercise with sequential 5-min stages of 25, 50, and 75% of $\dot{V}o_2max$. Oxygen uptake during this exercise in weightlessness was slightly but consistently less in all nine Skylab astronauts at the same absolute work rate on the cycle ergometer [75, 76, 85]. Slightly elevated expired carbon dioxide (from 2.58 ± 0.22 preflight to 2.60 ± 0.26 inflight) and respiratory exchange ratio (0.945 ± 0.081 preflight to 1.001 ± 0.089 inflight, $p < 0.05$) at the 75% $\dot{V}o_2max$ level were reported [75]. The greater recovery oxygen uptake of 742 ± 63 ml/min following exercise in microgravity compared to 678 ± 44 ml/min before flight supports the notion that a greater proportion of energy demand was required from anaerobiosis [59, 76]. Increased inflight recovery oxygen uptake has been associated with fatigue observed during work in space [59].

The only measurement of $\dot{V}o_2$ during maximal exercise in weightlessness was reported in the three Skylab-4 astronauts who were in space for 84 days [76]. During their personal exercise periods in flight, each crew member chose certain days throughout the flight to perform maximal exercise. The attainment of maximal work levels during flight was verified by heart rates above 183 bpm; these were slightly greater than their preflight and age-predicted maximal heart rates. The average values for $\dot{V}o_2max$ preflight and at progressive time intervals during flight are plotted in Figure 4.3. Despite the volume of data from ground-based human experiments demonstrating the consistent reduction of $\dot{V}_{O_2}$max following exposure to simulated microgravity [19–24, 86], it is surprising that the $\dot{V}_{O_2}$max of all three astronauts actually increased from a mean (±SE) of 3.11 ± 0.21 liters/min before flight to 3.37 ± 0.25 liters/min during the flight after 79–83 days of exposure. It is clear that, through an intense exercise program during flight, this crew was able to improve their aerobic capacity during the course of the mission.

The average daily energy expenditure during spaceflight (Soyuz-9) has been reported to be approximately 2500 kcal/day or an average oxygen uptake of 320 ml/min [18]. Average energy expenditure is probably higher than this because body weight is maintained or lost with daily dietary intakes that range from 2500 to 3000 kcal during long exposures to weightlessness [48, 102]. These energy costs during spaceflight are at the higher range of normal daily energy costs in 1g. This is surprising because one might suspect a significant reduction in metabolism inflight due to the lower muscular force requirements to perform a work task in the absence of gravity. The relatively high cost of energy in a lower force environment may be used to argue for a reduction in mechanical effi-

FIGURE 4.3

Maximal oxygen uptakes ($\dot{V}_{O_2}$max) of three astronauts before and during the 84-day Skylab-4 mission. Circles *and* lines *represent mean ± SE, respectively.* Asterisks *indicate that all subjects changed in the same direction. (Data plotted from Michel EL, Rummel JA, Sawin CF, Buderer MC, Lem JD: Results of Skylab medical experiment M171—metabolic activity. In Johnston RS, Dietlein LF (eds):* Biomedical Results from Skylab. *NASA SP-377, 1977, pp 372–387.)*

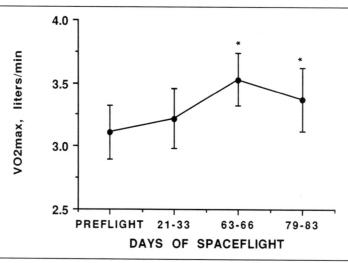

ciency to perform exercise or work. This notion is supported by the observation that cosmonauts on the Salyut-6 missions and astronauts on the U.S. Skylab missions appeared to require greater muscular effort during movement in the cabin and a longer time to perform certain working operations [64, 103].

The test for mechanical efficiency during spaceflight compared to 1g can be assessed from metabolic and work rate data collected from the nine astronauts who participated in the three U.S. Skylab missions [76]. A standardized exercise bout at an intensity of 150 W (918 kgm/min) was performed on a cycle ergometer by each astronaut before and during spaceflight. Therefore, the energy of work was maintained constant at 2.15 kcal/min. The average energy expenditure required to perform this work was 10.2 ± 0.1 kcal/min preflight and 9.3 ± 0.1 inflight ($\dot{V}o_2$ = 2.04 ± 0.02 and 1.86 ± 0.02 liters/min, respectively). Therefore, the mechanical efficiency of performing cycle ergometer exercise during flight (23%) was not significantly different from 1g (21%). Average data for daily exercise levels, energy expenditures, and mechanical efficiency during cycle-ergometry from three Skylab-4 astronauts [76] and from two cosmonauts on the 175-day Soviet Salyut-6 mission [88] are presented in Table 4.3. The Soviet data are consistent with the Skylab findings. The $\dot{V}o_2$ predicted during cycle exercise inflight (975 kg/min) was 2.25 liters/min (11.3 kcal/min) compared to the actual measured $\dot{V}o_2$ of 2.31 liters/min (approximately 20% mechanical efficiency). Thus, efficiency of performing exercise or work in a mechanical, stabilized device such as the cycle ergometer is unaltered by weightlessness.

In contrast to the maintenance of work efficiency on a controlled mechanical device, the energy cost of locomotion and work in weightlessness may be much higher when the body cannot be stabilized by

TABLE 4.3
Characteristics of Physical Training and Estimated Energy Expenditures during Each Exercise Session of the 175-Day Soviet Salyut-6 Mission (N = 2) and the 84-Day U.S. Skylab-4 Mission (N = 3)

Variables	Salyut-6 Cycle Ergometer	Salyut-6 Treadmill	Skylab-4 Cycle Ergometer
Average exercise volume	39,414 kgm	4,115 m	39,450 kgm
Average work rate	975 kgm/min	120 m/min	918 kgm/min
Average exercise duration	40.4 min	34.3 min	43.0 min
Daily exercise sessions	2	2	1
Total energy expenditure	467 kcal	255 kcal	
Average rate of energy expenditure	11.6 kcal/min	7.4 kcal/min	9.4 kcal/min
Actual oxygen uptake	2.31 liters/min	1.50 liters/min	1.87 liters/min
Predicted oxygen uptake	2.25 liters/min	1.10 liters/min	2.00 liters/min
Estimated mechanical efficiency	20%	15%	23%

Values represent daily averages. Salyut data are derived from Siminov and Kasyan [88] and Skylab data are derived from Michel et al. [76].

postural muscles in terrestrial gravity. This point is emphasized by the data in Table 4.3, which presents the average work rate and metabolic cost of exercise on the cycle compared to the treadmill during the 175-day Salyut-6 mission [88]. The two cosmonauts who flew on this flight exercised on the treadmill twice daily for about 34 min each at a speed of 120 m/min (about 4.5 mph). A system of "bungee-cords" provided a pull to the long axis of the body, which resulted in a force equivalent to 50 kg [43, 103]. Under these conditions, the energy expenditure of treadmill walking/running in Earth gravity would be predicted at approximately 5.7 kcal/min (1.15 liters/min $\dot{V}O_2$). However, their measured energy expenditure to treadmill exercise was 7.4 kcal/min (1.50 liters/min $\dot{V}O_2$). This calculates a reduction in mechanical efficiency from a predicted 20% in $1g$ to an actual 15% in weightlessness. These results were corroborated by the responses to cycle and treadmill exercise on cosmonaut Romanenko who was the first person to be in space for 1 year. During each inflight exercise session, this cosmonaut exercised for about 30 min on the treadmill at an average speed of 125 m/min (combined walking and running) and for 26.5 min on the cycle ergometer at 800 kgm/min. Based on prediction equations from $1g$, this cosmonaut would have required an oxygen uptake of about 1.9 liters/min on each exercise device, or approximately 570 kcal during treadmill and 500 kcal during cycling. Thus, the total predicted energy expenditure per exercise session would be 1070 kcal (20% mechanical efficiency). However, an average energy cost of 1460 kcal (1400–1520) was actually reported, indicating a reduction in mechanical efficiency of the total exercise session to 15% (Second US/USSR Joint Working Group on Space Biology and Medicine, Washington, D.C., September, 1988). If we assume that the mechanical efficiency of cycle ergometry was not altered from $1g$ as previously indicated [76, 88], then it can be estimated that 960 kcal were required to perform treadmill exercise rather than the predicted 570 kcal, a reduction in mechanical efficiency from 20 to 11%.

Biomechanical analysis of treadmill exercise during spaceflight also supports the notion that there is a reduced mechanical efficiency [14]. Running, i.e., both feet leaving the ground at the same time, is nearly impossible because of the spring-loaded harness pulling the astronaut toward the treadmill surface. Further, the motion of walking and running is performed on tiptoe during treadmill in space in contrast to heel-to-toe in $1g$ [14, 101]. The proposal that the use of the treadmill and harness-device currently being used on U.S. Space Shuttle flights will provide the greatest forces and best protection to muscle and bone of the lower extremities may be tenuous because small forces may be applied to the long bones without heel strike and without the body leaving the ground surface. It therefore appears that a human loses some mechanical advantage of using gravity during exercise and work with the lower extremities in a weightless environment.

The issue of mechanical efficiency loss in weightlessness presents several relevant implications. From the viewpoint of mission operations, it may be important to consider apparatus designed to stabilize the body during operational work tasks to optimize mechanical efficiency during flight. In addition, the treadmill has been advanced as a necessary exercise device to provide the muscular forces and impact to bone that will help defend against musculoskeletal deterioration during spaceflight [95]. However, the metabolic data from treadmill exercise may suggest as much as a 50% reduction in mechanical efficiency. Operationally, this implies that treadmill exercise performed at 75% $\dot{V}o_2$max may provide only half the mechanical work output that can be realized in 1g. This may result in forces that may not be great enough to maintain musculoskeletal integrity during long-duration missions. Clearly, new methods for providing mechanical stability during walking and running in weightlessness must be investigated if treadmill exercise is to provide forces to muscle and bones of the lower extremities in a similar fashion to that in terrestrial gravity.

WORK PERFORMANCE IN WEIGHTLESSNESS

Extravehicular Activity

The first extravehicular activity (EVA) performed by a man in a spacesuit (Voskhod-2) revealed that respiration rate increased to 26–36 breaths/min compared to 10–15 on Earth, and heart rate reached 152–162 bpm. Although some degree of anxiety may have contributed to the elevation of heart rate, the data suggested a moderate to high energy cost requirement for physical work in a spacesuit [59].

The astronauts of Gemini 9 and 10 not only had high respiration and heart rate during EVA, but displayed profuse perspiration, excessive accumulation of heat, and signs of fatigue during "space walks." It was estimated that performance of operations in space required four to five times more exertion than similar tasks on Earth, resulting in limitation or cancellation of planned operations during these missions. During these Gemini EVAs, heart rates were maintained from 130 to 170 bpm while energy expenditure exceeded 500 kcal/hr ($\dot{V}o_2$ approximately 1.7 liters/min) [9].

When astronaut Michael Collins performed EVA during Gemini 10, his respiration rate rose to 36 breaths/min and heart rate was 160 bpm; as a result, duration of his activity was reduced due to development of fatigue. Similarly, the EVA of Richard Gordon (Gemini 11) was curtailed due to severe perspiration and overheating. His respiration rate rose to 36–40 breaths/min during EVA and perspiration was excessive (500 kcal/hr). Although energy expenditure by these astronauts was not measured directly, it was apparent that heat production (estimated to be as much as 860 kcal/hr) was greater during EVA than the efficiency of the spacesuit cooling systems [9]. As a result, progressive elevations in body temperature were observed and work rates had to be limited. Thus, body heat produced from EVA in the Gemini spacesuit microenvironment represented a limitation to work performance.

During the Apollo program, metabolic rates during EVA were calculated based on heart rate, oxygen usage from the decrease in oxygen bottle pressure, and differences between temperatures of the coolant water flowing into and out from the astronauts' liquid cooling garments [104]. Average metabolic rate of seven astronauts (Apollo 9, 15, 16, and 17) during EVAs in weightlessness was approximately 240 kcal/hr (range 115–500 kcal/hr) or an average $\dot{V}O_2$ of about 0.8 liter/min over an average duration of EVA of about 1 hr [104]. These data indicate that the crew members were able to work at moderate levels with no limitations.

With refinement of the design of U.S. spacesuits, there was decreased cardiorespiratory responses and energy expenditure during EVA in the Skylab missions [105]. Average energy expenditure was about 230 kcal/hr ($\dot{V}O_2$ = 0.8 liter/min) during EVAs of Skylab astronauts, ranging from 260–330 kcal/hr for the first Skylab crew, 180—310 kcal/hr for the second crew, and 145–250 kcal/hr for the third crew. The highest level of 500 kcal/hr was recorded for the commander of the first crew, when he tried to cut a bracing that was preventing the deployment of a large solar energy panel [105]. At no time was EVA limited in these astronauts.

The mean oxygen uptake over 3–6 hr of EVA during various Space Shuttle missions was approximately 0.8 liters/min, similar to that of both Apollo and Skylab missions [104, 105]. The $\dot{V}O_2$ required during peak work of short duration (minutes) during nine shuttle EVAs (averaged over six missions) was about 1.6 liters/min. To provide some perspective on the relative energy cost for work during these EVAs, it should be appreciated that muscular work during EVA requires predominantly arm and upper body activity. Because the $\dot{V}O_2max$ of the arms and upper body for individuals at similar aerobic fitness levels as the astronauts is approximately 1.8 liters/min [61], astronauts may be functioning for hours at an average intensity of 45–50% of arm $\dot{V}O_2max$ with short periods requiring as much as 80% of the maximal working capacity of the arms and upper body muscle groups. Shuttle astronauts have expressed some degree of fatigue following these long activities. Based on these estimations, endurance and strength capacities of the arms and upper body may become limiting factors to EVA performance.

Analogous data of heart rate, respiration rate, and energy expenditure were obtained from the two cosmonauts on the Soviet Soyuz-32-Salyut-6 orbital complex who performed extensive extravehicular work on day 172 of that mission [59]. During EVA, respiration rate ranged from 16 to 28 breaths/min while moving over a distance of 28 m in a spacesuit, using hand rails, and disconnecting the radiotelescope antenna. Cardiorespiratory and metabolic responses during two EVAs performed by the crew for 170 min on day 128 and 175 min on day 130 of the 150-day mission of Salyut-7/Soyuz-T were reported [102]. Heart rate ranged from about 80–120 bpm during the first EVA to 70–108 bpm during the second. Respiration rate ranged from 30–42 and 20–38 breaths/min during the two EVA tasks. Mean energy expenditure was 3.8 kcal/min in the commander and 4.9 kcal/min in the flight engineer during the first EVA and 3.3 and 4.3 kcal/min, respectively, during the second. Maximum energy expenditure of 6–7 kcal/min (approximately 1.2–1.4 liters/min $\dot{V}_{O_2}$) were reported during performance of final operations to open a solar battery and close the exit hatch. During the 170 and 175 min of EVA, total oxygen uptake ranged from 107 to 127 liters, constituting a mean of about 0.7 liters/min, similar to the average of 0.8 liters/min reported from U.S. Apollo, Skylab, and Space Shuttle EVAs.

Physical Activity on the Moon

Total energy expenditure of 12 astronauts (Apollo 11, 12, 14, 15, 16, and 17) averaged 200–300 kcal/hr ($\dot{V}_{O_2}$ = 0.7–1.0 liters/min) during 28 lunar surface EVAs involving deployment of scientific packages, geological station activity, overhead work (lunar module egress and ingress, lunar sample stowage, etc.), and lunar rover vehicle operations [104]. These lunar EVAs ranged from 2.5 to 7.5 hr in duration. The energy expenditure levels are about the same as walking on Earth at the rate of 5 km/hr without using any gear or when moving in a spacesuit at the rate of 1 km/hr. The average walking rate over a distance of 2.9 km on the moon surface was about 2.4 km/hr with energy expenditure of about 300 kcal/hr. Maximum energy expenditure of 350–450 kcal/hr was related to performance of discrete operations: walking up steep inclines, carrying and installing scientific equipment, and drilling. A lower metabolic rate was recorded while driving the lunar rover. Thus, there appears to be little limitation to performing basic physical activities of movement on the moon in a one-sixth gravity environment. However, more tasking operations such as building structures for lunar stations may involve greater limits to productivity and should be tested.

POSTFLIGHT RESPONSES TO EXERCISE

Cardiovascular Responses

Following 6 days of spaceflight, selected physiological responses to 450 kgm/min on a supine and upright (sitting) cycle ergometer were compared to preflight responses in the two crew members of the Soyuz-19 orbital mission [100]. Following flight, exercise heart rate was 12% higher in supine and 17% higher in upright cycling compared to pre-flight responses. These results are similar to those reported from groundbase studies [19, 24], suggesting that higher supine heart rate after flight probably represented the effect of reduced blood volume while the additional tachycardia in the upright posture probably represented the added influence of the orthostatic effect of 1g on end-diastolic filling volume and stroke volume. Further, average upright exercise stroke volume was reduced by 24 ml in the three astronauts of Skylab 4 while supine stroke volume was decreased by only 5 ml [76]. These data support the notion that elevated heart rate during terrestrial exercise following spaceflight is a compensatory response to reduced stroke volume, a response that is exaggerated in the upright orthostatic posture compared to the supine position.

Cardiovascular responses during supine cycle exercise at 600 kgm/min for 7 min performed preflight and 3–7 days postflight are presented in Table 4.4. These data represent the average data of two cosmonauts from each of four Soviet space missions: (a) the 30-day Soyuz-17 flight, (b) the 63-day Soyuz-18 mission in the Salyut-4 orbital station, (c) the 96-day Soyuz-26/ Salyut-6 mission, and (d) the 140-day Soyuz-29/Salyut-6 flight [7, 8]. In the postflight supine resting state, stroke volume was reduced but cardiac output was maintained as a result of an increased heart rate. After flight, exercise stroke volume was reduced an average of 20% and cardiac output fell an average of 10% despite an average elevated exercise heart rate of 15 bpm.

Similar observations were reported in the three Skylab 4 astronauts whose hemodynamic responses were measured at 75% $\dot{V}o_2$max before and after their 84-day spaceflight. Mean heart rate increased from 103 bpm preflight to 114 bpm postflight in response to a reduction in stroke volume from 110 ml preflight to 97 ml postflight [76]. Although diastolic pressure was unaltered during rest or exercise following return to earth from prolonged exposure to microgravity in both U.S. and Soviet flights, exercise systolic blood pressure was elevated in all cosmonauts after flight compared to their preflight responses. The increase in both resting and exercise heart rates and systolic pressure resulted in an average elevation of 25% in their product, an indication of a significant elevation in myocardial oxygen demand after returning to 1g from spaceflight [8]. Because there is no apparent cardiovascular dysfunction in flight during rest [32, 36, 48, 81] or exercise [13, 35, 38, 101], Beregovkin et al. [8] interpreted the postflight increase in myocardial and hemodynamic responses during rest and exercise as resulting primarily from a change in the regulation at rest due to blood volume reduction rather than a sign of myocardial dysfunction.

Thus, upon return to terrestrial gravity following prolonged exposure to weightlessness, we find lower stroke volume and cardiac output at

TABLE 4.4
Cardiac and Hemodynamic Responses to a Standardized Exercise (600 kgm/min for 3 min) before and after Spaceflight

Variables	30-Day Salyut-4 Flight		63-Day Salyut-4 Flight		96-Day Salyut-6 Flight		140-Day Salyut-6 Flight	
	Rest	Exercise	Rest	Exercise	Rest	Exercise	Rest	Exercise
Heart rate, bpm								
Preflight	60	112	69	120	67	112	61	104
Postflight	67*	131*	76*	136*	73*	119*	84*	119*
Oxygen uptake, ml/min								
Preflight	270	1538	268	1469	246	1326	305	1286
Postflight	283*	1498*	293*	1428*	259*	1272*	305	1335
Systolic blood pressure, mm Hg								
Preflight	129	138	125	132	137	155	113	155
Postflight	140*	158*	127	143*	130	173*	130*	170*
Diastolic blood pressure, mm Hg								
Preflight	71	80	73	76	73	93	65	83
Postflight	73	77	70	73	78	85	78*	93*
Stroke volume, ml								
Preflight	98	142	92	133	87	149		
Postflight	86*	96*	85*	116*	72*	131*		
Cardiac output, liters/min								
Preflight	5.9	15.9	6.3	16.0	5.7	16.6		
Postflight	5.8	12.6*	6.4	15.7*	5.2*	15.6*		
Rate pressure product, bpm-mm Hg								
Preflight	7,740	15,456	8,625	15,840	9,179	17,360	6,893	16,120
Postflight	9,380*	20,698*	9,652*	19,448*	9,490*	20,587*	10,920*	20,230*

Values represent mean ± SE ($N = 2$). Asterisk indicates that all cosmonauts changed in the same direction compared to preflight values. Salyut-4 data, taken 3 days postflight, are derived from Beregovkin et al. [7] and Salyut-6 data, taken 7 days postflight, are derived from Beregovkin et al. [8].

rest, during standing, and during a standardized work rate despite higher heart rate and systolic blood pressures. Reduced size of the left ventricle has been reported following flight [5] and has been implicated as a deconditioning effect on the cardiovascular system [3, 4, 101]. However, maintained or improved cardiac performance during rest and exercise during and after flight, as indicated by increased ejection fractions and aortic pulse wave propagation velocities, refutes the notion that cardiovascular deconditioning occurs and limits the capacity to perform physical exercise. It appears more likely that blood volume reduction, which occurs in weightlessness, contributes most significantly to the limitation of the cardiovascular system to meet the demands of exercise and work performance during and after spaceflight.

Metabolic Responses

Preflight and postflight metabolic responses during submaximal cycle ergometer exercise were measured and compared from the U.S. Apollo 7–11 and Apollo 14–17 flights [82–84]. Oxygen uptake was measured at heart rates of 120, 140, and 160 bpm at minutes 6, 9, and 12 of a continuous graded cycle ergometer exercise protocol. These heart rates corresponded to average work intensities of 25, 50, and 75%, respectively, of the astronauts' preflight peak oxygen uptake (average 45 ml/kg/min) [11]. Results from the Apollo 7–11 astronauts ($N = 15$) indicated that the mean oxygen uptake at 160 bpm decreased from the preflight level of 2.44 ± 0.09 liters/min to 1.93 ± 0.09 liters/min (−21%, $p < 0.05$) on the 1st day of return and returned to 2.34 ± 0.13 liters/min (−4%, not significant) by 24–36 hr postflight [82, 84]. Comparable results from Apollo 14–17 astronauts ($N = 12$) were that oxygen uptake at 160 bpm decreased from a preflight level of 2.68 ± 0.14 liters/min to 2.23 ± 0.12 liters/min (−17%, $p < 0.05$) on the 1st day postflight and returned to 2.49 ± 0.11 (−7%, not significant) 24–36 hr after flight [83, 84]. The rapid reduction (within 15 days) and restoration (24–36 hr) of oxygen uptake and work rate seem to support groundbase data suggesting that changes in vascular volume represent an important contributing factor to the reduction in work capacity following exposure to microgravity [20, 24].

The 17–21% reduction in exercise intensity at a given heart rate following spaceflights of less than 15 days observed in the Apollo program may suggest that maximal work and aerobic capacity were reduced with exposure to microgravity. However, because maximal heart rate is elevated following exposure to simulated microgravity of similar duration [19, 20, 22, 24, 25], the Apollo metabolic data obtained during exercise at standardized submaximal heart rates do not assure than maximal capacity has been reduced. In fact, the increase in heart rate during submaximal graded exercise after spaceflight in the Skylab 4 astronauts with an increased inflight $\dot{V}o_2$max [76] argues for an uncoupling between aerobic capacity and cardiovascular adjustments postflight. Unfortunately, there are no available flight studies in which maximal capacities have been measured upon return to Earth. Without such data, it is difficult to interpret what lower oxygen uptakes at standard heart rates mean with regard to limits of exercise and work performance following return to gravity. Such studies are sorely needed.

Metabolic responses during supine cycle exercise at 600 kg/min for 7 min performed preflight and 3–7 days after 30–140-day spaceflights are presented in Table 4.4. These data represent the average of two cosmonauts from each of four Soviet space missions as described earlier [7, 8]. In the postflight supine resting state, oxygen uptake was elevated slightly but consistently in all but the two cosmonauts who flew the 140-day mission. Postflight exercise $\dot{V}o_2$ lagged appreciably behind the preflight levels, suggesting a slowing of $\dot{V}o_2$ kinetics. Also, greater $\dot{V}o_2$ during recovery from exercise was reported in cosmonauts after these and other flights [7, 100]. In the three Skylab 4 astronauts, average postflight $\dot{V}o_2$ during 5 min of recovery from exercise was also elevated ($p < 0.05$) from 678 ml/min preflight to 776 ml/min postflight [76]. Slower exercise $\dot{V}o_2$ kinetics and recovery $\dot{V}o_2$ have also been reported in groundbase experiments [21]. These changes in $\dot{V}o_2$ dynamics during and after exercise may reflect a greater requirement for anaerobic metabolism following spaceflight to provide for the energy demand of exercise in terrestrial gravity. This is further supported by higher blood lactate and ventilation and respiratory exchange ratio following exposure to groundbase simulations of microgravity [22, 86, 106].

Neuromuscular Changes

It is evident that the neuromuscular system undergoes adaptation to weightlessness, which affects function upon return to Earth. Indices of neuromuscular function were measured before and after the 18-day Soyuz-9 mission in two cosmonauts [17]. Patellar reflex excitability, determined by recording the electrical activity of the muscles involved in the reflex, increased from an average of 65 μV before flight to 205 μV postflight when a standardized force was applied, but had recovered by 11 days postflight. These findings were corroborated by electromyography (EMG) data collected from the gastrocnemius muscle of the three astronauts who flew on the Skylab 3 59-day mission and from the biceps brachii in one astronaut on the Apollo-Soyuz 9-day flight [65, 66]. Frequency of impulse propagation was increased in both muscle groups as evidenced by a significant shift of the predominant firing frequency into higher bands. In the gastrocnemius, there was a shift of approximately

25% from the base preflight level. A shift to higher frequencies indicates relatively more use of fast muscle, which is inefficient from a neuromuscular point of view when the same load is acted against.

The measurement of muscle tone or firmness has been used by the Soviets as another indication of neuromuscular integrity. The loss of muscle tone and greater reflex excitability in resting muscle must be a rapid adaptation because these changes were observed in flights of only 2–5 days duration in 12 cosmonauts who flew Soyuz-3, -4, -5, -6, -7 and -8 [55, 56], after 9 days in one U.S. astronaut [66], and after 18 days in two Soyuz-9 cosmonauts [17]. In the Soviet Soyuz flights, the magnitude of decrease in muscle tone in relative units from preflight to postflight was 103 ± 1 to 95 ± 2 (8%, $p < 0.05$) in the tibialis anterior and 77 ± 2 to 69 ± 2 (10%, $p < 0.05$) in the quadriceps muscles, with virtually no change in the biceps brachii. Reflex excitability was increased from 58 μV preflight to 76 μV postflight using the muscle electrical (EMG) response to the patellar reflex.

Muscle electrical efficiency, measured by the ratio of electrical activity to unit of force, was found to decrease in the gastrocnemius of Apollo astronauts as a result of weightlessness [66], a finding similar to that reported in Soviet cosmonauts after short and long duration flights and presented in Figure 4.4 [62]. However, the electrical efficiency of the biceps brachii was increased after weightlessness [66]. Elevated EMG activity has also been observed during a standardized walk test following Soviet spaceflight [16]. Following the Soyuz-3, -4 and -5 flights, electrical activity of the leg muscles was elevated from preflight to postflight during graded exercise from 68 ± 14 μV to 85 ± 10 μV ($p < 0.05$) at 600 kgm/min and from 126 ± 12 μV to 163 ± 13 μV ($p < 0.05$) at 1000 kgm/min [55]. Thus, following short-term spaceflight, there is decreased firmness of the muscles and increased reflex excitability of the neuromuscular system at rest, which gradually increases in severity as the weightlessness continues. Taken together, muscle tone, excitability, and electrical efficiency data from both U.S. and Soviet spaceflights reinforced that the greatest loss of neuromuscular function during weightlessness occurs in the lower extremities with little change in the upper extremities. The greater use of arms rather than legs in normal mission operations and mobility in the spacecraft, and the possibility that the arm muscles that generate relatively small forces on Earth are less affected by the absence of gravity than the antigravity muscles of the lower extremities, could account for postflight neuromuscular maintenance in the arm muscles.

The mechanisms associated with these changes in neuromuscular excitability and efficiency are unclear. Kakurin et al. [56] have proposed that impulses from the central nervous system to the muscles are reduced during exposure to weightlessness. According to this hypothesis, central command impulses would dramatically increase upon return to terrestrial gravitation and become a stronger stimulus of the muscular

FIGURE 4.4

Ratio of EMG activity to force development during maximal ankle extension (calf muscle contraction) performed at four standard angular velocities before (open bars) *and after* (hatched bars) *7 days of spaceflight.* Bars and lines *represent mean ± SE from 11 Salyut-6 cosmonauts. Asterisks indicate significantly greater* (p < 0.05) *postflight values compared to preflight. (Modified data were analyzed and plotted from Kozlovskaya IB, Grigoryeva LS, Gevlich GI: Comparative analysis of effects of weightlessness and its models on velocity and strength properties and tone of human skeletal muscles. Kosm Biol Aviakosm Med 18(6):22–26, 1984.)*

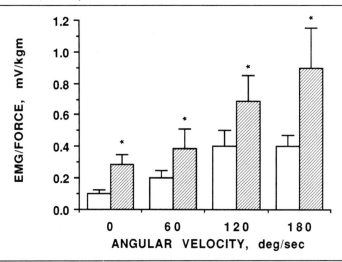

gravireceptor system compared to microgravity. This scenario could explain the postflight increase in reflex excitability observed at rest and during exercise. These changes may affect work performance following return from spaceflight to terrestrial gravitation and may indicate the involvement of impaired somatic neural activity.

Because most human activity on Earth is performed in a vertical posture, any change in the regulation of the erect position would impair physical performance. The erect posture of the seven cosmonauts from the 5-day missions of Soyuz-6-Soyuz-8 and two Soyuz-9 crew members who underwent an 18-day mission was investigated before and after their flights [78, 79]. Using a "stabilographic" method, which provides a picture of movement of the body's center of gravity in the sagittal and frontal planes, the cosmonauts after landing were tested with eyes open and head erect, eyes closed, head backward, and head tilted down. Most cosmonauts expressed that while standing it was difficult for them to maintain equilibrium. This characteristic was supported by the stabilographic data, which revealed a considerable decrease in the vertical stability of these subjects. During the stand maneuvers, the amplitude of center of gravity oscillations was increased and the frequency of oscillations was reduced. This translates into movements of greater swaying back and forth with slower response for correction. In addition, cosmonauts often complained of leg muscle pain, a sensation of "weight of the entire body," and a considerable increase in the weight of all objects after landing [78, 79, 101]. These data were interpreted as indicating a considerable impairment in the coordinating system regulating erect posture following spaceflight, although loss of strength in the muscles of the lower extremities may also contribute to postural instability. The alteration in control of posture was virtually recovered by 10 days postflight.

In addition to the problems of maintaining the erect posture following spaceflight, some Soviet and U.S. astronauts have exhibited an unstable gait during the first hours after landing. Using a cyclogrammetric method, the structure of walking was examined in the two crew members of the Soyuz-9 18-day mission [15]. The first period after landing, which lasted about 2 days, was characterized by distinct changes in gait. The cosmonauts deviated from a straight trajectory and frequently extended their arms to either side for greater stability. Walking was in short steps of unstable length. The height to which the knee of the striding leg was raised during movement was reduced. It was characteristic that while taking a forward step the cosmonaut did not put down his foot, but thrust it onto the support, creating the impression of a "stamping" gait. These cosmonauts described terrestrial gravitation as an unusual and unaccustomed weight and demonstrated a poor perception of the muscular efforts developed in walking. Impairment in their perception of the relative position of individual links in the legs during walking was evident by the fact that the leg grazed a step when they were climbing stairs. Subjectively the cosmonauts sensed the height of raising their leg to be adequate, although in reality the angle of flexion in the coxofemoral and knee joints was inadequate. Accordingly, weightlessness, becoming the customary environment during the 18-day flight, caused an impairment in perception of the relative position of body parts upon return to terrestrial conditions. In addition, a dramatic restructuring of motor skill of walking was evidenced by increases in the horizontal velocity components of the knee (14%) and talocalcaneal (39%) joints. In a later flight of longer duration (63 days), distances of long and high jumps were reduced by an average of 11 and 14% in two cosmonauts and associated with about 10% reduction in force characteristics [16].

During experiments on the U.S. Spacelab 1 10-day mission, thresholds for mass discrimination under microgravity during flight were found to be nearly 2-fold higher than those for weight discrimination before flight [80]. This suggests that sensitivity to inertial mass of objects is lost during flight and may impair the capacity to work with tools and equipment in space. Further, weight discrimination thresholds remain elevated for 2–3 days after flight, an effect which may limit physical working mechanics during the first days following return to Earth.

Muscle Function: Strength and Fatigability

Clearly, the ability to develop and maintain forces with dynamic muscular contractions will affect exercise and work performance. Because skeletal muscles provide the force for moving the body and external objects against Earth's gravity, the absence of gravity removes a major stimulus to maintain normal strength and endurance in microgravity. Although this may not be detrimental to work and exercise performance in weightlessness, it seems to be a significant limiting factor upon safe return and normal productivity in 1g following prolonged spaceflight.

The loss of strength in postural muscles has been reported following only 2–5 days of exposure to weightlessness in 12 cosmonauts during the Soyuz-3 through Soyuz-8 missions [55, 56]. Back strength (in relative units), measured by dynamometry, was reported to decrease from 137 ± 6 preflight to 116 ± 5 postflight (−15%). Such rapid and dramatic changes may reduce work output and predispose individuals to back injuries upon return to a gravity environment.

Strength of the muscles activating the elbow, and the knee flexors and extensors was measured preflight and postflight on all three U.S. Skylab missions using isokinetic dynamometry in the supine posture at an angular rate of 45°/s [95]. Average peak torque was reduced in knee extensors by 20 and 21%, and in knee flexors by 10 and 19% following 28 and 59 days of spaceflight, respectively. There was less strength loss in elbow flexors and extensors. The loss in strength of these muscle was minimized in the 84-day Skylab 4 mission, with no change in knee extensors. However, comparisons of these data from the three different flights is difficult because exercise countermeasures were significantly increased with subsequent flights. In addition, strength measurements were not angle-specific and were limited to only one speed. However, the general conclusion was that weightlessness reduced muscle strength primarily in the legs and that the magnitude of strength loss was directly associated with body weight and leg volume reduction, and inversely related to volume of exercise performed inflight [95].

Using isokinetic dynamometry, the force-velocity relationship of the ankle flexors (anterior tibialis) and extensors (calf muscles) was measured in crew members before and after participation in short (7 days) and long (110–237 days) missions on the Soviet Salyut space station [47]. The data demonstrated that spaceflight reduces static and dynamic strength of the ankle flexors and extensors during both short and long missions (Fig. 4.5). An effect of duration of weightlessness exposure was demonstrated by the reduction of strength across the entire range of

FIGURE 4.5

Torque-velocity relationship of the calf (upper curves) and anterior tibialis (lower curves) muscles before (open circles) and after (closed circles) short-term (left panel) and long-term (right panel) spaceflight. Circles and bars represent mean ± SE values from 12 cosmonauts on Salyut-6 (7 days) and six cosmonauts on Salyut-7 (110–237 days). Asterisks indicate significantly greater (p < 0.05) preflight values compared to postflight. (Modified data from Grigoryeva LS, Kozlovskaya IB: Effect of weightlessness and hypokinesia on velocity and strength properties of human muscles. Kosm Biol Aviakosm Med 21(1):27–30, 1987.)

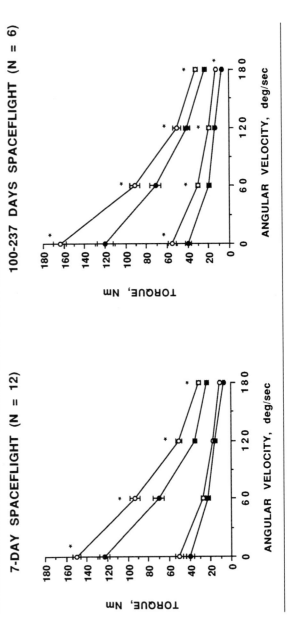

velocities for ankle flexors that was significant only after the longer flights. It is interesting to note that the decline of dynamic strength in the ankle extensors was similar after short and long duration flight while torque development in the isometric mode was greater after the long-term (27%) compared to the 7-day (18%) flights. It was suggested that these results reflected a greater amount of dynamic physical exercise with the calf muscles during the 110–237-day flights [47].

The mechanisms involved in the loss of muscle strength during exposure to weightlessness are unclear. The loss of load-bearing input to muscle proprioception has been viewed as a primary factor in the development of motor disturbances, particularly during brief exposure to weightlessness. The possible contribution of impaired neuromotor mechanisms to the limitation of force development after exposure to weightlessness was suggested by a high correlation (0.81–0.86) between the reduction in muscle tone (rigidity) and force development in anti-gravity muscles [62]. Because this relationship was observed after only 7 days of weightlessness, it was presumed that muscle atrophy was not a significant factor in the diminished isokinetic muscle force development over a range of 0–180° of limb motion.

Muscle atrophy resulting from unloading and relative disuse has been proposed as a primary contributing factor to the cause of postflight loss in muscle strength [47, 97]. The reduction of limb size during space-flight has been well documented and used as an indication of muscle atrophy [17, 50, 54, 97]. Unfortunately, except for these gross anthropometric measurements, which are influenced by fluid shifts, there are no data from human muscle samples to substantiate an atrophic process at the cellular level during or after spaceflight. However, recent ground-base studies using human subjects in bed rest revealed a significant atrophy of both fast-twitch (18%) and slow-twitch (11%) fibers [49]. Ultra-structural analyses revealed cellular edema, disorganized myofibrils, irregular Z-bodies, and fiber necrosis (disrupted fiber membranes) as indicated by disrupted sarcolemma, abnormal mitochondria, disrupted striation patterns, and mitochondria located in the intercellular spaces. These structural changes were associated with reduction in the force-velocity relation [39] similar in magnitude to that reported following spaceflight [47, 62, 97], suggesting that similar structural alterations in muscle may occur during weightlessness. However, the data from these groundbase studies underscore the importance of obtaining muscle samples from space travelers in order to identify the mechanisms associated with loss of muscle strength.

Data regarding the fatigability characteristics of muscle groups in humans following spaceflight are limited. Using spectral power analysis from EMG, LaFevers et al. [66] reported significantly increased fatigability in the gastrocnemius muscles following flight as evidenced by a shift of spectral power to the lower frequencies in response to maintaining a tension equal to 50% of maximum voluntary contraction for 1 min (Fig. 4.6). Significant fatigability was not evident in the biceps brachii. Although it appears that weightlessness increases postflight muscle fatigability in the lower extremities, the mechanism is not obvious. LaFevers et al. [66] suggested that more fatigable muscle fibers with higher excitation thresholds become more excitable (lowered threshold) after spaceflight and are therefore recruited at lower tensions. It is generally agreed that the stronger the contraction of a muscle, the higher its discharge frequency until fatigue develops. Therefore, more fibers are used for a given tension, which implies that a greater proportion of the muscle's contractile capacity is being used. The intensity of the contraction of a muscle exposed to weightlessness is proportionately greater than that of a normal muscle to achieve or maintain a given tension, leading to earlier fatigue. Compared to preflight, increased EMG amplitude per unit of force developed in calf muscles during postflight tests argues for this notion even for short-duration contractions [62]. However, this hypothesis remains speculative. Reductions in muscle oxygen delivery (arterial blood flow) and/or oxygen consumption may contribute to increased fatigability because decreased capillary-to-fiber ratios and enzyme activities of aerobic metabolic pathways have been reported

FIGURE 4.6

Plots of fatigue data for the gastrocnemius muscle obtained from EMG activity during a 1-min isometric contraction at 50% maximum voluntary contraction showing spectral power shifts from before (solid line) *to after* (broken line) *9 days of spaceflight. (Data modified from LaFevers EV, Nicogossian AE, Hursta WN: Electromyographic analysis of skeletal muscle changes arising from 9 days of weightlessness in the Apollo-Soyuz space mission. NASA Technical Memorandum. NASA TM X-58177, 1976, pp 1–30.)*

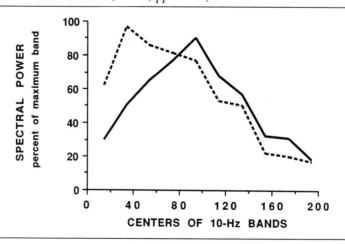

in humans exposed to groundbase analogs of microgravity [49]. Future spaceflight research should include studies designed to determine the etiology of both nerve and muscle in neuromuscular dysfunction attributable to weightlessness and to investigate the practical consequences of postflight muscle dysfunction on work performance capability.

OTHER CONTRIBUTING FACTORS

The Space Environment

Environmental factors such as temperature, humidity, and partial pressure of oxygen can affect work and exercise performance. Atmospheric composition of the spacecrafts in the U.S. program has evolved from 100% oxygen at 260 torr in the Mercury, Gemini, and Apollo capsules [74] to close to ambient earth in the shuttle orbiter [70]. The design range for ambient temperature and humidity in the Apollo Command modules was maintained between 21 and 27°C with a relative humidity of 40–70% [74]. Composition of the atmosphere in the living compartments of the Soviet spaceships is close to ambient earth with total pressure between 735 and 811 mm Hg with partial pressures of oxygen at 175–235 mm Hg, carbon dioxide at 1.6–10.7 mm Hg, and water vapor at 7.0–12.8 mm Hg [48, 100, 101, 103]. Air temperature was maintained between 18 and 25°C. Thus, the environments of current U.S. and Soviet spacecrafts are maintained within environmental limits that should not limit physiological capacity to perform physical work or exercise during flight.

Although not a major concern for acute effects on work performance in space, the daily intensity of the dose caused by galactic cosmic radiation and the influence of the Earth's radiation belts is a concern. At routine flight altitudes (about 350 km), the mean levels of radiation are about 14–15 mrad [100, 101]. During the entire 63-day flight of Salyut-4, the level of radiation on the station crew was approximately 1.2–2.0 rem; this was much lower than the admissible dose (15 rem) for similar flights [100, 101]. Similar data from the three U.S. Skylab missions corroborate that the dose equivalents for crew members were well below the threshold of significant clinical effect and constituted no danger for the crew's health or limitation to the crew's ability to live for long periods in space or perform physical tasks in space [2].

Fluid and Electrolyte Changes

One of the most consistent and rapid adaptations to microgravity is the loss of body fluids. Reduction of total body water was measured in all three Skylab 2 astronauts averaging from 47.5 ± 3.1 liters before flight to 46.3 ± 2.8 liters following 28 days of spaceflight [68]. Approximately 300 ml of this fluid came from the plasma compartment, decreasing from 3.34 liters preflight to 3.05 liters postflight (−8.4 ± 3.0%) [52]. Plasma volume measurements made after Gemini 4, Gemini 5, and three Apollo missions of shorter duration than Skylab 2 (4–11 days) demonstrated that 12 of 13 crew members had similar relative reductions of their plasma volume by an average of 8.6 ± 1.3% (range from −4 to −16%) [41]. Plasma volume decreased by 6% after 10 days on the U.S. Spacelab 1 shuttle mission [71]. The average reduction of plasma volume was greater in three Skylab 3 (13%) and three Skylab 4 (16%) astronauts after longer durations of spaceflight (59 and 84 days) [53]. Taken together, these data suggest an early reduction in plasma and blood volume followed by a gradual stabilization sometime between 30 and 60 days of flight (Fig. 4.7). Interestingly, plasma concentrations of sodium and osmolality were not altered following flights as long as 63 days [63]. These findings suggest that there is a proportionate loss of fluid and electrolytes, i.e., isotonic, from the body during flight, which acts to protect the interior milieu.

The reduction in body fluids and electrolytes, particularly within the vascular space, might contribute to the limitation of hemodynamic responses required to support adequate blood flow and thermoregulation accompanying moderate to heavy work during or following spaceflight. Groundbase data have demonstrated a high correlation between the amount of plasma volume reduction and the reduction in $\dot{V}o_2max$ following simulated microgravity [24]. However, plasma volume was reduced by nearly 16% in the Skylab 4 astronauts after 84 days of spaceflight (Fig. 4.7), but inflight $\dot{V}o_2max$ was increased [76]. Although hypovolemia induced by microgravity may contribute to reduced work performance in weightlessness, other factors must be involved.

Red Blood Cell and Hemoglobin Changes

A consistent influence of weightlessness reported in both U.S. and Soviet astronauts has been a reduction in circulating hemoglobin and red cell mass [71]. From two cosmonauts on Soyuz-9 mission (18 days), hemoglobin concentration decreased from 16.4 g/dl preflight to 13.7 g/dl postflight while erythrocytes number per volume of blood remained constant (from 4,570,000 preflight to 4,625,000 postflight) [72]. These results were corroborated by data on the two crew members of the 16-day Salyut-3 mission and the crews of the 30-day and 63-day missions of Salyut-4, in which significant reductions in total circulating hemoglobin were reported [73]. The constant erythrocyte concentration in light of a reduction in total circulating blood volume indicates a loss in total red cells as well as hemoglobin. Red cell mass measurements made after

FIGURE 4.7

Percent changes in plasma volume, red cell mass, and total hemoglobin as a function of spaceflight duration. Bars *represent mean values and* lines *represent standard errors. (Data were extracted and plotted from: Spacelab 1 (Leach CS, Johnson PC: Influence of spaceflight on erythrokinetics in man.* Science *225:216–218, 1984); Skylab-2, Skylab-3, and Skylab-4 (Johnson PC, Driscoll TB, LeBlanc AD: Blood volume changes. In Johnston RS, Dietlein LF (eds):* Biomedical Results from Skylab. *NASA SP-377, 1977, pp 235–241); and Salyut-3, 4, and 6 missions (Legenkov VI, Kiselev RK, Gudim VI, Moskaleva GP: Changes in peripheral blood of crew members of the Salyut-4 orbital station.* Kosm Biol Aviakosm Med *11(6):3–12, 1977).)*

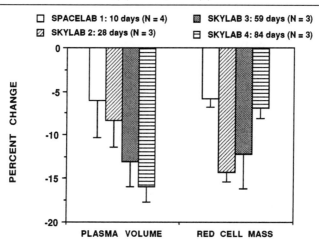

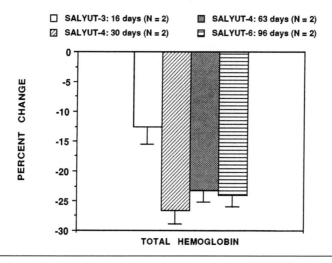

three Gemini (4–14 days) and three Apollo missions (7–11 days) demonstrated that 13 of 15 crew members had reduced their red blood cell mass by an average of 10.1 ± 1.9% (range from −1 to −22%) [41]. Erythrocytes show normal life span in weightlessness and there is no evidence of loss of red cells through hemorrhage or hemolysis [57]. Although the hyperoxic spacecraft atmosphere of the early Mercury, Gemini, Apollo, and Skylab flights may have contributed to some observations [41], the decrease in red cells and hemoglobin appears to be due primarily to impaired hemopoiesis (regeneration) because erythropoietin decreased concomitant with a reduction in erythrocytes in all crew members of the U.S. Spacelab 1 mission in a normoxic environment [57, 71].

In the 30-day and 63-day missions of Salyut-4, the magnitude of hemoglobin loss was 12.5% for the 16-day mission and decreased to 26 and 23% [72], and 24% in the Salyut-6 96-day mission [103]. Reduction in red cell mass showed a similar pattern, decreasing by 6% after the 10-day U.S. Spacelab 1 mission [71] and continuing to 14 and 12% after the 28- and 59-day Skylab missions [52]. As presented in Figure 4.7, the U.S. Skylab and Spacelab 1 and Soviet data suggest an early reduction in red cells and hemoglobin with a plateau by 30 days of flight [52, 71, 73]. This represents an approximate 25% reduction in oxygen-carrying capacity of the blood, which could contribute to the limitation of exercise and work capacity during and following short and prolonged flights. It is interesting to note that the prevention of red cell loss in Skylab 4 astronauts after 84 days of spaceflight (Fig. 4.7) with high levels of inflight exercise was associated with maintenance of inflight $\dot{V}o_2max$ [76].

Leg Compliance Changes

Increased leg (venous) compliance has been reported in both U.S. astronauts [96] and Soviet cosmonauts [109]. The mechanism(s) of the increased compliance in weightlessness is unclear, but is related to the size (cross-sectional area) and tone of the muscle compartment [26, 60]. Calf compliance is increased early in actual and simulated microgravity [28, 96], suggesting that interstitial fluid shifts out of the leg may contribute. When the muscle compartment is reduced during simulated microgravity, compliance increases [27, 28]; when the muscle compartment loss is attenuated with routine muscular activity during bed rest, the compliance changes are eliminated [40]. These data indicate that the loss of muscle composition and activity that occur during weightlessness are important factors contributing to the increase in venous compliance in the lower extremities.

In addition to the effect of plasma and blood volume reduction, more compliant veins can exaggerate reduced venous return, stroke volume, and cardiac output during exercise in weightlessness and after flight by providing a greater capacity to pool blood in the lower extremities under the same hydrostatic pressure [50, 54]. This notion is supported by the observation that lower venous return and stroke volume during exercise in spaceflight has been associated with increased venous compliance in the legs [108]. Thus, the increase in venous compliance may contribute to reduced work performance, particularly after return to terrestrial gravity.

Pulmonary Function

Although changes in pulmonary ventilation in microgravity could limit gas exchange and affect work performance, there is little evidence to support this notion. Resting vital capacity, residual volume, total lung capacity, tidal volume, alveolar ventilation, forced expiratory volume, maximum voluntary ventilation, and closing volume were not altered following spaceflight [77, 87]. Whereas resting vital capacity was lower during weightlessness [87], exercise levels were well within preflight values ranging from 4458 to 4600 ml [59]. In the nine Skylab astronauts, pulmonary efficiency measured as ventilation volume during exercise at an oxygen uptake of 2.0 liters/min, was essentially unaltered from 55.4 ± 1.5 liters/min on the ground to 58.6 ± 2.2 liters/min during weightlessness [76]. Average ventilation volume during 75% $\dot{V}o_2max$ in the three Skylab 4 astronauts was reported as 82.4 ± 9.9 liters/min preflight compared to 83.3 ± 10.8 liters/min inflight [76]. Similar results have been reported in cosmonauts [59]. Although the slightly increased work of respiration may add to the metabolic cost of work during weightlessness, these data suggest that pulmonary function per se does not represent a limiting factor to gas exchange during exercise in a microgravity environment or upon return to terrestrial gravity.

Thermoregulation

There are few data regarding the effects of weightlessness on thermoregulatory responses to physical work and exercise during and after flight. Daily evaporative water losses during the three U.S. Skylab missions were measured indirectly using mass and water-balance techniques [69]. Although it was expected that evaporative water losses would increase in the hypobaric environment of the Skylab spacecraft (one-third atmosphere), the mean daily values for the nine crew members who averaged 1 hr of daily exercise decreased from 1750 ± 37 ml preflight to 1560 ± 26 ml during flight ($p < 0.05$). The results suggest that weightlessness decreased sweat losses during exercise and possibly reduced insensible skin losses as well. The weightlessness environment apparently promotes the formation of an observed sweat film on the skin surface during exercise by reducing convective flow and sweat drippage.

This apparently results in high levels of sustained skin wetness that acts to suppress sweating [69].

Data from groundbase studies showed excessive elevation in rectal temperature (0.2–0.4°C) in seven men during 70 min of submaximal supine cycle ergometry (45–48% $\dot{V}o_2max$) performed in ambient temperature of 22°C after 14 days of simulated microgravity [46]. This exercise hyperthermia was greater than the pre-bedrest ambulatory control level, suggesting a reduced capacity to dissipate heat. No significant differences in total body sweat production were observed, suggesting an inhibition of sweating from the same core temperature stimulus. Thus, data from flight and groundbase models indicate that weightlessness causes some impairment in thermoregulation during exercise, which could be limiting to work performance of extended duration such as EVA. However, this problem may be removed or mitigated during work or exercise inside the spacecraft habitat area by the use of high volume air movement in the area of the exercise equipment.

Substrate Availability and Its Control

Although the availability of substrates carried in the blood to working muscles may be one limiting factor to work performance during spaceflight, the evidence does not strongly support this notion. Blood glucose levels were not altered in cosmonauts who flew in missions of 15, 24, 29, and 63 days [6] and were slightly elevated postflight compared to preflight in the 63-day Salyut-4 mission [98]. However, in the three U.S. Skylab missions, fasting blood glucose was slightly elevated initially and then decreased slightly below preflight levels for the remainder of the flight [70]. It is interesting that plasma insulin also decreased during the Skylab missions [70]. The reduction of the insulin response to glucose load following exposure to simulated microgravity (bed rest) [37] may suggest decreased sensitivity of the stimulus-response relation for the control of circulating glucose during weightlessness. However, the consequence of insulin-glucose changes on the metabolic response to exercise in weightlessness and after return to earth is unclear and warrants further investigation.

Significantly increased levels of both thyroxine-stimulating hormone and thyroxine have been reported after spaceflight [70]. Increased thyroid hormone levels cause increased oxygen consumption, heat production, and increased metabolism of protein, carbohydrates, and fats. Elevated thyroxine may have contributed to increased resting oxygen uptake reported during spaceflight [76]. The possible role of this hormone in the control of metabolism during exercise in weightlessness has not been studied.

Plasma catecholamines were not altered from preflight to postflight in the 63-day Salyut-4 mission [98]. However, epinephrine and norepinephrine excretion were decreased during the 84-day Skylab mission [70], perhaps suggesting a reduction in autonomic response to the weightless environment, which may affect the control of substrate mobilization. Results from groundbase studies show that this decreased norepinephrine response can be prevented by exercise [67], suggesting that physical activity may be important in providing an adequate maintenance of sympathetic control for metabolism. However, the role that catecholamines play in energy production and substrate availability during exercise and work in weightlessness is only speculative and has not been satisfactorily examined.

Although plasma concentrations of circulating free fatty acids at rest have not been reported for spaceflight, groundbase studies suggest no change [106]. It should be appreciated that the maintenance of the concentration of these potential substrate fuels indicates that the total amount of circulating substrate available to the working muscle is proportionately reduced with the reduction in plasma and blood volume. This reduction in absolute amount of circulating substrate could be on the same order as the 5–15% plasma volume reductions, depending on the duration of the mission (Fig. 4.7), and could therefore represent a limiting factor to work performance, particularly if the work in space involves moderate intensities of EVA for 3–6 hr. Finally, the possible limitation of total circulating substrates associated with lower plasma and blood volumes may reflect impaired mobilization and/or utilization of substrates as a result of reduced total body muscular activity in weightlessness.

Substrate availability is also dependent upon adequate dietary intake. The diets of both U.S. and Soviet space missions have been relatively high in carbohydrate: 60–67% carbohydrate, 16–19% fat, and 19–24% protein by weight [48, 89, 103]. The average caloric content of the daily diet consumed by the 24 astronauts of Apollo 7 through 14 was 1745 kcal. However, it should be noted that the average weights of these astronauts decreased from 166.5 ± 2.6 pounds preflight to 160.0 ± 2.7 pounds postflight ($p < 0.05$). As spaceflights became longer and required more inflight exercise in the Soviet program, caloric intake was increased from about 2600 kcal during flights of 2–8 days to the present 3150 kcal consumed on past and current Salyut and Mir orbiting space station missions of greater than 16 days [48, 103]. Water consumption is approximately 1,500–2000 ml per person per day [48]. These diets appear to be adequate in maintaining circulating substrate availability for inflight and postflight exercise and work. However, the consistent observation of weight loss in weightlessness despite high caloric intake and aerobic exercise may be related to muscle atrophy and the requirement for more protein in the diet. The effect of diet composition on circulating substrates, substrate stores, muscle growth, and work performance in weightlessness is unclear.

Muscle Pain

The astronauts of Apollo-7 complained of pain in muscles of the back, which developed (in the opinion of the astronauts) because of the need to constantly maintain the body and limbs in an unusual position in weightlessness, even at rest. It is noteworthy that this pain disappeared after exercising. On the day following flight, cosmonauts have reported painful feelings in the gastrocnemius and femoral muscles similar to those that occur after intensive physical training [43].

Repeated Exposures to Microgravity

Although 100 astronauts and cosmonauts have flown in space at least two times, there are few data available to describe the effects of repeated exposure in microgravity on exercise and work performance during and after flight. Cosmonaut V.V. Ryumin made his 185-day flight 6 months after a previous 175-day flight. In both missions it was reported that his work capacity remained essentially identical, indicating a complete recovery to his normal state during the intervening 6-month period [103]. Although there are limited data suggesting the recovery of cardiovascular, fluid-electrolyte, and metabolic capacities to preflight levels by about 2 weeks after return to Earth [7], data are not available to show conclusively whether full recovery of muscle takes place or the time course of such recovery.

EXERCISE AS A COUNTERMEASURE

Past and Present Exercise Prescriptions

The use of exercise during spaceflight as a countermeasure to attenuate specific adaptations to weightlessness such as reduced cardiovascular and work capacity, muscle atrophy, and bone demineralization has been employed in both the U.S. and Soviet space programs.

The medical report of the two cosmonauts of the Soyuz-14-Salyut-3 16-day orbital mission showed insignificant reductions in muscle tone and limb circumference; strength of the muscles did not change [48]. It was suggested that these protective effects were associated with inflight use of a physical trainer (resistance pulling device) and the wearing of spring-loaded suits (Penguin suits) during waking hours (8 hr/day). The Penguin suit provided consistent resistance (axial loads) up to 50% of body mass to the major muscles of the arms, legs, and torso. However, it was not possible to quantify the specificity and amount of "exercise" performed by these crew members during flight, and the lack of change in muscle size and function may have been merely a result of the shortness of the exposure to microgravity.

By 1975, with flight durations increasing, the recommended inflight regimen for Soviet cosmonauts prescribed two to three exercise periods daily for a total of 2.5 hr. The prophylactic means employed during the Salyut-4 30-day and 63-day orbital flights included a treadmill-complex trainer with a system for harnessing and holding the cosmonaut. For exercise on the treadmill, the cosmonauts donned a special load suit, which together with the harnessing system ensured that they would remain on the track. This system simulated a weight load of approximately 50 kg along the longitudinal axis of the body and also a static load on the principal groups of antigravitational muscles [101, 103]. A diagram of the Soviet space treadmill is presented in Figure 4.8. The cycle ergometer was also used at graded loads of 440, 585, 790, 980, 1160, and 1350 kgm/min at 60 rpm. The two cosmonauts exercised about 2 hr/day using both apparatus. In addition, both cosmonauts wore the Penguin spring-loaded suits 10–12 hours daily. These exercise regimens during

FIGURE 4.8
Diagram depicting the Soviet space treadmill with harness designed to keep a person on the belt and provide a load of approximately 50 kg on the longitudinal axis of the body.

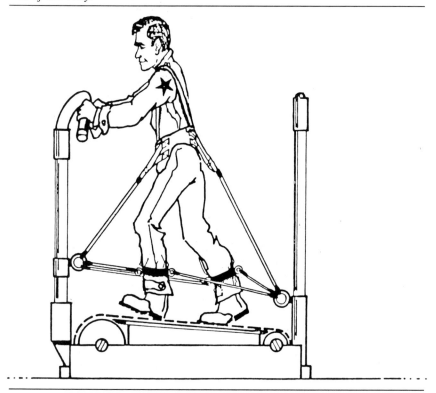

flight maintained a normal heart rate (Fig. 4.1) and stroke volume response to 440 kgm/min ($\dot{V}o_2$ = 1.2 liters/min), but did not protect against the onset of inflight and postflight orthostatic intolerance.

A similar exercise regimen was employed during the 1977–1981 era of the Soviet Salyut-6 space station. Beginning with mission days 4–7, crew members were scheduled to exercise every morning and evening using a bicycle ergometer and a treadmill equipped with a pulling harness that provided approximately 50 kg directed parallel to the long axis of the body [103]. The exercises were performed on a cyclic basis, i.e., for 3 days, according to a specially developed program and the 4th day was ad libitum. Additionally, crew members donned the Penguin spring-loaded suits that provided an axial load upon the musculoskeletal system. These suits were removed before sleep periods.

During the early part of the 96-day flight aboard the Soviet Salyut-6 space station, poorer endurance to a standardized exercise test (750 kgm/min for 5 min at 60 rpm) was reported in the two crew members [44]. This response was presumed to be caused by physical deconditioning, which was manifested by increased heart rate, elevated arterial pressure, and reduced stroke volume to lesser work intensity and an inability to complete the 5-min exercise bout on the 24th day of flight. This stage of the mission was characterized by an increase in volume of work related to operation of the station and a subsequent disruption of the work and rest daily schedule and a reduction in the prescribed daily exercise. Although it was unclear what the daily exercise prescription was for these cosmonauts, the return to normal scheduled work-rest cycles and exercise regimens improved the hemodynamic responses and exercise endurance by day 70 through the remainder of the flight. These observations indicate the importance of regular physical loading for the maintenance of work capacity during prolonged exposure to a microgravity environment.

Because the magnitude of cardiac and hemodynamic responses was similar in cosmonauts who were in space from 30 to 140 days despite differences in the duration of exposure (Table 4.4), it was proposed that the similar exercise responses in cosmonauts who flew on missions of longer duration may reflect improvement of protective effects from more extensive exercise training programs that were implemented during subsequent flights [8]. This thesis is best supported by the results of the three U.S. Skylab missions. On the 28-day Skylab mission, only the cycle ergometer was used for inflight exercise [95]. Daily exercise was performed at approximately 70 W (430 kgm/min, $\dot{V}o_2$ = 1.2 liters/min) for an average of 30 min. Heart rate was greater and cardiac output less during postflight exercise compared to preflight responses, suggesting reduced cardiovascular reserve [75]. Arm and leg strength decreased by 15–20% [95]. After this flight, a device called the Mini Gym, which provided concentric resistive isokinetic exercise for the arms and trunk, was added to the second 59-day flight [95]. Also, the average amount of work performed on the cycle ergometer was more than doubled on this flight so that total daily exercise was about 1 hr in duration. Arm strength was preserved following the Skylab 3 mission. However, despite the significant increase in volume and mode of exercise during the second Skylab mission, postflight cardiovascular responses to dynamic exercise and loss of leg strength were similar to that of Skylab 2 [75, 95]. On the 84-day Skylab 4 mission, a Teflon-coated plate used as a treadmill was added to the exercise arsenal used on the previous Skylab flights and total daily exercise time was increased to about 1.5 hr [95]. It seems that the treadmill was used very little for walking or running, but its tethering harness device was used for jumping and toe rises [76]. Following flight, the reduction in exercise stroke volume and cardiac output, and loss of body weight, leg volume, and leg strength were less than half that of the previous two missions [76, 95]. These observations indicate the possibility of effective prevention of physical deconditioning by using exercise during long-term spaceflights. However, some degree of diminished cardiovascular reserve to exercise and loss of muscle strength in terrestrial gravity after flight indicates a need for further refinement of exercise regimens to safely conduct longer space missions.

It is difficult to assess the current effect of the volume of exercise performed during spaceflight because the regimens are not standardized and rarely is all activity reported. However, recent Soviet data presented in Table 4.3 describe the average exercise costs during the Soviet 175-day Salyut-6 mission [88]. Several basic observations can be made from this table. Both cycle ergometer and treadmill exercise were used during each exercise session on this mission. There were two sessions of exercise daily, each session consisting of an average 40 min on the cycle ergometer and 34 min on the treadmill. Cycle exercise consisted of an average 975 kgm/min workrate ($\dot{V}O_2$ = 2.3 liters/min). Treadmill exercise consisted of an average locomotion speed of 120 m/min (4.5 mph) with about one-third the distance spent walking and two-thirds spent running (average $\dot{V}O_2$ = 1.5 liters/min). The average volume of exercise performed (39,414 kgm and 4,115 m per session) was greater than originally planned (20,080 kgm and 4,074 m), increasing in the second half of flight compared to the first half. Based on exercise heart rate responses and oxygen uptakes, it can be concluded that exercise used during this mission represented a training regimen of approximately 50–75% $\dot{V}O_2$max performed for 2.5 hr daily, 6 days/week. This activity was effective in nearly eliminating cardiovascular and musculoskeletal adaptations to microgravity [88, 99]. It is clear from these and other U.S. and Soviet experiences with long-duration spaceflight that as the exposure to weightlessness increases with longer visits to orbiting space and planetary stations so must the volume of exercise in order to prevent physical deconditioning.

Considerations for Future Exercise Prescriptions

The requirement for greater volume of exercise during spaceflight is the product of intensity, duration, and frequency. Work rates and metabolic costs of inflight exercise presented in this review indicate that an emphasis has been placed on aerobic conditioning with greater duration and moderate intensity. Unfortunately, the resulting 2–4 hr of daily exercise is extremely costly to the operational work day and in caloric expenditure. For instance, the average daily metabolic cost of 1,450 kcal for 2.5 hr of exercise currently performed during Soviet missions represents about half of the total 3,150 kcal intake on these missions [103]. If the combination of exercise intensity, duration, and frequency could be optimized to reduce the total exercise volume in half, this could save approximately 225,000 kcal over a 6-month mission, or enough to feed one astronaut for an additional 75 days. Finally, long laborious exercise regimens may cause difficulty in compliance because the Soviets have reported that some crew members resist exercising during their mission. Because productive working time and life support (oxygen, water, food) are at a premium during spaceflight, it is paramount to design efficient exercise prescriptions.

There is evidence to suggest that the use of graded maximal exercise can acutely restore some of the cardiovascular and metabolic capacities attenuated following exposures to simulated microgravity or physical deconditioning. One bout of maximal exercise at the end of 10 days of bedrest restored $\dot{V}o_2max$, heart rate, blood pressures, rate-pressure-product, oxygen pulse, and endurance time on a treadmill to pre-bed-rest levels within 2 hr of ambulation [25]. Maximal exercise can acutely expand plasma volume by 12% [45], a response that has acutely reversed the effects of detraining on reduced stroke volume during exercise and aerobic capacity [31]. Maximal exercise may act as a possible inflight countermeasure against orthostatic intolerance. Extensive aerobic exercise of moderate intensity and long duration performed during both U.S. and Soviet space missions failed to provide complete protection against postflight orthostatic hypotension [33, 34, 50, 54, 58, 101, 103]. Two primary mechanisms associated with the development of postflight orthostatic hypotension appear to be reduced blood volume [4] and impaired baroreflex activity [29]. In addition to the acute expansion of blood volume induced by maximal exercise [45], a single bout of maximal exercise has increased the responsiveness of the arterial baroreflexes [30, 91] and reversed fainting episodes following acute exposure to simulated microgravity [92].

The reasons for maximal exercise being more effective than the submaximal levels used in spaceflight in restoring $\dot{V}o_2max$, plasma volume, cardiovascular capacity, baroreflex function, and orthostatic tolerance after exposure to simulated microgravity are not clear. However, the use of less frequent and more intense exercise as a possible countermeasure against the loss of cardiovascular and metabolic capacities during exercise and development of postflight orthostatic hypotension should be thoroughly explored. Such an exercise prescription would be maximally cost effective by enhancing crew health maintenance and postflight recovery while minimizing inflight use of work time, food, water, and oxygen for exercise activities [25].

Another consideration for the development of future exercise countermeasure programs is the use of a resistive mode designed to eliminate or minimize muscle atrophy and reduced muscle strength. Except for the resistive loads provided by the Penguin suits in the Soviet space program and the Mini Gym in the U.S. Skylab program, the use of resistive exercise has received little attention. There are several issues that need to be addressed. First, the consistent reduction in strength of the lower extremities following spaceflight [47, 62, 95] despite the use of extensive dynamic exercise suggests that greater resistances are required to preserve muscle function. An equally important factor may be the absence of eccentric movements in the weightless environment as well as in exercise activity during spaceflight. Because eccentric movement is an integral part of our daily activities in terrestrial gravity, its absence in weightlessness may contribute significantly more to muscle atrophy and dysfunction. Resistive training on Earth, which involves performance of eccentric and concentric muscle actions, induces approximately twice the increase in strength as training with only concentric actions [93, 94]. In addition, the incorporation of eccentric actions in resistive training did not appreciably increase the energy cost of exercise with greater force development (G.A. Dudley, unpublished data). Clearly, the advantages of incorporating eccentric resistive training as a countermeasure during spaceflight include lower energy cost and less muscular fatigue at similar or greater forces as those developed by concentric actions. The role of eccentric movements in the preservation of muscle structure and function in weightlessness needs to be better defined and understood. This mode of exercise might provide a greater preventative measure against muscle atrophy and loss of strength during spaceflight at less time and energy cost to the crew.

The use of further groundbase and inflight experiments designed to identify the specificity of various modes, intensity, duration, and frequency of exercise should provide a more effective countermeasure prescription that requires significantly less time and energy expenditure than the regimens currently in use.

SUMMARY

Data describing the physiological adaptations to weightlessness and their effects on exercise and work performance during and after spaceflight have been accumulated from a limited number of subjects. However, some conclusions can be drawn based on certain consistent findings. Some degree of physical deconditioning, particularly apparent during postflight testing, is manifested by alterations in cardiovascular and metabolic responses to dynamic exercise and by reduced strength and greater fatigability of skeletal muscles. Deconditioning effects are more pronounced for activities involving muscle groups of the legs. Impaired cardiovascular performance is primarily the result of reduced blood volume rather than myocardial dysfunction. Altered fluid electrolytes, hemoglobin, leg compliance, thermoregulation, and substrate availability may contribute to the limitation of long-duration, submaximal work during and after spaceflight. Long periods of daily exercise performed during spaceflight have provided some protection against physical deconditioning, especially for cardiovascular and metabolic systems. Groundbase experiments on physiological responses to exercise have provided similar results as data from spaceflight, indicating the usefulness of using analogs of microgravity for future research. Future groundbase and flight studies should be designed to identify the mechanisms of cardiovascular, metabolic, and neuromuscular alterations induced by weightlessness and provide more efficient countermeasures that will preserve work capacity and minimize the use of crew work time and life-support resources.

ACKNOWLEDGMENTS

The author thanks Drs. Gary A. Dudley and Paul Buchanan for their valuable suggestions in the preparation of this manuscript, and Cynthia A. Thompson for her technical assistance in the gathering of research literature and presentation of data. Special thanks and appreciation is given to my wife Barbara who graciously accepted the burden and responsibilities of our home and family to provide me with the dedicated time and energy required to complete this manuscript.

REFERENCES

1. Atkov OY, Bednenko VS, Fomina GA: Ultrasound techniques in space medicine. *Aviat Space Environ Med* 58 (Suppl 9):A69–A73, 1987.
2. Bailey JV, Hoffman RA, English RA: Radiological protection and medical dosimetry for the Skylab crewmen. In Johnson RS, Dietlein LF (eds): *Biomedical Results from Skylab.* NASA SP-377, 1977, pp 64–69.
3. Bungo MW, Johnson PC: Cardiovascular examinations and observations of deconditioning during the Space Shuttle orbital flight test program. *Aviat Space Environ Med* 54:1001–1004, 1983.
4. Bungo MW, Charles JB, Johnson PC: Cardiovascular deconditioning during space flight and the use of saline as a countermeasure to orthostatic intolerance. *Aviat Space Environ Med* 56:985–990, 1985.

5. Bungo MW, Goldwater DJ, Popp RL, Sandler H: Echocardiographic evaluation of space shuttle crewmembers. *J Appl Physiol* 62:278–283, 1987.
6. Balakhovskiy IS, Orlova TA: Dynamics of cosmonauts' blood biochemistry during space missions. *Kosm Biol Aviakosm Med* 12(6):3–8, 1978.
7. Beregovkin AV, Vodolazov AS, Georgiyevskiy VS, Kalinichenko VV, Korelin NV, Mikhaylov VM, Pometov YD, Shchigolev VV, Katkovskiy BS: Reactions of the cardiorespiratory system to a dosed physical load in cosmonauts after 30- and 63-day flights in the 'Salyut-4' orbital station. *Kosm Biol Aviakosm Med* 10(5):24–29, 1976.
8. Beregovkin AV, Vodolazov AS, Georgiyevskiy VS, Kakurin LI, Kalinichenko VV, Korelin NV, Mikhaylov VM, Shchigolev VV: Cardiorespiratory system reactions of cosmonauts to exercise following long-term missions aboard the Salyut-6 orbital station. *Kosm Biol Aviakosm Med* 14(4):8–11, 1980.
9. Berry CA: Summary of medical experience in the Apollo 7 through Apollo 11 manned space flights. *Aerospace Med* 41:500–519, 1970.
10. Berry CA: Weightlessness. In Parker JF, West VR (eds): *Bioastronautics Data Book.* NASA SP-3006, 1974, pp 349–415.
11. Berry CA, Squires WG, Jackson AS: Fitness variables and the lipid profile in United States astronauts. *Aviat Space Environ Med* 51:1222–1226, 1980.
12. Biryukov YN, Krasnykh IG: Change in optical density of bone tissue and calcium metabolism in the cosmonauts A.G. Nikolayev and V.I. Sevastyanov. *Kosm Biol Med* 4(6):42–45, 1970.
13. Butusov AA, Lyamin VR, Lebedev AA, Polyakova AP, Svistunov IB, Tishler VA, Shulenin AP: Results of routine medical monitoring of cosmonauts during flight on the 'Soyuz-9' ship. *Kosm Biol Med* 4(6):35–39, 1970.
14. Cavanagh PR, Buczek FL, Milliron MJ: The kinematics of locomotion in space. *A Final Report to Krug International,* 1987, pp 1–126.
15. Chekirda IF, Bogdashevskiy RB, Yeremin AV, Kolosov IA: Coordination structure of walking of Soyuz-9 crew members before and after flight. *Kosm Biol Med* 5(6):48–52, 1971.
16. Chekirda IF, Yeremin AV: Dynamics of cyclic and acyclic locomotion of the Soyuz-18 crew after a 63-day space mission. *Kosm Biol Aviakosm Med* 11(4):9–13, 1977.
17. Cherepakhin MA, Pervushin VI: Space flight effect on the neuromuscular system on cosmonauts. *Kosm Biol Med* 4(6):46–49, 1970.
18. Chirkov BA: Energy expenditures of the crew during the eighteen-day flight of the "Soyuz-9" spaceship. *Kosm Biol Aviakosm Med* 9(1):48–51, 1975.
19. Convertino VA, Hung J, Goldwater DJ, DeBusk RF: Cardiovascular responses to exercise in middle-aged men following ten days of bed rest. *Circulation* 65:134–140, 1982.
20. Convertino VA, Sandler H, Webb P, Annis JF: Induced venous pooling and cardiorespiratory responses to exercise after bedrest. *J Appl Physiol* 52:1343–1348, 1982.
21. Convertino VA, Goldwater DJ, Sandler H: Vo_2 kinetics of constant-load exercise following bedrest-induced deconditioning. *J Appl Physiol* 57:1545–1550, 1984.
22. Convertino VA, Goldwater DJ, Sandler H: Bedrest-induced peak Vo_2 reduction associated with age, gender and aerobic capacity. *Aviat Space Environ Med* 57:17–22, 1986.
23. Convertino VA, Karst GM, Kirby CR, Goldwater DJ: Effect of simulated weightlessness on exercise-induced anaerobic threshold. *Aviat Space Environ Med* 57:325–331, 1986.
24. Convertino VA: Exercise responses after inactivity. In Sandler H, Vernikos-Danellis J (eds): *Inactivity: Physiological Effects.* New York, Academic Press, 1986, pp 149–191.
25. Convertino VA: Potential benefits of maximal exercise just prior to return from weightlessness. *Aviat Space Environ Med* 58:568–572, 1987.
26. Convertino VA, Doerr DF, Flores JF, Hoffler GW, Buchanan P: Leg size and muscle functions associated with leg compliance. *J Appl Physiol* 64:1017–1021, 1988.

27. Convertino VA, Doerr DF, Stein SF: Changes in size and compliance of the calf following 30 days of simulated microgravity. *J Appl Physiol* 66:1509–1512, 1989.

28. Convertino VA, Doerr DF, Mathes KL, Stein SL, Buchanan P: Changes in volume, muscle compartment, and compliance of the lower extremities in man following 30 days of exposure to simulated microgravity. *Aviat Space Environ Med* 60:653–658, 1989.

29. Convertino VA, Doerr DF, Eckberg DL, Fritsch JM, Vernikos-Danellis J: Bedrest impairs vagal baroreflex responses and provokes orthostatic hypotension. *J Appl Physiol* 68 (in press, 1989).

30. Convertino VA, Adams WC, Blamick CA: Carotid-cardiac baroreflex response during 24 hours after maximal exercise. *Aviat Space Environ Med* 60:501, 1989.

31. Coyle EF, Hemmert MK, Coggan AR: Effects of detraining on cardiovascular responses to exercise: role of blood volume. *J Appl Physiol* 60:95–99, 1986.

32. Degtyarev VA, Doroshev VG, Kalmykova ND, Kirillova ZA, Lapshina NA: Dynamics of circulatory indices in the crew of the Salyut orbital station during an examination under rest conditions. *Kosm Biol Aviakosm Med* 8(2):34–42, 1974.

33. Degtyarev VA, Doroshev VG, Kalmykova ND, Kirillova ZA, Kukushkin YA, Lapshina NA: Results of examination of the crew of the "Salyut" space station in a functional test with creation of negative pressure on the lower half of the body. *Kosm Biol Aviakosm Med* 8(3):47–52, 1974.

34. Degtyarev VA, Doroshev VG, Batenchuk-Tusko TV, Kirillova ZA, Lapshina NA, Ponamarev SI, Ragozin VN: Studies of circulation during LBNP test aboard Salyut-4 orbital station. *Kosm Biol Aviakosm Med* 11(3):26–31, 1977.

35. Degtyarev VA, Doroshev VG, Kalmykova ND, Kukushkin YA, Kirillova ZA, Lapshina NA, Popov II, Ragozin VN, Stepantsov VI: Dynamics of circulatory parameters of the crew of the Salyut space station in functional test with physical load. *Kosm Biol Aviakosm Med* 12(3):15–20, 1978.

36. Degtyarev VA, Doroshev VG, Kalmykova ND, Kirillova ZA, Lapshina NA, Lepskiy AA, Rabozin VN: Studies of hemodynamics and phase structure of cardiac cycle in the crew of Salyut-4. *Kosm Biol Aviakosm Med* 12(6):9–14, 1978.

37. Dolkas C, Greenleaf J: Insulin and glucose responses during bed rest with isotonic and isometric exercise. *J Appl Physiol* 43:1033–1038, 1977.

38. Doroshev VG, Batenchuk-Tusko TV, Lapshina NA, Kukushkin YA, Kalmykova ND, Ragozin VN: Changes in hemodynamics and phasic structure of the cardiac cycle in the crew on the second expedition of Salyut-4. *Kosm Biol Aviakosm Med* 11(2):26–31, 1977.

39. Dudley GA, Duvoisin MR, Convertino VA, Buchanan P: Alterations of the in vivo torque-velocity relationship of human skeletal muscle following 30 days exposure to simulated microgravity. *Aviat Space Environ Med* 60:659–663, 1989.

40. Duvoisin MR, Convertino VA, Buchanan P, Gollnick PD, Dudley GA: Characteristics and preliminary observations of the influence of electromyostimulation on the size and function of human skeletal muscle during 30 days of simulated microgravity. *Aviat Space Environ Med* 60:671–678, 1989.

41. Fischer CL, Johnson PC, Berry CA: Red blood cell and plasma volume changes in manned spaceflight. *JAMA* 200:579–583, 1967.

42. Garshnek V: Soviet space flight: the human element. *ASGSB Bulletin* 1:67–80, 1988.

43. Gazenko OG, Gurovsky NN, Genin AM, Bryanov II, Eryomin AV, Egorov AD: Results of medical investigations carried out on board the Salyut orbital stations. *Life Sci Space Res* 14:145–152, 1976.

44. Georgiyevskiy VS, Lapshina NA, Andriyako LY, Umnova LV, Doroshev VG, Alferova IV, Ragozin VN, Kobzev YA: Circulation in exercising crew members of the first main expedition aboard Salyut-6. *Kosm Biol Aviakosm Med* 14(3):15–18, 1980.

45. Green HJ, Thompson JA, Ball ME, Hughson RL, Houston ME, Sharratt MT: Alterations in blood volume following short-term supramaximal exercise. *J Appl Physiol* 56:683–689, 1985.
46. Greenleaf JE, Reese RD: Exercise thermoregulation after 14 days of bed rest. *J Appl Physiol* 48:72–78, 1980.
47. Grigoryeva LS, Kozlovskaya IB: Effect of weightlessness and hypokinesia on velocity and strength properties of human muscles. *Kosm Biol Aviakosm Med* 21(1):27–30, 1987.
48. Gurovskiy NN, Yeremin AV, Gazenko OG, Yegorov AD, Bryanov II, Genin AM: Medical investigations during flights of the spaceships 'Soyuz-12', 'Soyuz-13', 'Soyuz-14' and the 'Salyut-3' orbital station. *Kosm Biol Aviakosm Med* 9(2):48–54, 1975.
49. Hikida RS, Gollnick PD, Dudley GA, Convertino VA, Buchanan P: Structural and metabolic characteristics of human skeletal muscle following 30 days of simulated microgravity. *Aviat Space Environ Med* 60:664–670, 1989.
50. Hoffler GW: Cardiovascular studies of U.S. space crews: an overview and perspective. In Hwang NHC, Normann NA (eds): *Cardiovascular Flow Dynamics and Measurements*. Baltimore, University Park Press, 1977, pp 335–363.
51. Hung J, Goldwater D, Convertino VA, McKillop JH, Goris ML, DeBusk RF: Mechanisms for decreased exercise capacity following bedrest in normal middle-aged men. *Am J Cardiol* 51:344–348, 1983.
52. Johnson PC, Kimzey SL, Driscoll TB: Postmission plasma volume and red-cell mass changes in the crews of the first two Skylab missions. *Acta Astronautica* 2:311–317, 1975.
53. Johnson PC, Driscoll TB, LeBlanc AD: Blood volume changes. In Johnston RS, Dietlein LF (eds): *Biomedical Results from Skylab*. NASA SP-377, 1977, pp. 235–241.
54. Johnson RL, Hoffler GW, Nicogossian A, Bergman SA: Skylab experiment M-092: results of the first manned mission. *Acta Astronautica* 2:265–296, 1975.
55. Kakurin LI, Cherepakhin MA, Pervushin VI: Effect of spaceflight factors on human muscle tone. *Kosm Biol Med* 5(2):63–68, 1971.
56. Kakurin LI, Cherepakhin MA, Pervushin VI: Effect of brief space flights on the human neuromuscular system. *Kosm Biol Med* 5(6):53–56, 1971.
57. Kalandarova MP: Effect of spaceflight on hemopoiesis. *Kosm Biol Aviakosm Med*, 20(6):7–17, 1986.
58. Kalinichenko VV: Dynamics of orthostatic stability of cosmonauts following 2- to 63-day missions. *Kosm Biol Aviakosm Med* 11(3):31–37, 1977.
59. Kasyan II, Makarov GF: External respiration, gas exchange and energy expenditures of man in weightlessness. *Kosm Biol Aviakosm Med* 18(6):4–9, 1984.
60. Katkov VY, Kakurin LI: The role of skeletal muscle tone in regulation of orthostatic circulation. *Kosm Biol Aviakosm Med* 12(1):75–78, 1978.
61. Kinzer SM, Convertino VA: Role of leg vasculature in the response to arm work in wheelchair-dependent populations. *Clin Physiol* 9:525–533, 1989.
62. Kozlovskaya IB, Grigoryeva LS, Gevlich GI: Comparative analysis of effects of weightlessness and its models on velocity and strength properties and tone of human skeletal muscles. *Kosm Biol Aviakosm Med* 18(6):22–26, 1984.
63. Kozyrevskaya GI, Grigoryev AI, Dorokhova BR, Vatulya NM, Radchenko ND: Fluid-electrolyte metabolism in the crew of Salyut-4. *Kosm Biol Aviakosm Med* 13(4):12–18, 1979.
64. Kubis JF, McLaughlin EJ: Skylab task and work performance (experiment M-151—time and motion study). *Acta Astronautica* 2:337–349, 1975.
65. LaFevers EV, Nicogossian AE, Hoffler GW, Hursta W, Baker J: Spectral analysis of skeletal muscle changes resulting from 59 days of weightlessness in Skylab II. *NASA Technical Memorandum*. NASA TM X-58171, 1975, pp 1–19.

66. LaFevers EV, Nicogossian AE, Hursta WN: Electromyographic analysis of skeletal muscle changes arising from 9 days of weightlessness in the Apollo-Soyuz space mission. *NASA Technical Memorandum.* NASA TM X-58177, 1976, pp 1–30.

67. Leach CS, Hulley SB, Rambaut PC, Dietlein LF: The effects of bed rest on adrenal function. *Space Life Sci* 4:415–423, 1973.

68. Leach CS, Rambaut PC: Endocrine responses in long-duration manned space flight. *Acta Astronautica* 2:115–127, 1975.

69. Leach CS, Leonard JI, Rambaut PC, Johnson PC: Evaporative water loss in man in a gravity-free environment. *J Appl Physiol* 45:430–436, 1978.

70. Leach CS, Altchuler SI, Cintron-Trevino NM: The endocrine and metabolic responses to space flight. *Med Sci Sports Exerc* 15:432–440, 1983.

71. Leach CS, Johnson PC: Influence of spaceflight on erythrokinetics in man. *Science* 225:216–218, 1984.

72. Legenkov VI, Balskhovskiy IS, Beregovkin AV, Moshkalo ZS, Sorokina GV: Changes in composition of the peripheral blood during 18- and 24-day space flights. *Kosm Biol Med* 7(1):39–45, 1973.

73. Legenkov VI, Kiselev RK, Gudim VI, Moskaleva GP: Changes in peripheral blood of crew members of the Salyut-4 orbital station. *Kosm Biol Aviakosm Med* 11(6):3–12, 1977.

74. Michel EL, Waligora JM, Horrigan DJ, Shumate WH: Environmental factors. In Johnson RS, Dietlein LF, Berry CA (eds): *Biomedical Results of Apollo.* NASA SP-368, 1975, pp 129–139.

75. Michel EL, Rummel JA, Sawin CF: Skylab experiment M-171 "metabolic activity"—results of the first manned mission. *Acta Astronautica* 2:351–365, 1975.

76. Michel EL, Rummel JA, Sawin CF, Buderer MC, Lem JD: Results of Skylab medical experiment M171 —metabolic activity. In Johnston RS, Dietlein LF (eds): *Biomedical Results from Skylab.* NASA SP-377, 1977, pp 372–387.

77. Nicogossian AE, Sawin CF, Bartelloni PJ: Results of pulmonary function tests. In Nicogossian AE (ed): *The Apollo-Soyuz Test Project Medical Report.* NASA SP-411, 1977, pp 25–28.

78. Petukhov BN, Purakhin YN, Georgiyevskiy VS, Mikhaylov VM, Smyshlyayeva VV, Fatyanova LI: Regulation of erect posture of cosmonauts after an 18-day orbital flight. *Kosm Biol Med* 4(6):50–54, 1970.

79. Purakhin YN, Kakurin LI, Georgiyevskiy VS, Petukhov BN, Mikhaylov VM: Regulation of vertical posture after flight on the 'Soyuz-6' to 'Soyuz-8' ships and 120-day hypokinesia. *Kosm Biol Med* 6(6):47–53, 1972.

80. Ross H, Brodie E, Benson A: Mass discrimination during prolonged weightlessness. *Science* 225:219–221, 1984.

81. Rudnyy NM, Gazenko OG, Gozulov SA, Pestov ID, Vasilyev PV, Yeremin AV, Degtyarev VA, Balakhovskiy IS, Bayevskiy RM, Syrykh GD: Main results of medical research conducted during the flight of two crews on the Salyut-5 orbital station. *Kosm Biol Aviakosm Med* 11(5):33–41, 1977.

82. Rummel JA, Michel EL, Berry CA: Physiological responses to exercise after space flight—Apollo 7 to Apollo 11. *Aviat Space Environ Med* 44:235–238, 1973.

83. Rummel JA, Sawin CF, Buderer MC, Mauldin DG, Michel EL: Physiological responses to exercise after space flight—Apollo 14 through Apollo 17. *Aviat Space Environ Med* 46:679–683, 1975.

84. Rummel JA, Sawin CF, Michel EL: Exercise response. In: Johnson RS, Dietlein LF, Berry CA (eds): *Biomedical Results of Apollo.* NASA SP-368, 1975, pp 265–275.

85. Rummel JA, Michel EL, Sawin CF, Buderer MC: Medical experiment M-171: results from the second manned Skylab mission. *Aviat Space Environ Med* 47:1056–1060, 1976.

86. Saltin B, Blomqvist G, Mitchell JH, Johnson RL, Wildenthal K, Chapman CB: Response to exercise after bed rest and after training. *Circulation* 38 (suppl 7):1–78, 1968.
87. Sawin CF, Nicogossian AE, Schachter AP, Rummel JA, Michel EL: Pulmonary function evaluation during and following Skylab space flights. In Johnson RS, Dietlein LF, Berry CA (eds): *Biomedical Results from Skylab*. NASA SP-368, 1977, pp 388–394.
88. Siminov PV, Kasyan II (eds): *Physiological Investigations in Weightlessness*. Moscow, Medicine Publishers, 1983.
89. Smith MC, Rapp RM, Huber CS, Rambaut PC, Heidelbaugh ND: Apollo experience report—food systems. *NASA Technical Note*. NASA TN D-7720, 1974, pp 1–66.
90. Smith RF, Stanton K, Stoop D, Brown D, King PH: Quantitative electrocardiography during extended space flight. *Acta Astronautica* 2:89–102, 1975.
91. Somers VK, Conway J, LeWinter M, Sleight P: The role of baroreflex sensitivity in post-exercise hypotension. *J Hypertens* 3:S129-S130, 1985.
92. Stegemann J, Meier U, Skipka W, Hartlieb W, Hemme B, Tibes U: Effects of multi-hour immersion with intermittent exercise on urinary excretion and tilt table tolerance in athletes and nonathletes. *Aviat Space Environ Med* 46:26–29, 1975.
93. Tesch PA, Colliander EB: Effects of eccentric and concentric resistance training on muscular strength. *Med Sci Sports Exerc* 21 (Suppl):S88, 1989.
94. Tesch PA, Buchanan P, Dudley GA: An approach to counteracting long-term microgravity-induced muscle atrophy. *Physiologist* 33 (in press, 1990).
95. Thornton WE, Rummel JA: Muscular deconditioning and its prevention in space flight. In Johnson RS, Dietlein LF (eds): *Biomedical Results from Skylab*. NASA SP-377, 1977, pp 191–197.
96. Thornton WE, Hoffler GW: Hemodynamic studies of the legs under weightlessness. In Johnson RS, Dietlein LF (eds): *Biomedical Results from Skylab*. NASA SP-377, 1977, pp 324–329.
97. Thornton WE, Hoffler GW, Rummel JA: Anthropometric changes and fluid shifts. In Johnson RS, Dietlein LF (eds): *Biomedical Results from Skylab*. NASA SP-377, 1977, pp 330–338.
98. Tigranyan RA, Popova IA, Belyakova MI, Kalita NF, Tuzova YG, Sochilina LB, Davydova NA: Results of metabolic studies on the crew of the second expedition of the Salyut-4 orbital station. *Kosm Biol Aviakosm Med* 11(2):48–53, 1977.
99. Tishler VA, Yeremin AV, Stepantsov VI, Funtova II: Evaluation of physical work capacity of cosmonauts aboard Salyut-6 station. *Kosm Biol Aviakosm Med* 20(3):31–35, 1986.
100. Vorobyev YI, Gazenko OG, Gurovskiy NN, Nefedov YG, Yegorov BB, Spitsa II, Biryukov YN, Bryanov II, Yeremin AV, Yegorov AD: Experimental 'Soyuz'-'Apollo' flight. Preliminary results of biomedical investigations carried out during flight of the 'Soyuz-19' ship. *Kosm Biol Aviakosm Med* 10(1):15–22, 1976.
101. Vorobyev YI, Gazenko OG, Gurovskiy NN, Nefedov YG, Yegorov BB, Bayevskiy RM, Bryanov II, Genin AM, Degtyarev VA, Yegorov AD, Yeremin AV, Pestov ID: Preliminary results of medical investigations carried out during flight of the second expedition of the 'Salyut-4' orbital station. *Kosm Biol Aviakosm Med* 10(5):3–18, 1976.
102. Vorobyev YI, Gazenko OG, Shulzhenko YB, Grigoryev AI, Barer AS, Yegorov AD, Skiba AI: Preliminary results of medical investigations during 5-month spaceflight aboard Salyut-7-Soyuz-T orbital complex. *Kosm Biol Aviakosm Med* 20(2):27–34, 1986.
103. Vorobyov EI, Gazenko OG, Genin AM, Egorov AD: Medical results of Salyut-6 manned space flights. *Aviat Space Environ Med* 54:S31-S40, 1983.
104. Waligora JM, Horrigan DJ: Metabolism and heat dissipation during Apollo EVA periods. In Johnson RS, Dietlein LF, Berry CA (eds): *Biomedical Results of Apollo*. NASA SP-368, 1975, pp 115–128.

105. Waligora JM, Horrigan DJ: Metabolic cost of extravehicular activities. In Johnson RS, Dietlein LF (eds): *Biomedical Results from Skylab* NASA SP-377, 1977, pp 395–399.
106. Williams DA, Convertino VA: Circulating lactate and FFA during exercise: effect of reduction in plasma volume following simulated microgravity. *Aviat Space Environ Med* 59:1042–1046, 1988.
107. Yegorov AD, Itsekhovskiy OG, Polyakova AP, Turchaninova VF, Alferova IV, Savelyeva VG, Domracheva MV, Batenchuk-Tusko TV, Doroshev VG, Kobzev YA: Results of studies of hemodynamics and phase structure of the cardiac cycle during functional test with graded exercise during 140-day flight aboard the Salyut-6 station. *Kosm Biol Aviakosm Med* 15(3):18–22, 1981.
108. Yegorov AD, Itsekhovskiy OG: Study of cardiovascular system during long-term spaceflights. *Kosm Biol Aviakosm Med* 17(5):4–6, 1983.

5
Biomechanical Response of Bone to Weightlessness

RONALD F. ZERNICKE, Ph.D.
ARTHUR C. VAILAS, Ph.D.
GEORGE J. SALEM, M.S.

"Our job is not only to make sure astronauts can function adequately in space, but also that they can function on their return to earth."

DR. FRANK SULZMAN
NASA Space Medicine Branch

Significant physiological adjustments occur in response to short- and intermediate-duration weightlessness. Areas of concern include motion-sickness, cardiovascular deconditioning, hematological and immunological alterations, and musculoskeletal adaptations. Future space mission proposals that include flights carrying humans to Mars and a space station with a human crew will require astronauts to remain in microgravity conditions for 18 months or longer. The exacerbation of physiological adaptations during these substantially longer missions may prove hazardous to astronauts, either in space or after returning to Earth. Because of the risk of fracture in osteopenic bones upon return to Earth, skeletal degeneration and calcium loss from the body could be a major factor limiting the duration of a mission [23, 33, 50].

Theoretical predictions of spaceflight-induced bone mineral loss were confirmed as early as 1963, when Vostoks 2 and 3 cosmonauts had increased levels of urinary calcium excretion during their spaceflights [14]. Other calcium-balance studies in the Gemini, Apollo, Skylab, and Salyut-6/Soyuz astronauts and cosmonauts yielded similar findings of negative calcium balance through increased urinary and fecal calcium excretion [8, 20, 21, 24, 27, 29, 38, 58–61] (Fig. 5.1). In the 28-day Skylab 2 and the 59-day Skylab 3 missions, astronauts lost an average of 140–184 mg of calcium and 220–400 mg of phosphorus/day, with urinary excretion exceeding fecal excretion. Urinary excretion of hydroxyproline also increased, suggesting increased bone resorption [21]. Preflight and postflight roentgenological evaluations of Gemini 4, 5, and 7 astronauts indicated that significant bone mass loss occurred in the calcaneus, talus, and hand phalanges during orbit [27–30]. The duration of

167

FIGURE 5.1

Mean calcium balance of all astronauts on Skylab missions. (From Rambaut PC, Goode AW: Skeletal changes during space flight. Lancet 2:1050–1052, 1985.)

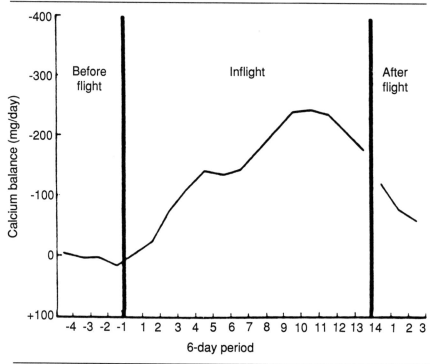

spaceflight, however, did not correlate significantly with the amount of bone mass loss; thus, dietary and exercise influences [10] must also be taken into consideration [26].

Enhanced bone-density measurements, via photon absorptiometry, quantified changes in the radius, ulna, and calcaneus during Apollo, Skylab, Spacelab, and Salyut-6/Soyuz missions, and although significant bone density changes were not seen in the nonweightbearing radius and ulna, decreases of 3–8% were seen in the calcaneus [14, 20, 21, 58]. Weightbearing trabecular bone, therefore, may be particularly sensitive to spaceflight effects. Soviet scientists suggest that bone demineralization may plateau during extended spaceflight [33], but the possibility of irreversible osteoporotic changes persists.

To help understand the underlying mechanisms of osteopenia and the potential changes in bone composition and structure in response to spaceflight, rats have been sent into orbit and analyzed extensively using invasive techniques. For example, 56-day-old rats orbited 7 days aboard Spacelab 3 had significantly reduced cortical and trabecular bone mass, mineral content, osteocalcin production, periosteal bone formation, growth hormone secretion, bone growth turnover, and vertebral apatite crystal size/perfection [15, 35, 43, 47, 63]. Also, 83-day-old rats flown for 18.5 days aboard the Cosmos 1129 Biosatellite had decreases in bone formation and calcification in weightbearing bones, bone mass in trabecular bone, vertebral bone formation, periosteal bone formation in the tibia and humerus, and alterations in bone mineral ratios [11, 19, 41, 48, 64]. In these same rats, increases were found in trabecular-bone fat content, while bone *resorption* remained constant in both the ribs and lumbar vertebrae [6, 11]. Others report retarded bone *formation* as a result of spaceflight [34], suggesting that during spaceflight, bone formation and bone resorption are uncoupled, and the difference in their rates may lead to significant reductions in bone mass. Subsequent spaceflight studies (Cosmos 1514 and 1667) tend to support those earlier findings, but alterations to bone remodeling may be sensitive to both spaceflight duration and anatomical site [54–56].

What are the consequences of the spaceflight-related structural and compositional changes to bone? Because a bone's ultimate strength and stiffness will affect its predisposition to injury, spaceflight-related adaptations in bone biology can have important implications. Although the biological adaptations may be consistent with the functional demands in a microgravity environment, such changes may have maladaptive consequences with the return to normal gravitational conditions on Earth. Here, we primarily review information related to the biomechanical adaptations of rat bone to weightlessness and simulated weightlessness to provide a context for future proposals to examine the effects of exercise, diet, and pharmacological agents to ameliorate the deleterious effects of spaceflight on bone.

EFFECTS OF WEIGHTLESSNESS ON BONE MECHANICS

Even with the tremendous monetary cost involved, the limited availability of orbiter space, and the significant demands on crew and experimenter time, spaceflight experiments are best for examining the effects of weightlessness on the mechanics of bone. In space, factors associated with Earth-bound, simulated weightlessness experiments are eliminated; on the other hand, with spaceflight experiments there are circumstances and experimental factors that can confound anticipated results. For example, animals, ideally, should be killed and frozen within 6 hr after return from space, as significant changes in protein synthesis can occur within this period [4]. With unanticipated reentry locations or times in some of the spaceflights, however, animals were killed as soon as feasible after return to Earth, but that may have been 12 hr or 2 days after landing. Whether significant changes in mechanical properties of rat bones occur during the wait between the time of reentry and the tissue harvest is not known. But despite the variations in the spaceflight durations and the limitations imposed on the interpretation of findings because of different flight protocols, current data clearly suggest that significant changes occur in rat bone mechanical properties as a consequence of spaceflight.

Cortical Bone

Spengler et al. [49] investigated the mechanical properties of rat femurs from the Cosmos 936 mission. Forty male, 63-day-old, Czechoslovakian Wistar rats (202 g) were divided into four groups: two flight groups and two control groups. The two flight groups were stationary rats or centrifuged rats (1*g*). The control, ground-based groups had vivarium rats and simulated-flight rats. The simulated flight group was exposed to noise levels, vibration stresses, accelerations, and reentry stresses similar to those of the flight groups. Half of the animals from each group were killed immediately after the 18.5-day flight and half were killed 25 days after reentry. Femurs were removed from all animals and tested via torsional loading.

Stationary flight rats had significantly lower femur failure torque, torsional stiffness, and energy than either vivarium controls or flight-centrifuged rats. By 25 days postflight, nevertheless, femoral mechanical properties of the stationary-flight rats had returned to normal. Mechanical properties of the centrifuged-flight rat femurs were not different from Earth controls either at reentry or 25 days postflight. To parcel out geometrical from material changes in the rat femur, the investigators generated hollow, elliptical stress-analysis models of femurs from the data of weight-matched stationary flight and vivarium rats [42]. Their theoretical results suggested that geometrical differences alone could not account for the differences in mechanical properties and that material properties of the femurs were also compromised with spaceflight. Density measurements of vivarium and stationary-flight femurs indicated a notable, but not statistically significant, deficit in matrix composition of the flight rats. Thus, Spengler and colleagues concluded that bone-matrix maturation was impaired during spaceflight in growing animals.

Later, Patterson-Buckendahl and coworkers [36] examined the mechanical properties of the humerus after 7 days spaceflight (Spacelab 3). Eighteen rats were equally divided into preflight, flight control, and flight groups. The preflight rats were killed the day the space shuttle was launched. Flight animals were killed 11 hr after the orbiter landed, and flight control rats were killed 48 hr later. Osteocalcin (OC) levels were measured in serum and vertebrae, and serum OC levels were correlated with humerus breaking strength. Stiffness, ultimate load, and work-to-ultimate load were significantly reduced in humerus of the flight rats when compared to flight control rats. Serum OC levels and vertebral OC content were significantly reduced in the flight animals, even when adjusted for age-related differences. Furthermore, the ultimate load and work-to-ultimate load were significantly correlated with serum OC. Thus spaceflight significantly effects OC levels and humerus strength, and OC content appears to be a sensitive indicator of spaceflight affects on bone metabolism.

In a companion report, Shaw et al. [45] compared the effects of the 7-day Spacelab 3 flight on the geometry and mechanics of rat tibia and humerus. The preflight, flight control, and flight paradigm, described by Patterson-Buckendahl et al. (36), was the same for Shaw and colleagues, but the specific methods to test the samples were the following.

On the day of mechanical testing, bones were thawed at room temperature and were equilibrated for a minimum of 1 hr in a buffered solution (50 mM potassium phosphate, 37°C, pH 7.4). Prior to mechanical testing, lengths were measured with calipers. Temperature-equilibrated tibias and humeri were subjected to three-point bending loads until fracture with servo-controlled electromechanical testing system (Fig. 5.2). Bending tests were performed with the bones submerged in the

FIGURE 5.2

Three-point bending test set-up for tibia and humerus. (From Matsuda JJ, Zernicke RF, Vailas AC, Pedrini VA, Pedrini-Mille A, Maynard JA: Morphological and mechanical adaptation of immature bone to strenuous exercise. J. Appl Physiol 60:2028–2034, 1986.)

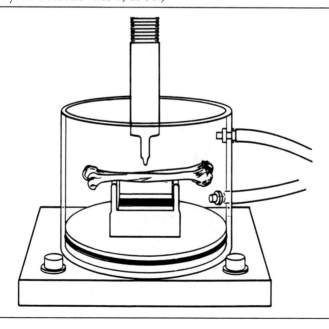

circulating buffered solution. Each tibia was loaded in a medial-to-lateral direction (about the anterior/posterior axis), and the humerus was loaded in a lateral-to-medial direction (about the anterior/posterior axis). Load-deflection records of mechanical tests were digitized to determine load, deformation, and energy at the proportional limit, maximum, and fracture points, flexural rigidity, elastic modulus, tensile stress (determined at proportional limit), and nonlinear displacement. Tensile stress was calculated as MC/I, where M = bending moment at yield (0.5 force at proportional limit × 0.5 intersupport distance), C = distance from centroid to tensile periosteal surface, and I = area moment of inertia about the bending axis translated to the centroid. Flexural rigidity $(EI) = (d^3/48) (\Delta F/\Delta L)$, where E = elastic modulus, and $\Delta F/\Delta L$ = slope of the linear region of the load-deflection curve. The elastic modulus was calculated as $E = EI/I$. Nonlinear displacement was the amount of deformation that occurred between the proportional limit and maximum load.

Significant mechanical deficits occurred in both the tibia and humerus in response to spaceflight, even when results were corrected for age differences between the groups. Tibial flexural rigidity for the flight group was significantly less (19%) than the flight control group and was similar to the preflight groups (Fig. 5.3). Although not statistically significant, tibial elastic modulus was less (13%) for the flight group than the flight control group (Fig. 5.4). Flight-rat tibias had significantly greater

FIGURE 5.3
Flexural rigidity for tibia (TIB) *and humerus* (HUM). *Mean values and SD error bars are indicated. Statistically significant (p ≤ 0.05) relationships include the following: for tibia,* b > a; *humerus,* y > x. (*From Shaw SR, Vailas AC, Grindeland RE, Zernicke RF: Effects of a 1-wk spaceflight on the morphological and mechanical properties of growing bone. Am J Physiol 254:R78–R83, 1988.*)

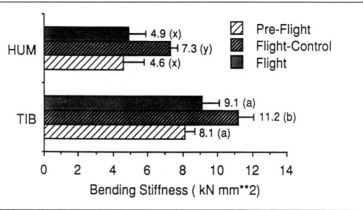

FIGURE 5.4

Elastic modulus for tibia and humerus. Mean values and SD error bars are indicated. By use of Duncan's multiple range test (SAS, Cary, NC), statistically significant (p ≤ 0.05) relationships include the following: for tibia, b > a; humerus, y > x. (From Shaw SR, Vailas AC, Grindeland RE, Zernicke RF: Effects of a 1-wk spaceflight on the morphological and mechanical properties of growing bone. Am J Physiol 254:R78–R83, 1988.)

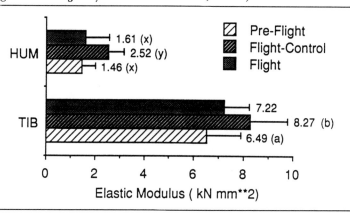

energy to the proportional limit than did flight control rats, which may have been related to the significantly greater bending displacement that occurred in the flight rats. Flight rats had significantly less tibial maximum load than flight control rats (Fig. 5.5). Humeral flexural rigidity (Fig. 5.3), elastic modulus (Fig. 5.4), load at the proportional limit, tensile stress, and maximum load (Fig. 5.5) were all significantly greater in the flight control rats than either flight or preflight animals.

Bone geometry measurements indicated that significant decreases in humeral length occurred in the flight rats compared to flight control rats. Tibial diaphysial cross-sectional densities (mass/unit dry volume) were also significantly smaller (22%) in the flight rats than in flight controls. Thus, the 7-day spaceflight prevented or delayed normal maturational changes in geometry and mechanical strength in the rat tibia and humerus.

In 1989, Vailas and colleagues [52] reported the geometry, biomechanics, and biochemistry of humeri from rats flown on the 12.5-day Cosmos 1887 Biosatellite. The *flight* animals were compared with *basal, synchronous,* and *vivarium* controls (5/group, 90-day-old at the beginning of the flight, male specific-pathogen-free rats, Czechoslovakian Wistar). The flight rats were housed 10 rats/cage and were fed a paste diet of 55 g/day/rat. Because of reentry difficulties, the biosatellite landed in Siberia rather than at the designated site. The biosatellite was found within 3 hr of landing, and a heated (23°C) tent protected the animals; the satel-

FIGURE 5.5

Maximum load for tibia and humerus. Mean values and SD error bars are indicated. Statistically significant (p ≤ 0.05) relationships include the following: for tibia, b > c > a; humerus, y > x. (From Shaw SR, Vailas AC, Grindeland RE, Zernicke RF: Effects of a 1-wk spaceflight on the morphological and mechanical properties of growing bone. Am J Physiol 254:R78–R83, 1988.)

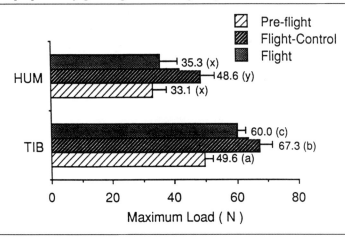

lite interior temperature did not fall lower than 12°C. All flight rats appeared healthy and injury-free when examined on removal from the flight cage. The following morning the rats were placed in transport cages and taken to Moscow. Fifty-three hours elapsed between reentry and killing of the flight rats.

Basal rats were put into flight-type cages and on a paste diet 19 days prior to their killing on the day of the biosatellite lift-off. Temperature, humidity, and light-dark cycles were similar to inflight conditions. Synchronous controls were maintained in flight-type cages and on the paste diet. These rats were exposed to the launch forces and vibrations and exposed to the same regimen and temperature as flight rats after landing. After their simulated flight, killing was delayed the same period as for flight rats. The reentry forces and postflight transportation conditions of the flight animals were not mimicked for the synchronous control group. Vivarium controls were kept in standard vivarium rat cages and fed once/day. Postflight conditions (e.g., temperature) were not mimicked for this group.

Findings suggest that the 12.5-day spaceflight significantly affected humerus geometry and mechanical properties. The spaceflight humeri had less cortical cross-sectional area, periosteal circumference, and second moment of area with respect to bending and nonbending axes. The flexural rigidity of the flight humeri was significantly less than synchronous and vivarium control rats and comparable to the younger basal-control rats. Elastic modulus and matrix biochemistry were not significantly different among the groups. The data suggest that normal bone resorption may have occurred during the 12.5-day spaceflight, but periosteal bone formation may have been slowed. Further, the spaceflight differences in humeral mechanical strength and flexural rigidity were likely the result of geometry changes rather than material property changes, because the material characteristics (e.g., elastic modulus and matrix biochemistry) of the flight humeri were not affected.

Trabecular Bone

The compressional strength of vertebral-body bone was examined by Kazarian [22] after a 18.5-day spaceflight aboard Cosmos 1129. Wistar rats were divided ($n = 25$) into flight, synchronous control, and vivarium control groups. These were subdivided into groups of animals killed at spacecraft recovery (R), recovery plus 6 days (R + 6), and recovery plus 29 days (R + 29), to study the readaptation of bone to 1g.

The R (no days of recovery) flight rats had significantly less vertebral body ultimate load and energy to ultimate load than either vivarium or simulated control animals. Vertebral displacement to ultimate load was significantly greater in the vivarium rats but similar in the flight and synchronous rats. Vertebral body stiffness, however, was significantly greater in the flight and synchronous rats than in the vivarium animals. At R + 29, flight rat vertebral body ultimate load approached the levels of the vivarium and synchronous control groups. Thus, Kazarian concluded that spaceflight increased the susceptibility of vertebral body fracture.

Zernicke et al. [68] also examined the effects of 12.5-day spaceflight on the biomechanical properties of the sixth lumbar vertebrae [L6) of Czechoslovakian Wistar rats flown on the Cosmos 1887 Biosatellite. The vertebrae came from the same rats—basal control, synchronous control, vivarium control, and flight groups—as described earlier for the humerus data of Vailas et al. [52]. As described by Zernicke et al. [68], the following methods were used to test the vertebral specimens.

Immediately after being killed, L6 of the rats was dissected and removed. Bones were hermetically wrapped and frozen ($-70°C$) until the day of mechanical testing. The freezing of rat bone has been shown not to affect bone mechanical properties [37]. While still sealed, the L6 vertebra thawed ($7°C$) for 16 hr prior to mechanical testing, and on the day of testing, the body of L6 was isolated from the vertebral pedicles. Care was taken to avoid damage to the centrum cortical shell because of its potential contribution to the specimen's mechanical properties (40). The average height of L6 was determined for each group. The caudal face of each vertebral body was fixed with cyanoacrylate cement to the surface of a machined stainless steel cylindrical test plate (Fig. 5.6). While fixed

FIGURE 5.6

Set-up for the rat vertebral body compression tests. The vertebral body is shown fixed to a cylindrical stainless steel plate while immersed in a warmed, circulating buffer solution. (From Salem GS, Zernicke RF, Vailas AC, Martinez DA: Determination of biomechanical and biochemical differences in lumbar vertebrae of rapidly growing rats. Am J Physiol 256:R259–R263, 1989.)

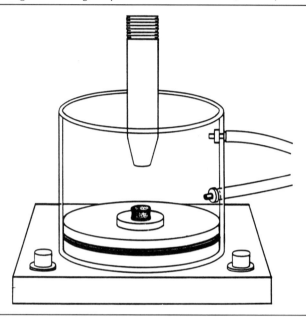

to the stainless steel plate, the rostral surface of each vertebral body was cut so the height of each L6 test specimen was 80% of the average vertebral body height for each respective group. Because the natural caudal and rostral surfaces of the vertebral bodies are not parallel, the specimen preparation assured parallel superior and inferior surfaces of the vertebral body. During the cutting process, the vertebral bodies were bathed in buffer solution. After cutting, each test specimen, while still fixed to the stainless steel plate, was immersed and temperature equilibrated in physiological buffer solution (37°C) for at least 1 hr prior to the compression testing.

Using procedures modified from Salem et al. [44], the vertebral bodies were compressed to a nominal 50% strain at a fast strain rate (50%/s) using a servo-controlled electromechanical testing system (Instron 1122). Figure 5.6 illustrates the compression testing set-up. While fixed to a cylindrical stainless steel base, each vertebral body was compressed with a flat-surfaced stainless steel probe. Specimens were tested while immersed in a buffered solution (37°C) that circulated through the test chamber. Analog load-time data were converted to digital data, and a custom-designed program was used to quantify the structural and material properties of the vertebral bodies. The program used interactive computer graphics, and for each L6 test, five points were marked: initial load, two points in the linear-load region, proportional limit, and 50% strain. A program computed bone structural properties including: load, displacement, and energy at the proportional limit, initial maximum, and 50% strain marks. The compressional stiffness was the slope of a regression line fitted to the linear region of the load-deformation curve.

Mechanical properties of the flight group were consistently lower than those of the other groups. For example, the flight group L6 stiffness was

FIGURE 5.7

Compressional stiffness and normalized stiffness (per unit vertebral body weight) for rat L6. Mean and SD values are indicated for the flight, vivarium, synchronous, and basal control groups. (From Zernicke RF, Vailas AC, Grindeland RE, Kaplansky A, Salem GJ, Martinez DA: Spaceflight effects on biomechanical and biochemical properties of vertebrae in rapidly-growing rats. Am J Physiol (in press).)

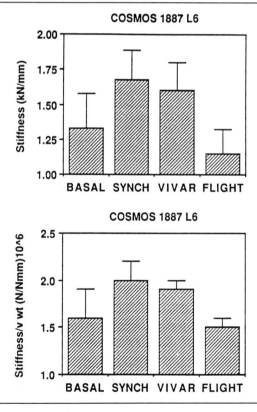

39% less than that of the vivarium, 46% less than that of the synchronous, and 16% less than that of the basal control. When normalized for L6 vertebral body weight, the flight group's L6 stiffness was 27% less than that of the vivarium, 33% less than that of the synchronous, and 7% less than that of the basal control (Fig. 5.7). The average initial maximum load of the flight group was 22% that of the vivarium, 18% that of the synchronous, and 5% that of the basal control. When normalized for vertebral body weight, the initial maximum load of the flight group was 11% that of the vivarium and synchronous controls, but did not differ from that of the basal controls Fig. 5.8). The load at the proportional

FIGURE 5.8

Initial-maximum load and normalized initial-maximum load (per unit vertebral body weight) for rat L6. Mean and SD values are indicated for the flight, vivarium, synchronous, and basal control groups. (Zernicke RF, Vailas AC, Grindeland RE, Kaplansky A, Salem GJ, Martinez DA: Spaceflight effects on biomechanical and biochemical properties of vertebrae in rapidly-growing rats. Am J Physiol (in press).)

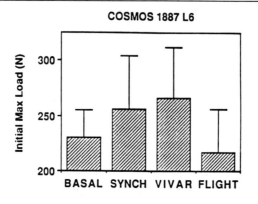

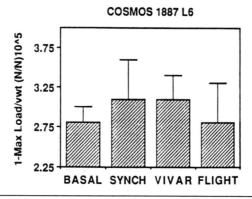

limit for the flight group was significantly (34%) less than that of the vivarium, 25% less than that of the synchronous, and 4% less than that of the basal control. When normalized for vertebral body weight, the flight group was still 22% less than that of the vivarium, 17% less than that of the synchronous, and the same as that of the basal control. Although the calcium, phosphorous, and hydroxyproline concentrations did not differ between groups, the hydroxypyridinoline content of the flight groups was significantly (35%) less than that of the vivarium, 17% less than that of the synchronous, and 15% less than that of the basal control.

Because of these biomechanical and matrix-biochemistry findings, decreases in vertebral-body strength were likely a consequence of changes in bone material as well as structural properties. The lack of strength and development of stiffness, in conjunction with the greater proportion of immature hydroxypyridinoline cross-links, suggested that the 12.5-day spaceflight slowed the maturation of vertebral bone in the rat.

SIMULATED WEIGHTLESSNESS MODELS

Simulated weightlessness models were developed to overcome the infrequency, prohibitive expense, and spatial restrictions associated with spaceflight experiments. Typical simulated weightlessness models include immobilization or bed rest studies with human subjects or animal immobilization, nerve sectioning, or suspension models. Bed rest or immobilization induces negative calcium balance in humans [3, 5, 9, 18, 25, 57]. Estimates of total body calcium loss through excretion range from 0.5% after 2 weeks of bed rest [57] to 1–2% after 6 weeks in a body cast [9]. These estimates, however, usually exclude sweat calcium [16], which may be significant [7], and may underestimate calcium loss. Roentgenological examinations of fracture and paralyzed patients clearly show evidence of osteopenia [13, 17], but some reports indicate no significant radiographic changes following immobilization for 6 weeks [5, 9]. Other studies report no significant decreases in bone mass with 4 months of bed rest, despite increases in indicators of osteoclastic activity and decreases in mineralization rate [53]. These findings emphasize the difficulties of developing reliable and valid Earth-bound models of the effects of spaceflight and substantiate the need for directly measuring the geometrical, biomechanical, and biochemical changes in bone, as can be done only with animal models.

Simulated weightlessness models using animals generally can be categorized as: immobilization, nerve transection, or suspension [1, 2, 35, 39, 46, 51, 64–66]. Because of the introduction of confounding variables with the nerve transection or immobilization, the suspension technique generally is the preferred model for simulated weightlessness [35]. According to Morey et al. [35], requirements for an acceptable model include: (*a*) allowing the animal to exercise using only the front limbs (in a pulling, but nonweightbearing mode); (*b*) total unloading of the rear limbs without paralysis; (*c*) a fluid shift mimicking that seen during space missions; (*d*) allowing the animal to eat, drink, and groom as normally as possible; and (*e*) causing a minimum of stress to the animal.

In 1979 Morey et al. [35] developed a rat suspension model to mimic the effects of microgravity on bone. As described by Morey and coworkers, the model allows the animal to move about a 360° arc and pull itself along a mesh cage with its front paws to reach food and water. The rear limbs are totally nonweightbearing and unrestrained. A harness is made of a perforated, orthopedic casting material, Hexcelite, which is like plastic wrap when placed in hot water but regains its semi-rigid structure when cooled. The harness design can be precut, warmed, molded to the contour of the shaved back of a rat, and then bonded in place with RTV silicone rubber. Additional silicone rubber is applied to encapsulate the Hexcelite so that the animal does not catch its nails or teeth in the mesh. The bond remains functional for about 2 weeks. After 2 weeks, the harness can be removed by cutting through the new-grown hair and replaced if desired. A paper clip through the Hexcelite harness at the posterior end provides a system for quickly attaching or disconnecting the rat. The paper clip is positioned through the harness so that the animal, when connected to the model, maintains about a 30° head-down tilt to shift fluids, intestines, and organs toward the chest. This innovation was suggested when Soviet scientists reported that head-down tilt in humans simulated weightlessness more closely than did horizontal bedrest.

Suspended rats, regardless of initial age, lost weight the first 2–4 days on the harness. Within another 7–10 days, animals had returned to their initial weight. Control animals consistently gained 20% more in weight and gained more weight per gram of food consumed than suspended rats. Comparisons with Cosmos flight rats indicated that the model was useful in predicting some of the metabolic costs of spaceflight. Some caution, however, is warranted, because differences between Soviet Cosmos and U.S. rat diets, strain of rat, and caging environments make weight gain comparisons tentative [69]. Examination of the tibiofibular junctions, nevertheless, revealed that the suspended rats had decreases in periosteal bone formation rates of 37 and 44% when compared to weight-matched and pair fed controls. Cosmos 936 and Cosmos 782 also showed inhibition of periosteal formation of 43 and 47%. Thus, the model appeared to mimic the retardation of weight gain and periosteal bone formation effects of spaceflight in the growing rat.

Wunder et al. [65] examined the effects of both high and low gravitational accelerations on the femur bending properties of 117 Sprague-

Dawley rats. Animals were divided into control, harnessed control, harness suspended, and centrifuged (3.1g) groups. Here, the suspended animals were harnessed, so that all four limbs remained nonweight-bearing. The changes in body mass were attributed more to the harness itself than to the suspension as both harnessed groups experienced significantly less weight gain throughout the 40 days of exposure than did the control animals. Biomechanical measures included displacement of the femur at failure (h_u), stress at failure (u), and strain at failure (E_u). Only the suspended animals between 27 and 34 days of age showed a significant decrease in h_u compared to controls. After suspension, the youngest rats showed less-than-normal E_u; but, when deviations were regressed as a function of gravitational field g (0.0, 1.0, 1.2, and 3.1g, respectively, for suspended, control, harnessed control, and centrifuged rats) the result was an insignificant $1 \pm 4\%/g$ effect on E_u. In contrast, the regression coefficient showed a $19 \pm 1\%/g$ effect on h_u, indicating that this variable was more sensitive to changes in gravitational field.

The first data on the mechanical adaptations of hindlimb tibia and femora to suspension and exercise in the young-adult rat were reported by Shaw et al. [46]. Female Sprague-Dawley rats (120-days-old) were divided into control, sedentary-suspended, or exercise-suspended groups. The suspension method used was a modification of the Morey technique [35]. The sedentary-suspension group remained suspended for the entire 4-week experimental period, while the exercise-suspended animals experienced ground reaction forces only during treadmill training sessions (7 days/week). Training sessions were begun at 10 min/session at 30% grade (33.5 cm/s) on a motor-driven treadmill, and sessions were gradually increased in duration by 5 min/day, such that at the end of the experimental period, the animals were running for 1.5 hr/day, approximately 80% of maximum aerobic capacity. During the training periods, the suspension harness was clipped to the treadmill cover rails, allowing it to slide freely so that hindlimb weightbearing was unimpaired.

At the time of killing, the sedentary suspended group mean body mass was significantly less than the control group. The exercise suspended rats, however, had a group mean mass that was the same as for the control rats. Mechanical test data for femora and tibia are provided in Tables 5.1 and 5.2. The data reveal that the hindlimb suspension significantly decreased the femoral mechanical properties, while the tibial mechanical properties were largely unaffected. Flexural rigidity, however, was significantly reduced in both the femora and tibia as a result of suspension. In general, the exercise protocol did not produce significant differences between suspension groups. In addition, bone geometry was altered by suspension as indicated by region-specific cortical thinning and endosteal resorption in both the tibia and femora. These effects alone, however, cannot completely account for the changes in mechani-

TABLE 5.1
Mechanical Characteristics of Femur

	Control (n = 8)	Sedentary Suspended (n = 8)	Exercise Suspended (n = 7)
Flexural rigidity (kN·mm²)	25.5 ± 2.8*	20.8 ± 3.2	17.5 ± 4.2
Tensile stress (N/mm²)	260.0 ± 26.0*	210.0 ± 26.0	225.0 ± 43.0
Load at proportional limit (N)	120.5 ± 7.6*	93.9 ± 12.5	89.5 ± 17.0
Energy at proportional limit (mJ)	15.6 ± 2.2*	12.4 ± 3.8	12.8 ± 3.1
Nonlinear displacement (μm)	440.0 ± 80.0	350.0 ± 170.0	200.0 ± 170.0†
Maximum load (N)	160.5 ± 9.8*	128.5 ± 17.4	110.7 ± 23.0
Energy at maximum load (mJ)	81.5 ± 11.3*	53.3 ± 27.6	33.3 ± 19.8
Load at failure (N)	159.6 ± 9.8*	127.2 ± 16.9	107.7 ± 21.6
Energy at failure (mJ)	85.4 ± 15.6*	56.3 ± 29.1	41.1 ± 33.0

* Indicates that the control group mean (±SD) is significantly ($p \leq 0.05$) different from the sedentary suspended and exercise suspended group means.
† Indicates that the exercise suspended group is significantly ($p \leq 0.05$) different from the control group.
Adapted from Shaw SR, Zernicke RF, Vailas AC, DeLuna D, Thomason DB, Baldwin KM: Mechanical morphological and biochemical adaptations of bone and muscle to hindlimb suspension and exercise. *J Biomech* 20:225–234, 1987.

cal properties. As indicated by suspension-related changes in tensile stress at the proportional limit, the quality of the femoral material was also compromised. The regionally specific bone geometry changes were likely a result of both selective muscle atrophy and the elimination of ground reaction forces. Although strenuous exercise partially counteracted the suspension atrophic effects on muscle, it did not ameliorate the detrimental effects on bone cross-sectional geometry or mechanical properties. The intensity of the exercise itself, however, may have been

TABLE 5.2
Mechanical Characteristics of Tibia

	Control (n = 8)	Sedentary Suspended (n = 8)	Exercise Suspended (n = 7)
Flexural rigidity (kN·mm²)	19.9 ± 1.2*	18.6 ± 1.4	18.0 ± 0.8
Tensile stress (N/mm²)	201.0 ± 35.0	203.0 ± 38.0	220.0 ± 22.0
Load at proportional limit (N)	75.6 ± 8.1	71.6 ± 5.8	66.6 ± 7.1
Energy at proportional limit (mJ)	8.3 ± 1.3	7.8 ± 1.3	7.0 ± 1.3
Nonlinear displacement (μm)	270.0 ± 50.0	270.0 ± 70.0	270.0 ± 70.0
Maximum load (N)	108.8 ± 7.9	102.2 ± 3.7	98.0 ± 11.3
Energy at maximum load (mJ)	34.2 ± 4.0	32.1 ± 5.9	30.5 ± 10.2
Load at failure (N)	82.3 ± 12.2	76.6 ± 18.2	79.9 ± 15.0
Energy at failure (mJ)	74.8 ± 22.9	67.9 ± 23.2	55.8 ± 30.7

* Indicates that the control group mean (±SD) is significantly ($p \leq 0.05$) different from the sedentary suspended and exercise suspended group means.
Adapted from Shaw SR, Zernicke RF, Vailas AC, DeLuna D, Thomason DB, Baldwin KM: Mechanical, morphological and biochemical adaptations of bone and muscle to hindlimb suspension and exercise. *J Biomech* 20:225–234, 1987.

detrimental to the mechanical properties of the rats—regardless of the suspension effects. For example, Zernicke and coworkers [67] report that intense exercise can deleteriously affect the biomechanical and morphological properties of immature rat cortical and trabecular bones.

Abram and coworkers [1] also used a model similar to that of Morey et al. [35] to study the effects of suspension on the rat femur. Three groups of 42-day-old male Sprague-Dawley rats were suspended for periods of 1, 2, or 3 weeks while a fourth recovery group was suspended for 2 weeks followed by 2 weeks of normal activity. The right femora were tested using nonfailure bending, nonfailure torsion, and failure torsion tests. Although femora growth rate (GR) decreased with age for both control and suspension animals, the suspension (GR) was significantly less than controls after 1, 2, and 3 weeks of suspension. After the 2-week recovery period, GR stabilized at the 2-week suspension level (Fig. 5.9). Bone cross-sectional area, second moment of inertia, and polar moment of area showed similar trends. The second moment of inertia

FIGURE 5.9

Growth rate versus age (lower abscissa) *or experimental hang time* (upper abscissa). Solid lines *connect consecutive age points.* Vertical cross-bars *indicate standard deviations, and* asterisks *indicate significant differences between experimentals and controls.* Dotted line *indicates 2-week recovery period. (From Abram AC, Keller TS, Spengler DM: The effects of simulated weightlessness on bone biomechanical and biochemical properties in the maturing rat.* J Biomech *21:755–767, 1988.)*

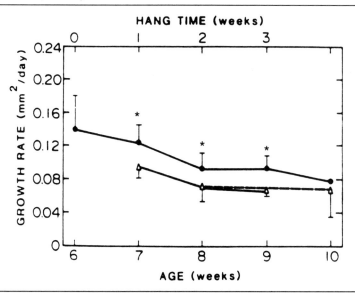

and polar moment of area, however, had a slower recovery and did not become significantly different from controls until the 3rd week of suspension. Cortical bone area of the 3-week experimentals was 18% lower than controls.

The ultimate sheer stress and percent calcium were significantly different from controls at 2 and 3 weeks. Although percent calcium (% ash weight) was initially higher in the control group, it became increasingly lower than experimentals at 2 and 3 weeks of suspension. Further, calcium content decreased for experimental animals but at a slower rate than ash weight, which may explain the increase in percent calcium (% ash weight) seen in the experimental groups. Ultimate sheer stress (τ) exhibited a significant degree of recovery following a return to normal activity (Fig. 5.10). Flexural rigidity and axial rigidity showed sharp and significant reductions in experimental animals after 3 weeks (Fig. 5.11). Ultimate torque was significantly reduced in the experimental animals after 2 and 3 weeks of hang time but showed good recovery, becoming equivalent to the 1-week hang time values and similar to controls after 2 weeks of recovery (Fig. 5.12).

Because control animal age was closely correlated ($r = 0.89$) with body weight times bone length (BWBL), Abram et al. [1] predicted animal age using the following equation.

$$\text{Age} = \text{BWBL} \times 0.040 + 23.64 \qquad (1)$$

Adjusted bone age (n Age) was then predicted from the equation:

$$n \text{ Age} = \text{Age}_i + 0.040 \, (724.8 - \text{BWBL}_i) \qquad (2)$$

where Age_i = measured age of specimen, 0.040 is the slope from Equation 1, 724.8 is the mean BWBL (g·cm), and BWBL_i is the body weight times bone length of the i-th specimen. Using equation 2, the authors determined that the experimental skeletal age was 4 days/week of suspension lower than the control. Thus, by the end of the 3rd week of suspension, the experimental animals were effectively 12 days skeletally less mature than controls (Fig. 5.13). After the 2-week recovery period, the adjusted experimental age difference between controls and recovery experimentals was maintained, indicating that full recovery takes longer than the suspension period in the growing rat. The observed bone structural hypotrophy was due to changes in bone geometry and bone quality. The 50% reduction in ultimate torque in the suspended rats was likely related to the 27% decrease in material and 29% decrease in geometric properties. Thus, the geometrical and material property contributions were essentially equivalent. Reambulation, they suggested, resulted in a slow recovery, taking longer than the suspension period.

FIGURE 5.10

Material properties versus animal age (lower abscissa) *or experimental hang time* (upper abscissa). *Percent change between ultimate shear stress (τ), calcium content (% CA$_{ASH}$), and mineral content (% ASH-α) are shown. Six-week points are control only, with* solid lines *connecting percent change between consecutive weekly data points.* Dotted lines *indicate the 2-week recovery periods. Asterisks above data points indicate significant differences between the experimental and control values.* Negative percent *change indicates control values greater than experimental. (From Abram AC, Keller TS, Spengler DM: The effects of simulated weightlessness on bone biomechanical and biochemical properties in the maturing rat.* J Biomech *21:755–767, 1988.)*

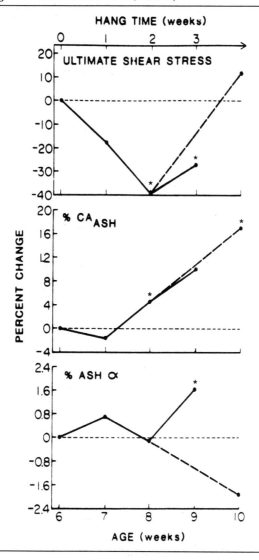

FIGURE 5.11

Structural properties versus animal age (lower abscissa) *or experimental hang time* (upper abscissa). *Percent changes between torsional rigidity* (GK), *flexural rigidity* (EI_{xx}), *and axial rigidity* (EA) *are shown. Six-week points are control only, with* solid lines *connection percent change between consecutive weekly data points.* Dotted lines *indicate the 2-week recovery periods.* Asterisks *above data points indicate significant differences between experimental and control values.* Negative percent *change indicates control value greater than experimental value. (From Abram AC, Keller TS, Spengler DM: The effects of simulated weightlessness on bone biomechanical properties in the maturing rat. J Biomech 21:755–767, 1988.)*

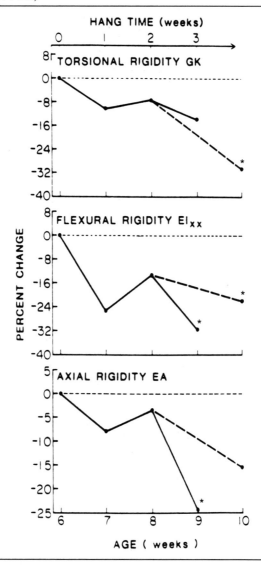

FIGURE 5.12

Ultimate torque (T_{ULT}) *versus age* (lower abscissa) *or experimental hang time* (upper abscissa). *Six-week point is control only with* solid lines *connecting percent change between consecutive weekly data points.* Asterisks *above data points indicate significant differences between experimental and control values.* Negative percent *change indicates control value greater than experimental value.* Dotted line *indicates the 2-week recovery period. (From Abram AC, Keller TS, Spengler DM: The effects of simulated weightlessness on bone biomechanical properties in the maturing rat.* J Biomech *21:755–767, 1988.)*

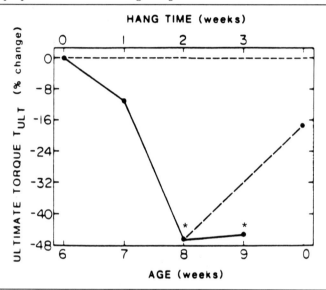

Wronski and Morey-Holton [64] compared Morey and coworkers' original simulated weightlessness model [35] with a new tail-suspension model. Male Munich Wistar rats (43 days old, 124 g) were subjected to tail suspension and compared with age-matched controls and back-suspended animals. As described by Wronski and Morey-Holton [64], conscious rats were loosely restrained in a towel while their tails were lightly abraded with gauze soaked in 70% ethanol. Tincture of benzoin was applied to the skin and allowed to dry. Orthopaedic tape, attached to a plastic suspension bar, was applied to the lateral sides of the tail. The tape was secured by wrapping a strip of stockette around the rail. Each rat was subsequently attached via the plastic suspension bar to a pulley system mounted on the top of a Plexiglas cage.

Although the rats subjected to back suspension weighed significantly less than controls at the end of the 2 weeks, tail suspension rats gained weight at a comparable weight to controls and were not significantly different from controls at the end of 2 weeks. Quantitative bone histomorphometry indicated that back suspension resulted in loss of trabecu-

FIGURE 5.13
Normalized age difference versus experimental hang time. Normalized age difference values indicate age difference between experimental and control rats with respect to the mean body weight times bone length (BWBL). Solid lines connect consecutive age points and dotted line indicates 2-week recovery period. (From Abram AC, Keller TS, Spengler DM: The effects of simulated weightlessness on bone biomechanical properties in the maturing rat. J Biomech 21:755–767, *1988.)*

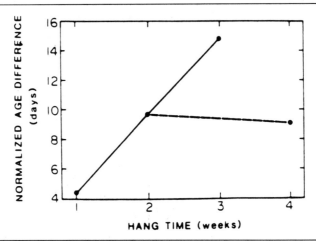

lar bone mass, an accumulation of marrow fat, a depressed rate of longitudinal bone growth, a decline in osteoblast population, and an increase in osteoclast population. Most bone histological parameters, however, were not influenced in tail suspended animals, but, tail-suspended rats did exhibit a significant reduction in trabecular bone volume. Trabecular bone volume loss in the back-suspended animals was 50%, while in the tail-suspended animals it was 20%.

The potentially more stressful back suspension method (lack of weight gain) resulted in systemic alterations, as well as mechanical unloading changes to the bone. The tail suspension model, arguably, minimized undesirable stress-induced side effects and resulted in a reduced systemic response. Thus, the tail suspension appears to be preferable to back suspension for evaluating the effects of simulated weightlessness on bone.

CONCLUDING COMMENTS

The rapidity of the alterations in both human and rat skeletal system homeostasis during weightlessness dramatically highlights the probity of the observation that "bone is a dynamic tissue." Calcium balance is negative during spaceflight, and increased bone resorption may occur, but, as stated earlier—what are the short-term and long-term consequences of the spaceflight-related structural and compositional changes to bone? The definitive answer to that question is unknown, but spaceflight and simulated-weightlessness experiments using rats have opened a window through which researchers can examine the mechanisms responsible for the dramatic changes in bone in microgravity. Simulated-weightlessness experiments, alone, however, do not duplicate the microgravity environment of space, and thus, although costly—in terms of money, available orbiter space, and demands on crew and experimenter time—spaceflight experiments remain essential for examining the specific effects of weightlessness on the biomechanical properties of bone.

ACKNOWLEDGMENTS

The authors' research discussed in this chapter was supported in part by grants and fellowships funded by the National Aeronautics and Space Administration (NAG-2-568, NAGT-70093, NCA2-390-501, NAC2-390-502, and A53749C), UCLA Biomedical Research Support Grant RR7009 from the U.S. Public Health Service, and the UCLA Academic Senate Research Committee.

REFERENCES

1. Abram AC, Keller TS, Spengler DM: The effects of simulated weightlessness on bone biomechanical and biochemical properties in the maturing rat. *J Biomech* 21:755–767, 1988.
2. Bikle DD, Holloran BP, Cone CM, Globus RK, Morey-Holton E: The effects of simulated weightlessness on bone maturation. *Endocrinology* 120:678–684, 1987.
3. Birkhead NC, Glizzard JJ, Daly JW, Haupt GJ, Issekutz B Jr, Myers RN, Rodahl K: Cardiodynamic metabolic effects of prolonged bed rest. Aerospace Medical Research Laboratories, Wright-Patterson Air Force Base, OH, Report No. AMRL-TDR, 1963, pp 63–67.
4. Booth FW, Musacchia XJ: The use of suspension models and comparison with true weightlessness, 'A résumé.' *Physiologist* 28:S237–S240, 1985.
5. Brannon EW, Rockwood CA Jr, Potts P: The influence of specific exercises in the prevention of debilitation musculoskeletal disorders: implication in physiological conditioning for prolonged weightlessness. *Aerospace Med* 34:900–906, 1963.
6. Cann CE, Adachi RR: Bone resorption and mineral excretion in rats during spaceflight. *Am J Physiol* 244:R327–R331, 1983.
7. Consolazio CF, Matoush LO, Nelson RA, Hackler LF, Preston EE: Relationship between calcium in sweat, calcium balance, and calcium requirements. *J Nutr* 78:78, 1962.
8. David H: Russians discuss space radiation findings in conference. *Missiles and Rockets*, Conference Proceedings, October 21, 1963, p 34.
9. Detrick P, Whedon GD, Shorr E: Effects of immobilization upon various metabolic and physiologic functions of normal man. *Am J Med* 4:3–36, 1948.

10. Dietlein LF, Rapp RM: Experiment M-3, Inflight exercise work tolerance. *Gemini Midprogram Conference Including Experiment Results,* NASA Manned Spacecraft Center, Houston, TX, NASA SP-121, 1966, pp 393–396.

11. Eurell JA, Kazarian LE: Quantitative histochemistry of rat lumbar vertebrae following spaceflight. *Am J Physiol* 244:R315-R318, 1983.

12. France EP, Oloff CM, Kazarian LE: Bone mineral analysis of rat vertebrae following space flight: Cosmos 1129. *U.S. Air Force Aerospace Medical Research Laboratory Report.* AFAMRL-TR-83-055, 1983.

13. Freeman LW: Metabolism of calcium in patients with spinal cord injuries. *Ann Surg* 129:177, 1949.

14. Goode AW, Rambaut PC: The skeleton in space. *Nature* 317:204–205, 1985.

15. Grindeland RE, Hymer WC, Ferrington M, Fast T, Hayes C, Motter K, Patil L, Vasques M: Changes in pituitary growth hormone cells prepared in rats flown on Spacelab-3. *Am J Physiol* 252:R209-R215, 1987.

16. Hattner RS, McMillan DE: Influence of weightlessness upon the skeleton: a review. *Aerospace Med* 39:849–855, 1968.

17. Howard JE, Parson W, Bigham RS: Studies on patients convalescent from fracture. *Bull Johns Hopkins Hosp* 77:291, 1945.

18. Issekutz B, Blizzard JJ, Birkhead NC, Rodahl K: Effect of prolonged bedrest on urinary calcium output. *J Appl Physiol* 21:1013, 1966.

19. Jee WSS, Wronski TJ, Morey ER, Kimmel DB: Effects of spaceflight on trabecular bone in rats. *Am J Physiol* 244:R310–R314, 1983.

20. Johnston FL, Dietlein LF, Berry CA: Biomedical results of Apollo. Washington, D.C., NASA, 1975.

21. Johnston FL, Dietlein LF: Biomedical results from Skylab. Washington, D.C., NASA, 1977.

22. Kazarian LE: Vertebral body strength of rat spinal columns. Final reports of U.S. rat experiments flown on the Soviet Satellite Cosmos 1129. In Henrich MA, Souza KA (eds): *NASA Technical Memorandum* 81289, 1981, pp 228–266.

23. Kummer B: The so-called Wolff's Law and the adaptation of bone to microgravity. *The Gravity Relevance in Bone Mineralisation Processes Conference (European Space Agency Workshop),* Brussels, Belgium 1984, pp 29–34.

24. Lutwak L: Chemical analysis of diet, urine, feces, and sweat parameters relating to the calcium and nitrogen balance studies during Gemini VII flight (Experiment M-7). *NASA Contractor Report,* NAS 9–5375, 1966.

25. Lynch TN, Jensen RL, Stevens PM, Johnson RL, Lamb LE: Metabolic effects of prolonged bed rest: their modification by simulated altitude. *Aerospace Med* 38:10–20, 1967.

26. Mack PB, LaChance PA, Vose GP, Vogt FB: Bone demineralization of foot and hand of Gemini-Titan IV, V, and VII astronauts during orbital flight. *Am J Roentgenol Rad Ther Nucl Med* 100:503–511, 1967.

27. Mack PB, LaChance PA: Effects of recumbency and space flight on bone density. *Second Annual Biomedical Research Conference,* Houston, TX, 1966, pp 407–415.

28. Mack PB, Vose GP, Vogt FB, LaChance PA: Experiment M-6 on bone demineralization, manned spaceflight experiments. *Proceedings of the Symposium on Gemini Missions III and IV,* Washington, D.C.: NASA, 1965, pp 61–80.

29. Mack PB, Vose GP, Vogt FB, LaChance PA: Experiment M-6 on bone demineralization. *Gemini VII Mission, Proceedings of the Gemini Midprogram Conference,* NASA SP-121, Houston, TX: NASA, February 23–25, 1966, pp 407–415.

30. Mack PB, Vose GP, Vogt FB, LaChance PA: Experiment M-6 on bone demineralization. *Proceedings of the Manned Spaceflight Experiments Interim Report, Gemini V Mission,* Washington, D.C.: NASA, 1966, pp 109–128.

31. Marwick C: Physicians called upon to help chart future space effort. *JAMA* 256:2015–2016, 2020, 1025, 1986.

32. Matsuda JJ, Zernicke RF, Vailas AC, Pedrini VA, Pedrini-Mille A, Maynard JA: Morphological and mechanical adaptation of immature bone to strenuous exercise. *J Appl Physiol* 60:2028–2034, 1986,

33. Merz B: The body pays a penalty for defying the law of gravity. *JAMA* 256:2040–2052, 1986.

34. Morey E: Spaceflight and bone turnover: correlation with a new rat model of weightlessness. *Bioscience* 29:168–172, 1979.

35. Morey E, Turner RT, Baylink DJ: Quantitative analysis of selected bone parameters. In Rosenzweig SN, Souza KA (eds): *Final Reports of U.S. Experiments Flown on the Soviet Satellite Cosmos 936.* Washington D.C.: NASA TM-78526, 1978, pp 135–178.

36. Patterson-Buckendahl P, Arnaud SB, Mechanic GL, Martin RB, Grindeland RE, Cann CE: Fragility and composition of growing rat bone after one week in spaceflight. *Am J Physiol* 252:R240-R246, 1987.

37. Pelker RR, Friedlaender GE, Markham TC, Panjabi MM, Moen CJ: Effects of freezing and freeze-drying on the biomechanical properties of rat bone. *J Orthop Res* 1:405–411, 1984.

38. Rambaut PC, Goode AW: Skeletal changes during space flight. *Lancet* 2:1050–1052, 1985.

39. Roberts WE, Morey-Holton E, Gonsalves MR: Sensitivity of bone cell populations to weightlessness and simulated weightlessness. *The Gravity Relevance in Bone Mineralisation Processes Conference (European Space Agency Workshop)*, Brussels, Belgium, 1984, pp 67–72.

40. Rockoff SD, Sweet E, Bleustein J: The relative contribution of trabecular and cortical bone to the strength of human lumbar vertebrae. *Calcif Tissue Res* 3:163–176, 1969.

41. Rogacheva IV, Stupakov GP, Voloshin AI, Pavlova MN, Polyakov AN: Rat bone tissue after flight aboard Cosmos 1129 Biosatellite. *Moscow Kosm Biol Aviakosm Med* 18:39–44, 1984.

42. Rorke W: *Formulas for Stress and Strain.* New York, McGraw-Hill, 1965.

43. Russell JE, Simmons DJ: Bone maturation in rats flown on the Spacelab-3 mission. *Physiologist* 28:S235–S236, 1985.

44. Salem GS, Zernicke, RF, Vailas AC, Martinez DA: Determination of biomechanical and biochemical differences in lumbar vertebrae of rapidly growing rats. *Am J Physiol* 256:R259–R263, 1989.

45. Shaw SR, Vailas AC, Grindeland RE, Zernicke RF: Effects of a 1-wk spaceflight on the morphological and mechanical properties of growing bone. *Am J Physiol* 254:R78–R83, 1988.

46. Shaw SR, Zernicke RF, Vailas AC, DeLuna D, Thomason DB, Baldwin KM: Mechanical, morphological and biochemical adaptations of bone and muscle to hindlimb suspension and exercise. *J Biomech* 20:225–234, 1987.

47. Simmons DJ, Russell JE, Grypas MD: Bone maturation and quality of bone material in rats flown on the space shuttle 'Spacelab-3 mission.' *Bone Mineral* 1:485–493, 1986.

48. Simmons DJ, Russell JE, Winter F, Tran Van P, Vignery A, Baron R, Rosenberg GD, Walker WV: Effect of spaceflight on the nonweightbearing bones of the rat skeleton. *Am J Physiol* 244:R319–R326, 1983.

49. Spengler DM, Morey ER, Carter DR, Turner RT, Baylink DJ: Effects of spaceflight on structural and material strength of growing bone. *Proc Soc Exp Biol Med* 174:224–228, 1983.

50. Tipton CM: Considerations for exercise prescriptions in future spaceflights. *Med Sci Sports Exerc* 15:441–444, 1983.

51. Uebelhart D, Very JM, Baud CA: Morphometric and biophysical study of bone tissue in immobilization-induced osteoporosis in the growing rat. *The Gravity Relevance in Bone Mineralisation Processes Conference (European Space Agency Workshop)*, Brussels, Belgium, 1984, pp 73–78.

52. Vailas AC, Zernicke RF, Grindeland RE, Kaplansky A, Durnova GN, Li K-C, Martinez DA: Effects of spaceflight on rat humerus geometry, biomechanics, and biochemistry. *FASEB J* 4:47–54, 1990.
53. Vico L, Chappard D, Alexandre C, Palle S, Minaire P, Riffat G, Morukov B, Rakhmanov S: Effects of a 120 day period of bed-rest on bone mass and bone cell activities in man: attempts of countermeasure. *Bone Mineral* 2:383–394, 1987.
54. Vico L, Chappard D, Alexandre C, Palle S, Minaire P, Riffat G, Novikov VE, Bakulin AV: Effects of weightlessness on bone mass and osteoclast number in pregnant rats after a five-day spaceflight (Cosmos 1514). *Bone* 8:95–103, 1987.
55. Vico L, Chappard D, Bakulin AV, Novikov VE, Alexandre C: Effects of 7-day space flight on weight-bearing and non-weightbearing bones in rats (Cosmos 1667) *Physiologist* 30:S45–S46, 1987.
56. Vico L, Chappard D, Palle S, Bakulin AV, Novikov VE, Alexandre C: Trabecular bone remodeling after seven days of weightlessness exposure (Biocosmos 1667). *Am J Physiol* 255:R243–R247, 1988.
57. Vogt FB, Mack PB, Bewasley WG, Spencer WA, Cardus D, Valbona C: The effect of bedrest on various parameters of physiological functions: XII. The effect of bedrest on bone mass and calcium balance. NASA Contractor Report, NASA CR-182, 1965.
58. Vorobyov EI, Gazenko OG, Genin AM, Egorov AD: Medical results of Salyut-6 manned spaceflights. *Aviat Space Environ Med* 54:S31–S40, 1983.
59. Whedon GD, Lutwak L, Neuman W: Calcium and nitrogen balance. A review of medical results of Gemini 7 and related flight. Kennedy Space Center, FL, 1966, p 127.
60. Whedon GD, Lutwak L, Neuman WF, LaChance PA: Experiment M-7, calcium and nitrogen balance. NASA SP-121, *Gemini Midprogram Conference*, Houston, TX, 1966, pp 417–421.
61. Whittle MW: Caloric and exercise requirements of space flight: biostereometric results from Skylab. *Aviat Space Environ Med* 50:163–167, 1979.
62. Wronski TJ, Morey ER: Effect of spaceflight on periosteal bone formation in rats. *Am J Physiol* 244:R305–R309, 1983.
63. Wronski TJ, Morey-Holton ER, Doty SB, Maese AC, Walsh CC: Histomorphometric analysis of rat skeleton following spaceflight. *Am J Physiol* 252:R252–R255, 1987.
64. Wronski TJ, Morey-Holton ER: Skeletal response to simulated weightlessness: a comparison of suspension techniques. *Aviat Space Environ Med* 58:63–68, 1987.
65. Wunder CC, Tipton CM, Cook KM: Femur-bending properties as influenced by gravity: IV. Limits after high and low weight-bearing. *Aviat Space Environ Med* 51:902–907, 1980.
66. Yamaguchi M, Ozaki K, Hoshi T: Simulated weightlessness and bone metabolism: decrease of alkaline phosphatase activity in the femoral diaphysis of rats. *Res Exp Med (Berl)* 189:9–14, 1989.
67. Zernicke RF, Barnard RJ, Li K-C, Salem GJ, Hou JC-H, Li AF-Y: Biomechanical and morphological response of immature cortical and trabecular bone to strenuous exercise. In Dillman CJ, Nelson RC, Nigg BM, Voy RO, Newson MM (eds): *Proceedings of the First World Congress on Sport Sciences,* Colorado Springs, CO, 1989).
68. Zernicke RF, Vailas AC, Grindeland RE, Kaplansky A, Salem GJ, Martinez DA: Spaceflight effects on biomechanical and biochemical properties of vertebrae in rapidly-growing rats. *Am J Physiol* (in press).
69. Zernicke RF, Vailas AC, Grindeland RE, Li K-C, Salem GJ: Interactive effects of nutrition, environment, and rat-strain on cortical and vertebral bone geometry and biomechanics. *Aviat Space Environ Med* (in press).

6
Bioelectric Impedance for Body Composition

RICHARD N. BAUMGARTNER, Ph.D.
Wm. CAMERON CHUMLEA, Ph.D.
ALEX F. ROCHE, M.D., Ph.D.

INTRODUCTION

During the last decade, there has been increased interest in the assessment of body composition in physiological and nutritional research and in sports medicine. Many methods are currently available, but none are wholly satisfactory for all purposes. Laboratory methods such as neutron activation, magnetic resonance imaging, computed tomography, whole-body counting of ^{40}K, dual-energy absorptiometry, and isotope dilution are very accurate but are expensive, cumbersome, and/or require sensitive instrumentation and highly trained technicians. Underwater weighing (body density) is less expensive, but difficult to apply to some groups such as children and the elderly. Furthermore, the body density approach requires certain assumptions regarding the densities of the fat and fat-free compartments that are now recognized as inappropriate for many individuals. Anthropometry, including skinfold thickness measurements from calipers or small, portable ultrasonic equipment is useful in field studies, but has limited accuracy.

Recently, there has been considerable interest in bioelectric impedance as an inexpensive, safe, portable method of estimating body composition that is applicable in field studies. Bioelectric impedance has considerable potential for estimating body composition when used alone or in combination with anthropometry, but the present use of the method represents something of a "black box." As a result, a naive use of the method can lead to misconceptions regarding its applicability and validity. A better understanding of the complexity of bioelectric impedance will lead to increased appreciation of the limitations of the current approach, as well as of possible approaches that may be developed for analyzing body composition using bioelectric impedance. This paper discusses the physical principles of the conduction of electrical currents in the human body, and critically reviews the literature on the use of bioelectric impedance for estimating body composition.

193

EARLY STUDIES OF BIOELECTRIC IMPEDANCE

Studies of bioelectric phenomena in human and animal tissues began in the late 19th century (see Refs. 84 and 85 for reviews). A considerable body of work in the 1930s–1950s established the basic uses of impedance for measuring aspects of human physiology [5–12, 17–19, 69, 97–100]. These early studies explored the relationships of bioelectric impedance and its parameters to physiological variables such as thyroid function, basal metabolic rate, hormone levels, and blood flow. Studies by Cole and Curtis [25] of the conduction of electricity in unicellular organisms and in suspensions of cells provided many of the basic concepts for interpreting bioelectric impedance in complex, multicellular tissues and organs.

In some of these early studies, impedance was measured in the arms when they were immersed in a saline bath through which an alternating current was passed [12, 17]. In other studies, direct and alternating currents were applied using two or more electrodes placed on or through the skin [5–11, 18]. Horton and Van Ravenswaay [51] were among the first to use a four-electrode system with an alternating current similar to the technique used presently for body composition analysis. The "tetrapolar" method was further developed and refined by Nyboer [84] to study blood flow. These early studies revealed many problems in the accurate measurement of impedance in biological tissues, such as polarization of the current in tissues or between electrodes, surface rather than deep conduction of the current, and stray reactances associated with the skin-electrode interface, unshielded cables, and other electronic components. The technology for measuring bioelectric impedance with a high degree of accuracy is a recent development [1].

Bioelectric impedance was first used for body composition analysis in the 1960s–1970s. Thomasset and his associates [16, 35, 55, 117–120] developed methods for estimating total body water (TBW) and extracellular fluid (ECF) using a two-needle electrode technique. This approach has not become popular probably because of problems with patient acceptance. Hoffer and associates [49, 50] applied the four-surface electrode method used in blood flow studies [84] for estimating TBW. This approach was extended by Nyboer [86] to estimating fat-free mass (FFM) and percent body fat (%BF). Recent scientific interest has been stimulated by the commercial availability of low-cost, accurate bioimpedance analyzers. The present use of bioelectric impedance to estimate body composition is based upon the greater electrolyte content and conductivity of FFM, compared to that of adipose tissue or bone [67, 97, 106] and upon the geometrical relationship between impedance and the volume of the conductor [84, 87].

PHYSICAL PRINCIPLES

Impedance (Z) is the frequency-dependent opposition of a conductor to the flow of an alternating electric current and is composed of two vectors, resistance (R) and reactance (Xc). Resistance is the pure opposition of the conductor to the current flow and is the reciprocal of conductance, or the ability of an object to convey an electric current. From Ohm's Law, resistance (R) is equal to the voltage (E) divided by the current (I), or $R = E/I$. In a biological conductor, the current is primarily carried by ions, and conductivity, or the amount of electricity that can be conducted, is proportional to the number of ions (N_i) per unit volume (V), or kN_i/V, and is temperature dependent [64]. Reactance is the reciprocal of capacitance, or the storage of voltage by a condenser for a brief moment in time, and is associated with several types of polarization processes that may be produced by cell membranes, tissue interfaces, and nonionic tissues [1, 12, 99]. Capacitance causes the current to lag behind the voltage, creating a phase shift that is quantified geometrically as the arctangent of the ratio of reactance to resistance, or the phase angle. Reactance and phase angle are small in most biological conductors, but may have considerable significance for the analysis of body composition as will be shown later.

The geometric relationships between impedance, resistance, reactance, and phase angle are frequency dependent as illustrated in the impedance plot in Figure 6.1. At very low frequencies (f_l) the impe-

FIGURE 6.1
Impedance plot. (From Baumgartner RN, Chumlea WC, Roche AF: Bioelectric impedance phase angle and body composition. Am J Clin Nutr *48:16–23, 1988.)*

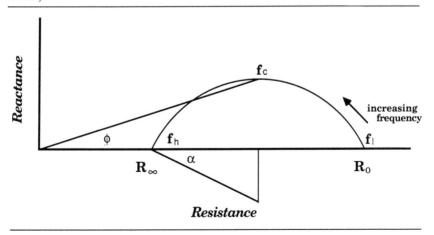

dance of the cell membranes and tissue interfaces is too high for conduction of the current. As a result, the current is conducted through the TBW only and the measured impedance is purely resistive (R_0). As the frequency is increased, the current penetrates the cell membranes and reactance (Xc) increases causing the phase angle (f) to open. The magnitude of the impedance is equal to the vector defined by the equation $Z^2 = R^2 + Xc^2$. The critical or characteristic frequency (f_c) is that at which Xc and f are maximal and is a specific electrical trait of the conducting medium. Above the characteristic frequency, the reactance decreases as the cell membranes and tissue interfaces lose their capacitive ability, and at very high frequencies (f_h) impedance is again equivalent to pure resistance (R_∞). In a biological conductor, the semicircular locus described by the change in impedance with change in frequency has a center below the x axis. This may occur because capacitance and intracellular resistance are not constant across all cells or tissues due to differences in membrane permeability, intracellular composition, size, shape, and orientation of cells, and tissue distribution [26, 59]. The amount to which the center of the locus is below the x axis is quantified as the depression angle (α) [1].

The "circuit-equivalent" model shown in Figure 6.2 corresponds to the impedance plot shown in Figure 6.1 [1, 59]. In this model, C_m and R_m

FIGURE 6.2

Circuit equivalent diagram for impedance in a cell or tissue.

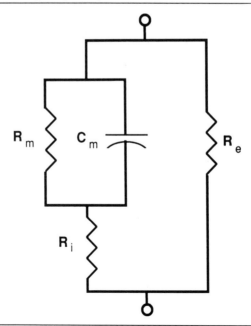

represent cell membrane capacitance and resistance, respectively. R_i and R_e correspond to intra- and extracellular resistances, respectively. At low frequency (f_l), the current primarily flows through the extracellular space and the impedance is equivalent to R_e. At high frequencies, the current fully penetrates the cell membranes and C_m and R_m are essentially short-circuited. Impedance at high frequency (f_h) is equivalent to $R_iR_e/(R_i + R_e)$ [59, 96].

For an isotropic conductor contacted uniformly by endplate electrodes, resistance is proportional to its length and inversely proportional to its cross-sectional area, or $R = \rho L/A$ [2]. Thus, for a cylindrical conductor with a uniform cross-section, the volume (V) of the conductor is proportional to its length (L) squared, divided by its resistance (R), or $V = \rho L^2/R$. Impedance (Z) may be substituted for R in this formula because the reactive component has a similar dependence upon the geometry of a capacitor when included in a conducting circuit [87]. The coefficient, ρ, in the above equations is called the *specific resistivity*. If Z is used in the formula, ζ is substituted for ρ and is called the specific impedivity [87]. In biological conductors, it is difficult to specify ζ because the nature of the capacitance is complex and uncertain [1] so ρ is preferred. In a homogeneous material with a constant cross-sectional area and uniform current density distribution, ρ is a constant physical property analogous to specific gravity [2, 39]. Specific resistivity is the reciprocal of conductivity and, therefore, is directly proportional to volume and inversely proportional to the number of electrolytic ions, or kV/N_i [64].

Considerable effort has been expended on the definition of specific resistivities for various biological tissues [18, 19, 39, 95, 97]. The present values for *tissue* resistivities, however, are not well-established, partly because of differences in the electrical techniques used for their measurement, but also because it is difficult to specify static homogeneous volumes and uniform current density distributions in biological conductors [2]. The resistivity of a tissue will vary depending upon its microstructure, level of hydration, and the concentration and types of electrolytic ions. The microstructure may produce anisotropy, or the dependence of the resistance on the direction of flow of the current in the conductor. Skeletal muscle is composed of elongated fibers, and resistance measured transversely to the fiber direction is considerably greater than resistance measured in the same direction [95]. Biological tissues resemble distributions of poorly conducting spheres and/or tubes filled and surrounded by electrolytic fluids. The relative volumes and electrolytic balances between the intra- and extracellular fluids will affect tissue resistivity. Because these factors may vary among individuals, *tissue* resistivities in biological conductors will be distributed continuously with mean and variance values. Figure 6.3 shows some mean values for tissue-specific resistivities reported in the literature [39, 85].

FIGURE 6.3
Geometric model of volume resistivities for a limb.

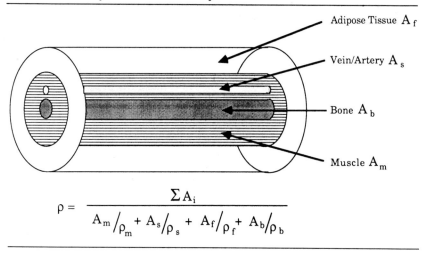

Adipose Tissue A_f

Vein/Artery A_s

Bone A_b

Muscle A_m

$$\rho = \frac{\Sigma A_i}{A_m/\rho_m + A_s/\rho_s + A_f/\rho_f + A_b/\rho_b}$$

The observed *volume* resistivity for a body segment or the whole body is the sum of the resistivities of all the tissues weighted by the relative amount of each tissue within the segment or the whole body [39, 85, 95]. Variation in *volume* resistivities among body segments and for the whole body occurs because of intra- and interindividual differences in tissue and fluid composition and the relative amounts of particular tissues and fluids present [95]. Figure 6.4 shows a geometric model illustrating the concept of *volume* resistivity as distinct from *tissue* resistivity for the arm or the leg. In this model, the concentric cylinders of bone, muscle, blood in veins or arteries, and adipose tissue act as parallel conductors. Theoretically, the *volume* resistivity is equal to the total cross-sectional area (or volume) of the segment divided by the cross-sectional area (or volume) of each tissue divided by the resistivity for that tissue. The high specific resistivities of bone (ρ_b) and adipose tissue (ρ_f) cause these fractions to approach zero, unless the amounts of these tissues are large. This may occur for adipose tissue and may explain inaccuracies in the use of bioelectric impedance for estimating FFM at extreme levels of adiposity [48]. Also, at higher levels of adiposity, relatively large amounts of water are contained in adipose tissue, which may affect volume resistivity. In terms of a circuit-equivalent model, bone and adipose tissue generally act as open parallel circuits due to their high resistivities and contribute little to the overall segment volume resistivity. Consequently, the effective measurable resistance is primarily determined by the muscle and blood tissues. This model is applicable to a limb but not to the trunk. The geometry, internal structure, and the orientation of tissues in the trunk are complex and produce nonuniform current density distributions and anistropic effects that are difficult to model.

The reactive component of bioelectric impedance (Xc) is very small (<3% of the resistance) in most biological conductors. Early studies suggested the importance of Xc, and especially the phase angle, for measuring certain aspects of body composition and physiological variables [6, 7, 9, 17, 112, 113]. Some recent studies have used Xc to differentiate among individuals in their amounts of TBW and ECF and have included Xc as an independent variable in predictions of FFM and TBW [74, 102, 112, 113].

The phase angle ($\tan^{-1}(Xc/R)$) was originally advanced as a tool for diagnosing metabolic disorders, particularly thyroid diseases [17, 51]. Variability in phase angles could be associated with variability in cell size, membrane permeability, or intracellular composition, which affect reactance and intracellular resistance. In addition, variation among individuals in the volume and electrolyte composition of the TBW and in the distribution of body fluids among tissues can affect the amount of "shunting" of the current through the interstitial spaces producing large changes in R in proportion to Xc. These changes increase the interindividual variability in the phase angles of specific tissues [1]. Relative changes in phase angles have been shown to be sensitive indicators of changes in body fluid distribution associated with dialysis and diuretic treatments [112, 113, 115, 116]. Phase angles for the trunk are corre-

FIGURE 6.4

Volume resistivities for selected tissues.

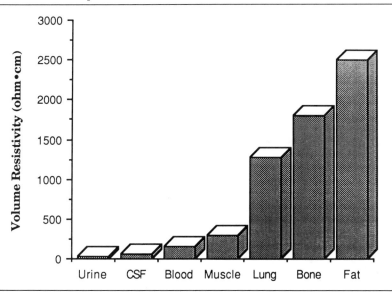

lated with %BF, possibly due to the increased water content of adipose tissue at higher levels of adiposity [14].

Low radiofrequency (1 kHz to 1 MHz) currents in the 500–800 μA range are used for body composition analysis. Most of the commercially available bioelectric impedance body composition analyzers operate at 50 kHz, which is the characteristic frequency for skeletal muscle tissue [59, 106]. It is assumed that the total conductive volume of the body is equivalent to that of TBW, most of which is contained in muscle tissue, and that the hydration of adipose tissue is minimal [16, 49, 50, 85]. Measures of bioelectric impedance at other frequencies, however, have been reported to discriminate the volumes of intracellular and TBW in the body [35, 55, 96]. The ratio of the resistance at 5 kHz to the resistance at 100 kHz has been reported to provide a good index of the proportion of TBW in extracellular fluids [55]. Higher frequency currents (1 MHz) may be preferred for TBW, although they may be more subject to technical problems involving sensitivity and stray capacitances [1]. The use of multiple frequency currents in bioelectric impedance analysis may have considerable value for exploring variations within and between individuals in levels of hydration [59]. Because the water content of FFM and adipose tissue is not constant [70, 90], studies of resistance at low and high frequencies could clarify the possible effects of different levels of hydration on estimates of FFM.

CURRENT METHODS OF ESTIMATING BODY COMPOSITION

Bioelectric Impedance Indices

Most recent studies using bioelectric impedance to estimate body composition have been based on the equation, $V = \rho S^2/R$, in which the conductive volume (V) is assumed to represent TBW, stature (S) is taken as an estimate of the length of the conductor, and whole body resistance (R) is measured between a wrist and ipsilateral or contralateral ankle using four surface electrodes. From the above discussion, it is apparent that the application of this equation to the human body is limited in principle, because it assumes a conductor of homogeneous composition and fixed cross-sectional area and a uniform current density distribution. These assumptions are not met when the human body is considered as a conductor. The cross-sectional area of the body is not constant, and the parts with the smallest cross-sectional areas will primarily determine the resistance [111]. Stature is not the actual length of the conductor. The specific resistivity (ρ) is unknown and will not be a constant for all individuals, but will vary depending upon the amounts and distributions of particular tissues and fluids present as illustrated above in Figure 6.4.

The implication is that S^2/R will not have the same relationship to TBW, or to other components of body composition, in all individuals, or even within individuals undergoing changes in body composition. The situation is more complicated with regard to body components such as the FFM because the level of hydration varies between and within individuals. A statistical association can be established between S^2/R and TBW or FFM for a sample of subjects. Estimates of FFM from densitometry or ^{40}K, or of TBW or ECF from chemical dilution have been regressed on S^2/R. The results of some of these studies are summarized in Table 6.1. Although very good R^2s and root mean squared errors (rmse) have been obtained, the regression coefficients (β) have varied among these studies, suggesting that ρ is not constant and its estimate, β, is sample-specific. Nonetheless, due to the high correlations reported, it is reasonable to consider S^2/R an "index" of TBW and FFM.

Prediction Equations

The statistical association between bioelectric impedance and body composition can be improved by the use of multivariate prediction equations that include additional measures of the size and shape of the conductor and factors such as age, sex, and ethnicity that may correlate with body composition. The addition of these predictor variables would be expected to help control for differences between individuals or groups in geometric and other factors affecting the relationship of resistance to body composition. The addition of independent variables, however, can increase the sample specificity of the equations. This problem can be reduced if certain procedures are applied in the development of the equations. Ideally, the sample from which the equations are developed should be selected randomly to be representative of the general popula-

TABLE 6.1

Selected Equations for the Prediction of Body Composition from Stature²/Resistance (S²/R)

Authors	Age (Years)	N	Regression Equations	rmse
TBW				
Lukaski et al. (1985)	19–42	37 men	$2.03 + 0.63\ (S^2/R)$	2.1 liters
Kushner and Schoeller (1986)	31.8–53.7	40 men and women	$0.83 + 0.714\ (S^2/R)$	2.5 liters
FFM				
Lukaski et al. (1985)	19–42	37 men	$3.04 + 0.85\ (S^2/R)$	2.6 kg
Lukaski et al. (1986)	18–50	84 men	$5.21 + 0.83\ (S^2/R)$	2.5 kg
		67 women	$4.92 + 0.82\ (S^2/R)$	2.0 kg
Chumlea et al. (1988)	9–62	24 boys	$-1.23 + 0.92\ (S^2/R)$	4.0 kg
		26 girls	$-1.38 + 0.96\ (S^2/R)$	4.2 kg
		28 men	$3.50 + 0.87\ (S^2/R)$	2.9 kg
		44 women	$11.55 + 0.69\ (S^2/R)$	2.7 kg
Cordain et al. (1988)	9–14	14 boys	$6.86 + 0.81\ (S^2/R)$	4.1 kg

tion and should be of sufficient size to allow the regression of several independent variables. It may be desirable to stratify selection to achieve overrepresentation of individuals who may have extreme values for the independent variables. The resulting equations will be weighted for these extremes. The equations developed should be cross-validated, preferrably using an independently selected sample. All-possible-subsets regression is preferred to stepwise regression, because the latter approach does not always select the best set of predictors. Ridge and robust regression procedures should be applied to increase the likelihood that the predictive equation will perform well when applied to other groups. These special regression techniques are needed because the independent variables may be expected to be highly intercorrelated producing multicollinearity that can make equations formed by ordinary least squares regression techniques highly unstable. Few studies have applied all these procedures.

The accuracy of prediction equations depends to some extent on the precision of measurement of the criterion or dependent variable. Thus, it is necessary that this be obtained by the best possible laboratory procedure. Criterion measures of FFM and %BF are often derived from body density. When using Siri's equation [108], age- and sex-specific values for the density of FFM should be used for children and adolescents due to their "chemical immaturity" [71]. Changes in body composition affecting the density of FFM also occur in aging, but corresponding density values needed for older ages are not available. Multicompartment models that include measures of TBW and total body mineral in addition to body density provide more accurate criterion estimates of FFM and %BF. FFM can be derived also from TBW or from ^{40}K counting, although the estimates may be inaccurate in some individuals. TBW can be obtained from dilution of deuterium oxide or tritium. Estimates of adipose and muscle tissue volumes can be obtained from computed tomography or magnetic resonance imaging, but the procedures are time-consuming and costly [121].

All these methods have "inescapable" or intrinsic errors ranging from about 1 to 3% when applied appropriately. This point is important because it means that, even when a prediction equation has a rmse approaching zero, some error in the estimation of body composition remains due to error in the criterion measurement. It is possible that, in the future, the current criterion methods will be replaced by newer procedures such as magnetic resonance imaging and dual energy absorptiometry. These procedures may not reduce the intrinsic errors substantially, but may be easier to apply because they do not require active participation by the subject and do not involve exposure to potentially toxic substances or much ionizing radiation.

Reported associations between resistance and anthropometric data can assist the selection of the independent variables to be included in predictive equations. Because electrical resistance is proportional to the length and cross-sectional area of a conductor, anthropometric measurement of body lengths and circumferences are desired. Significant correlations with resistance have been reported for stature, weight, upper arm and calf circumferences, upper arm and calf muscle areas, ratios of circumferences of limb segments to their lengths, and some skinfold thicknesses [13, 47, 49, 50, 57, 66, 76, 103, 109, 110, 119]. Baumgartner et al. [13] showed that 70% of the variance in resistance could be accounted for by a small set of anthropometric variables. The use of shoulder height plus arm length rather than stature as a measure of the length of the conductor improves the accuracy of prediction marginally [23, 53]. Anthropometric variables should be recorded using standard recommended procedures [73]. Age and age[2] should be included as possible predictors to make it likely so that the final equations will be applicable over a wide range of ages. There is an outstanding need for prediction equations for ethnic groups other than whites [125].

Factors Affecting the Measurement of Impedance

There is substantial evidence that impedance measurements are highly reliable based on interobserver and intraobserver comparisons with replacement of electrodes, and interday and interweek comparisons [36, 46, 47, 54, 62, 67, 68, 72, 76, 101, 109]. Because impedance analyzers from different manufacturers vary in the measures they provide even after calibration [27], it is recommended that impedance be measured using the type of analyzer employed to develop the prediction equation that will be applied.

The positioning of the electrodes is important for both whole body and segmental measurements. Displacement of the source electrodes proximally by 1 cm, on either the hand or the foot, reduces the measured resistance by 2.1%; if both are displaced, the reduction is 4.1% [36, 101]. Interobserver differences associated with the placement of electrodes can be reduced if the sites of electrode placement are marked [36].

If the source and receiving electrodes are placed closer together than 4–5 cm, electrode polarization may occur that will increase resistance. This problem may limit the application of bioelectric impedance methods to small children and infants. Barillas-Mury et al. [4] were able to separate the electrodes sufficiently to stabilize the measurement of resistance on the feet but not the hands of children aged 3–10 years. To overcome this problem with the hand, they placed one signal electrode on the dorsal wrist and placed one source electrode on the dorsal aspect of the forearm 6 cm proximal to the wrist. They state that a correction can be made for the reduction in the conductor length and volume but this is not easy. It would be necessary to develop prediction equations based on resistance measured with the altered placement and, as is well known, it is difficult to obtain accurate criterion values for body composition in young children.

The side on which impedance is measured must match the side measured during the development of the predictive equation. Resistance is systematically greater on the left side than the right side by about 8 ohms [41]. For example, the equations of Lukaski et al. [74] were derived from measurements on the right side but in their 1986 study these workers placed electrodes on both wrists and both ankles and used the combination for which the resistance was minimal, although the different combinations varied by less than 2%. The limbs should be positioned so that they are not in contact with each other, and they are slightly separated from the trunk. The greater their separation from the trunk, the higher the resistance. Schell and Gross [101] found that abducting the arm on which the electrodes were attached from 30 to 90° from the trunk resulted in a 12 ohm, or a 2%, increase in resistance.

RESULTS FOR WHOLE-BODY METHODS

Results of some studies using the conventional whole body method of measuring bioelectric impedance for predicting TBW and FFM are presented in Tables 6.1 and 6.2. The studies outlined below mostly employed S^2/R and additional anthropometry to develop multivariate equations predicting TBW, FFM, and %BF. It is clear that in multivariate equations the regression coefficient for the S^2/R term is no longer conceptually equivalent to a specific resistivity. It is also apparent that, although statistically significant, the gain in accuracy due to the inclusion of terms for age, sex, and additional anthropometric variables is small (i.e., <1 liter of TBW and <2 kg of FFM).

Total Body Water (TBW) and Extracellular Fluid (ECF)

It is generally assumed that the electrical current at 50 kHz is conducted by the electrolytes contained in the body water. As a result, S^2/R should be correlated more closely with this component of body composition than with any other. Studies have indeed shown that resistance is highly correlated with TBW [32, 49, 50, 76], but high correlations between a pair of variables does not mean that one is an efficient predictor of the other. The error of measurement of TBW by deuterium and tritium dilution is about 2–3%.

Equations supplied by the manufacturers of the presently available bioelectric impedance analyzers for prediction of TBW are generally considered unsatisfactory, because they systematically overpredict TBW [66]. Equations developed within studies have been reported to predict TBW from S^2/R with an rmse of 1.7 liters in 26 children [30] and with an

TABLE 6.2
Selected Equations, Which Have Been Cross-validated, for the Prediction of Body Composition Variables from Impedance and Anthropometric Variables

Authors	Age (Years)	N	Regression Equations	rmse
TBW				
Kushner and Schoeller (1986)	31.8–53.7 (means for groups differing by obesity and sex)	20 men	$0.396 (S^2/R) + 0.143 W + 8.399$	1.7 liters
		20 women	$0.382 (S^2/R) + 0.105 W + 8.315$	0.8 liters
Lukaski and Bolon-chuk (1988)	20–73	110 men and women	$0.377 (S^2/R) + 0.14 W - 0.08$ age $+ 2.9$ sex $+ 4.65$	1.5 liters
FFM				
Guo et al. (1989)	7–25	140 males	$-2.9316 + 0.6462 W - 0.1159$ Lat. Calf Skfd. -0.3753 Midax. Skfd. $+ 0.4754$ AMC $+0.1563 (S^2/R)$	2.3 kg
		110 females	$4.3383 + 0.6819 W - 0.1846$ Lat. Calf Skfd. -0.2436 Tric. Skfd. $- 0.2018$ Subscap. Skfd. $+0.1822 (S^2/R)$	
%BF				
Guo et al. (1987)	18–30	77 men	$1.5034 - 0.2790 (S^2/R) + 0.6316$ Tric. Skfd. $+ 0.3464 W$	3.3%
		71 women	$-8.4773 + 0.4296$ Bic. Skfd. $+ 1.3405$ Calf Circ. $- 0.8450 (S^2/R) + 0.3833 W$	3.2%

(S^2/R) = stature^2/resistance (cm^2/ohms); W = weight (kg); Lat. Calf Skfd. = lateral calf skinfold (mm); Midax. Skfd. = midaxillary skinfold (mm); AMC = arm muscle circumference (cm); Tric. Skfd. = triceps skinfold (mm); Subscap. Skfd. = subscapular skinfold (mm); Bic. Skfd. = biceps skinfold (mm); and Calf Circ. = calf circumference (cm).

rmse of 1.4 liters in 21 adults [28]. In 30 infants, an rmse of 0.4 liter (CV = 7.7%) was reported by Fjeld et al. [37] who successfully cross-validated their equation on 12 infants. In another study of 40 adults, the equations that were developed had an rmse of 1.75 liters and were equally accurate in the obese and the nonobese [67]. On cross-validation, these equations did not perform as well: the rmse were 2.3 liters for men and 2.9 liters for women. Lukaski and Bolonchuk [74] predicted TBW in 53 adults using S^2/R, sex, weight, and age as independent variables with an R^2 of 0.97 and rmse of 1.6 liters. The equation was cross-validated in a separate sample of 57 adults with excellent results. VanLoan and Mayclin [122] developed an equation for predicting TBW in 188 adults using S^2, weight, R, sex, and age that had an R^2 of 0.87 and rmse of 2.92 liters, but this equation was not cross-validated.

The authors of three studies concluded that impedance was satisfactory for estimating changes in TBW despite these rather high rmses [42, 67, 83]. There may be inaccuracies if the changes are interpreted as changes in FFM. As noted by Gray [42], there may be a greater loss of water than of FFM early in weight reduction by fasting and, as a result, impedance data may be misleading. This may explain why the apparent loss of FFM during weight loss is greater when calculated from body density than when calculated from S^2/R [33, 34].

A few studies have attempted to establish the relationship between ECF volume and impedance (Z) or resistance (R). In small samples, Joly [57], Thomasset et al. [117–120], Bolot et al. [16], and Gambini et al. [38] found correlations between ECF and Z ranging from 0.67 to 0.93. Lukaski and Bolonchuk [74] reported an R^2 of 0.86 and rmse of 1.17 liters for the prediction of ECF from S^2/R in 53 men and women. The prediction equation was improved slightly by the addition of weight and S^2/Xc and was cross-validated in a separate sample of 57 men and women with only a marginal loss of accuracy.

McDougall and Shizgal [77] reported significant associations between whole-body Xc and the ratios of extracellular to intracellular (E/I) mass and exchangeable sodium to potassium. Segal et al. [102] reported that Xc significantly discriminated between patients with normal E/I fluid distribution and patients with edema (abnormal overhydration of E). Lukaski and Bolonchuk [74] showed that S^2/Xc was correlated significantly with ECF ($r = 0.50$) after the association of ECF with TBW was partialled out.

Fat-free Mass (FFM)

In some studies, TBW has been estimated from S^2/R using a linear regression, and later FFM has been calculated using a constant value for the water content of FFM. Age- and sex-specific values for the water content of FFM should be applied, but the accuracy of these values is not

well-established. The use of TBW, estimated from bioelectric impedance, for calculating FFM is not recommended, because measurement
and estimation errors will be compounded. The correlations between
criterion and estimated values of FFM from these studies range from
0.70 to 0.93 [29, 62, 63, 85, 86, 103–105] with rmses from sample-
specific equations ranging from 2.7 to 4.4 kg in adults [29, 33, 34, 103–
105]. Segal et al. [103] improved their predictions by adding weight and
sex as independent variables; the rmse was then 3.1 kg. Much better
results were reported by Lukaski et al. [75] who obtained an rmse of 2.5
kg although they used only S^2/R as a predictor.

In other studies, FFM has been calculated from body density. It
should be remembered that the accuracy of the values calculated for
FFM depends on the validity of the assumption that the density of FFM
is 1.1 g/ml if Siri's equation is used. Bioelectric resistance is proportional
to the amount of water in FFM, but is independent of the amount of
bone because bone is a poor conductor. This may limit the accuracy of
estimation of FFM from body density and, consequently, the accuracy of
the prediction equation using bioelectric impedance and anthropometry. The use of multicompartment models that calculate FFM from body
density, TBW, and bone mineral to calculate criterion values for FFM
will improve accuracy.

Houtkooper et al. [52], using S^2/R to predict FFM, reported an rmse
of 2.6 kg in children aged 10–14 years. When anthropometric data were
used also, the rmse was 1.9 kg; when anthropometric data were used
alone, the rmse was 2.1 kg. This indicates that more information is
needed regarding the size and shape of the conductor than that provided
by stature. Segal et al. [105] reported a multilaboratory comparison of
the prediction of FFM from impedance and anthropometric variables in
1567 adults. The data collection procedures differed somewhat between
the laboratories, and the laboratory-specific groups differed in %BF.
Each laboratory used body density to calculate FFM and used sex-specific equations supplied by the manufacturer to predict it. These equations employed S^2/R and weight as independent variables. The rmses
were 3.7 kg for the men and 3.2 kg for the women with a systematic
overprediction of about 5.2 kg for the men and 2.7 kg for the women. In
other studies of the manufacturer's equations, Segal et al. [103] found an
rmse of 3.7 kg. Some other studies have shown that the manufacturer's
equations tend to underpredict FFM in the lean [62, 63, 103] and overestimate it in the elderly by a mean of about 6 kg [53, 110].

Segal et al. [105] also developed sex-specific equations for each laboratory sample. These workers reported that S^2 and R were better predictors as a pair than as a ratio. In the various laboratory groups, the rmse
ranged from 2.9 to 3.6 kg for men and from 2.2 to 2.5 kg for the women.
The results were good when each equation was cross-validated using
data from the other laboratories. These workers developed "obesity-

specific" equations to predict FFM in men with %BF > 20% and in women with %BF > 30%. When these equations were applied to the groups from different laboratories, the rmses were 2.4–2.5 kg for non-obese men, 3.0 kg for obese men, 1.0–2.0 kg for non-obese women, and 1.8–2.1 kg for obese women [105]. Segal and her coworkers realized that the obesity-specific equations would be difficult to apply, but they demonstrated that a preliminary categorization based on skinfold thicknesses was useful. These results can be compared with those of Hughes and Evans [53] who reported an rmse of 2.65 kg for a group of elderly subjects.

In other studies, values for FFM predicted from S^2/R have been compared with those calculated from total body potassium. Very high correlations between FFM and S^2/R values have been reported [29, 75, 76], but the values calculated from total body potassium are systematically higher than those predicted from S^2/R [29]. Presumably, this reflects the fact that FFM as predicted by S^2/R does not effectively include the skeleton.

Roche and Guo [93] derived an equation to predict FFM using data from 140 males aged 7–25 years. FFM was obtained from body density using age- and sex-specific densities [71]. All-possible-subsets regression was used to derive the prediction equation and the examination of R^2 and Mallow's Cp values showed that five independent variables should be retained in the final equation. The equation included S^2/R, weight, two skinfolds, and arm muscle circumference as independent variables. Ridge regression was used to stabilize the coefficients in the equation, and methods of robust regression were applied. This equation had an rmse of 2.31 kg and an R^2 value of 0.98.

Applying similar procedures to those of Roche and Guo [93], Guo et al. [44] used data from 140 males and 110 females, ages 7–25 years, to develop equations to predict FFM. The independent variables that were retained were weight, lateral calf skinfold, and S^2/R in each sex in addition to midaxillary skinfold and arm muscle circumference in the males and the triceps and subscapular skinfolds in the females. The equations had R^2 values of 0.98 and 0.95 and rmse values of 2.3 and 2.2 kg for the males and females, respectively. There was no tendency for these equations to overpredict or underpredict for different parts of the distribution of values for FFM. The rmses of the equations increased slightly (0.2–0.6 kg) when applied to two cross-validation groups.

Percent Body Fat (%BF)

If FFM can be estimated accurately from prediction equations using bioelectric impedance, %BF can be estimated indirectly by calculating 100 × (weight − estimated FFM)/weight. The error in this estimate of

%BF will, of course, be dependent on the error in the estimate of FFM. As an alternative, some investigators have developed equations predicting %BF directly from bioelectric impedance and anthropometry. In most of these studies, the dependent variable has been obtained from body density and is therefore affected by the amount of bone mineral present. As noted above, resistance is virtually independent of bone mineral because bone is a poor conductor of electrical currents. Furthermore, when judging the effectiveness of such predictive equations, it should be recalled that the inescapable error in the estimation of %BF from body density is about ±2.5% [70, 71].

To date, equations supplied by the manufacturers of the commercially available bioelectric impedance analyzer have been shown to perform poorly [60, 61, 68, 80, 81, 103]. These equations typically include S^2/R and weight as independent variables with equations for each sex but not for specific age groups. Some have used RW/S^2 as an index of %BF in their equations [54, 64, 103].

Lukaski et al. [75] estimated FFM from S^2/R and derived %BF. They reported rmses between %BF from body density and the derived values of 2.7 and 3.1% for men and women, respectively. Lukaski equations were applied to other groups by Jackson et al. [54] and by Colvin et al. [27] with markedly worse results. Segal et al. [103], using equations based on RW/S^2 that were supplied by the manufacturer of the impedance analyzer, reported an rmse of 6.1% for a sample of men and women. They reported lower rmses (4.4% men; 4.0% women) when they used equations that they developed [105]. These equations included R, stature, weight, and age as independent variables. Because the group studied by Segal and her coworkers included many obese individuals, they developed separate equations for the obese and the non-obese; the rmses were lower with the latter equations (3.3% men; 3.2% women). This directs attention to the fact that the reporting of results by rmse only may obscure tendencies of the equations to overestimate at low values of %BF and to underestimate at high values of %BF, as reported by several investigators [43, 47, 56, 103].

Khaled et al. [64] reported a very low rmse of 1.8% using ZW/S^2 and that the estimates from their equation using this index showed very little bias at the extremes of %BF. The use of this equation is based on the assumption that the whole body *volume* resistivity, ρ_w, is proportional to the amount of fat, or $\rho_w = \kappa F$. As noted in the discussion of physical principals above, large increases in the amount of fat will increase the total *volume* resistivity regardless of the high *tissue* resistivity of fat (see Fig. 6.4). Because $\rho_w \sim RV/L^2$, by substituting weight (W) for V, κF for ρ_w, and Z for R, the equation $ZW/L^2 \sim \kappa F$ is obtained. Through similar algebra, one can easily show that $ZW/L^2 \sim \gamma D$, where D is body density. Jackson et al. [54] considered the correlation of this index with %BF to be determined mostly by the association of body mass index, W/S^2, with %BF. Baumgartner et al. [15], however, showed that the index RW/S^2 explained a statistically significant percentage of the variance in %BF in samples of 63 men and 72 women after controlling for W/S^2. Although the coefficients of the prediction equation for the combined sexes in this study were closely similar to those reported by Khaled et al. [64], the rmse was about 5%.

Houtkooper et al. [52], in a sample of 103 children, found anthropometric variables alone or in combination with S^2/R predicted %BF with an rmse of 3.2%. Jones et al. [58], in 30 men and 29 women, predicted %BF from resistance, reactance, and hand-foot distance with an rmse of 3.2%. Guo et al. [43] developed equations using 16 possible independent variables recorded from 77 men and 71 women aged 18–30 years. Two sets of equations were developed: in one set only anthropometric variables were included and in the other set resistance was included as part of the ratio S^2/R. The final independent variables were selected by principal component analysis, followed by all-possible-subsets regression. The inclusion of S^2/R did not reduce the errors of prediction in the men, but it reduced the rmse marginally for the women from 3.8 to 3.2%. Thus, very little of the variance in %BF was explained by S^2/R after anthropometric variables had been entered. The equations of Guo et al. were applied to cross-validation groups with closely similar results. These results are similar to those reported by others [107] and suggest that %BF can be predicted with good accuracy from anthropometry alone and that the addition of S^2/R improves prediction only slightly.

Baumgartner et al. [14], using a unique approach, developed regression equations that included mean skinfold thickness, W/S^2, and the phase angle of the trunk as independent variables to predict %BF with rmses of 6% for males and 5% for females. The trunk phase angle explained a statistically significant percentage of the variance in %BF after mean skinfold thickness and W/S^2 had been entered. The bivariate correlation of %BF with trunk phase angle was as high or higher than the correlation with W/S^2 in each sex. The significance of this approach is that phase angle is independent of the geometry of the conductor. The association suggests that increased adiposity is associated with changes in cell membrane permeability or tissue interface capacitance that affect resistance and reactance differentially.

In summary, equations to predict %BF from anthropometry and resistance generally have rmses in the range 3.0–3.5%. These are quite good results considering the intrinsic error of about 2.5% that is associated with the dependent variable, but *they are not markedly better than those from anthropometry alone*. Equations using S^2/R or RW/S^2 alone have generally produced rmses of about 5%. Claims of considerably smaller rmses using these indices with no other anthropometry have not been supported by cross-validation results.

SEGMENTAL METHODS

The present whole-body bioelectric impedance methods of estimating body composition may be intrinsically prone to error due to violation of the several assumptions underlying the relation, $V = \rho L^2/R$. Even if the assumptions of uniform current distribution, isotropic structure, and homogeneous composition were met, error would arise because, given the placement of the electrodes, the conductive volume, V_c, for which R is measured is only a fraction of the target volume, V_t, of TBW or FFM. In other words, the relationship would be better expressed as, $V_t \sim (V_c/V_t)\rho S^2/R$, where the ratio V_c/V_t varies among individuals on the basis of body proportions and the amount of the total body within the electrical field. Body proportions, specifically variation between body segments in cross-sectional area, will affect this ratio because the resistance will be larger for the parts of the body with smallest circumferences [15, 89, 111]. The use of additional anthropometry in prediction equations can be seen as an attempt to correct for this problem, but alternative approaches may be available that have not been thoroughly explored. One approach is to divide the body into segments with simpler geometry (arm, leg, trunk) to which a more complete and uniform current field can be applied [111].

Specific Resistivity Approach

Chumlea et al. [21, 23, 24] have attempted to develop an alternative to the prediction equation approach that uses measurements of the lengths and resistances of the principal body segments and estimates of *volume* and *tissue* specific resistivities for these segments to directly calculate FFM. Excluding the head, the body consists of approximately five more-or-less cylindrical segments, two upper extremities (arms), two lower extremities (legs), and a trunk. Theoretically, the total conductive volume of the body can be derived from measures of the lengths of these segments and their biological resistance values according to the formula:

$$V_S = 2(\rho_a \times L_a{}^2/R_a) + 2(\rho_l \times L_l{}^2/R_l) + (\rho_t \times L_t{}^2/R_t)$$

where L_i is the length, R_i is the resistance, and ρ_i is the specific resistivity of each body segment (a = arm, l = leg, t = trunk). It is assumed that V_s will approximate total body volume more closely than the conductive volume, V_c, defined in the present whole-body method. Because the cross-sectional area varies substantially within each of these more-or-less cylindrical segments, Smith [111] suggested the addition to this equation of geometric weighting factors (G_i) for each segment. Accordingly, the equation would be rewritten as follows.

$$V_S = 2(\rho_a \times L_a{}^2/R_a)G_a + 2(\rho_l \times L_l{}^2/R_l)G_l + (\rho_t \times L_t{}^2/R_t)G_t$$

A method for the mathematical derivation of such weights, however, was not given.

Values for the segment-specific resistivities derived from anthropometric variables and taken from the previous literature [39] were used in the above equation to estimate FFM [23]. Mean absolute differences between the FFM estimated by this equation and FFM from densitometry were about 5–6 kg. The difference between the densitometric and bioelectric impedance estimates was primarily due to values used for the volume resistivity of the trunk and was correlated with %BF. Chumlea et al. [24] have also shown that an index of total subcutaneous fat mass can be calculated using a modification of this equation that takes into consideration differences between *volume-* and *muscle*-specific resistivities and proportional relationships between the body segments.

The merit of this approach is that it demonstrates the possibility of calculating body composition directly from anthropometric and bioelectric impedance measurements without the need of coefficients derived by regression procedures. A central problem is that it requires knowledge of the values of the specific resistivities ρ_i of the conductive volumes for each body segment. The assumption is made that these resistivities are constant or have very narrow ranges of variability with sex, ethnicity, and age. Theoretically, a resistivity ρ_i could be estimated for each body segment from the equation $\rho_i = V_i R_i / L_i^2$ if the true conductive volume could be accurately measured and the current was conducted uniformly. As noted in the previous discussion of tissue resistivities, this is very difficult, requiring complex geometric models and corrections for anisotropy and other effects. The present, published estimates for tissue resistivities were derived using a variety of nonstandardized and outmoded techniques from animal as well as human subjects and need to be updated [2]. Thus, the further application of this approach depends on the derivation of new estimates for tissue-specific resistivities.

Prediction from Body Segments

An alternative to the specific resistivity approach is the prediction of whole-body composition or the composition of body segments from measurements of the lengths and resistances of the segments. As in the whole body approach, this requires the formulation of regression prediction equations. The rationale for this approach was suggested by Settle et al. [106], who noted that 85% of the sum of the impedances of the arm, leg, and trunk was accounted for by the impedances for the arm and the leg, although these segments accounted for only 35% of the total body volume.

Going et al. [40] measured the lengths (L_i) and resistances (R_i) of the arm (a), leg (l), and trunk (t) and calculated indices of the form L_i^2/R for each body segment. The index for the arm (L_a^2/R_a) had the highest correlation with whole body FFM ($r > 0.93$), followed by indices for the leg (L_l^2/R_l) and the trunk (L_t^2/R_t). The sum of the segment indices was a better predictor of FFM than S^2/R (rmses 2.1 versus 3.2 kg). Baumgartner et al. [15] reported that the impedance index for the arm (L_a^2/R_a) predicted whole body FFM almost as accurately ($R^2 = 0.86$, rmse $= 4.25$ kg) as S^2/R ($R^2 = 0.90$, rmse 3.65 kg) in 135 men and women. In addition, an index of the form WR_a/L_a^2, where W is whole-body weight, predicted %BF with almost as good accuracy ($R^2s = 0.61-0.65$) as WR/S^2 ($R^2s = 0.61-0.74$).

The value of this approach is that it can be applied to individuals for whom accurate measurements of stature cannot be made, such as many elderly, chair- and bed-fast patients or amputees. Mitchell et al. [82] demonstrated the application of this approach for estimating TBW in elderly women and Vettorazzi et al. [123] have begun to develop equations for estimating body composition in amputees. Patterson et al. [89] reported that an equation including changes in impedance in each body segment predicted change in weight better than an equation based on change in impedance for the whole body.

EFFECTS OF PHYSIOLOGIC FACTORS

Although much of the early work using bioelectric impedance concerned associations with physiological factors such as basal metabolic rate and blood flow, little recent research has been directed toward the effects of physiological factors on bioelectric impedance estimates of body composition. Many physiological states, at least potentially, could alter measurements of resistance and few of these have been considered in the development of prediction equations.

Bioelectric impedance is temperature-dependent [39]. If measurements are made at 5-min intervals for 20 min, a change in the measured resistance is not noted if the subject is covered with a blanket, but there is a 2% decrease if this is not done [109]. Because in some studies, resistance is measured while the subject is wearing bathing clothes, it is important that the room be comfortably warm. If the ambient temperature is changed from 14.4 to 35°C, with corresponding skin temperatures of 24.1 and 33.4°C, there is a significant mean decrease in resistance of 35 ohms, which, using the manufacturer's equations, would decrease the predicted TBW by 2.5 liters [20]. These temperature-related effects may be due to a change in the volume of the conductor, an increase in subcutaneous blood flow, sweaty skin, or a change in the compartmental distribution of water when the temperature is raised [101]. If the measurements are made at a comfortable ambient temperature, these effects will not be present.

All the prediction equations were developed using data from individuals considered to be in a normal state of hydration. Several investigators have studied the effects of changes in hydration due to exercise and/or ingestion of water on impedance [34]. All measured whole-body resistance at 50 kHz. Stump et al. [114] found that strenuous exercise, followed by a period of fasting without water intake, increased resistance and reactance and that these changes were not reversed by drinking water during a subsequent 3-hr period. Khaled et al. [64], however, found that dehydration due to extended jogging decreased resistance and that overhydration due to ingestion of 1.2–1.8 liters of oral rehydration solution increased resistance. Guzman et al. [45] also reported that resistance was decreased when there was a loss of water due to exercise. Elsen et al. [36] found that drinking 1 liter of oral rehydration solution or electrolyte-free water or of donating 500 ml of blood did not alter substantially resistance at 50 kz. Kushner and Schoeller [67], however, found a marked decrease in resistance in one patient who developed nephrotic edema.

Hemodialysis and treatment with diuretics have been reported to produce disproportionate changes in resistance and reactance [112, 113, 124]. This suggests that phase angle may be a more sensitive indicator of acute changes in fluid volume and distribution than resistance or reactance alone. Tedner et al. [115, 116] have used impedance at 1.5 and 150 kHz to monitor changes in fluid distribution in patients during hemodialysis. In general, the use of bioelectric impedance at frequencies other than 50 kHz has not been studied with regard to differences or changes in fluid distribution that may affect body composition estimates.

There is no evidence of cyclical changes in resistance associated with menstruation, whether the subjects are taking oral contraceptives or not [22, 92, 109]. Nevertheless, because some store large amounts of water during the premenstrual period, it is good practice to avoid making measurements during the week before the expected commencement of the menstrual cycle. Diurnal differences in resistance are unimportant, as are those between values recorded during fasting and those measured 2 hr after lunch [31, 92]. Diurnal or cyclical changes in reactance and phase angle have not been studied.

The means of resistance values obtained in full inspiration are slightly higher than those obtained in full expiration [14, 36], but the differences are small and the measurements are usually made during quiet respiration.

DISCUSSION AND RECOMMENDATIONS

Baker [2], Patterson and coworkers [88, 89] and Smith [111] have outlined reasons why the current approach to using bioelectric impedance for estimating body composition has limited validity. According to electric field theory, the equation $R = \rho L/A$ is valid only for a homogenous isotropic material with a constant cross-sectional area and uniform current density distribution. Each of these assumptions is violated when the human body is the conductor. The body is a heterogeneous conductor and certain components, such as muscle tissue, are highly anisotropic. The body has a complex geometry and the cross-section, even of the limbs, is not constant. The inclusion of insulating bodies within some body segments, such as the lungs within the trunk, distorts the electrical field resulting in a nonuniform current density distribution that is very difficult to specify and which may vary among individuals. The use of "spot" electrodes may result in a nonuniform current density distribution unless the ratio of L/A is high. The source electrodes in the tetrapolar technique must be separated by a sufficient distance for deep tissue conduction of the current. If the source electrodes are too close, surface conduction may occur. Clearly, the equation $R = \rho L/A$ is not valid for the trunk, although the underlying assumptions may be met more closely for the limbs. Also, the impedance characteristics of the body segment with the smallest cross sectional area, or greatest ratio of L/A (i.e., the arm), will dominate determination of the whole-body resistance [15, 88, 106]. Arm and calf circumferences predict nearly half the variance in whole-body impedance measurements in men and women [13]. Thus, the empirical correlations demonstrated between S^2/R and TBW or FFM may be largely due to a fortuitous correlation between the impedance characteristics of the arm and/or leg and whole-body composition [15, 106].

These basic considerations and the preceding review of the literature on the theory and use of bioelectric methods allow the evaluation of current and potential approaches for estimating body composition from bioelectric impedance.

Current Whole-Body Methods

IMPEDANCE INDICES. Despite the limitations outlined by Baker [2], there is considerable evidence that, at 50 kHz, S^2/R, L_a^2/R_a, WR/S^2, WR_a/L_a^2, and phase angle have good empirical relationships to whole-body composition and can be used as indices of TBW, FFM, TBF, and %BF. Although they have limited accuracy for estimating body composition in all individuals, they may be used to grade body composition within groups in population studies. In this situation, their usefulness should be compared with that of limited anthropometry. When used as simple indices, they are more sensitive and specific in grading body composition than some other indices, such as W/S^2 [14, 15]. This approach may be most useful in epidemiologic studies and may eventually supplant the use of body mass indices, circumferences, or skinfold thicknesses for grading levels of adiposity.

PREDICTION EQUATIONS. More accurate estimates of body composition can be obtained in population studies through the use of prediction equations including anthropometry and impedance measurements rather than the use of simple impedance indices. These equations can be developed from measurements for the whole body or for a body segment, making the method applicable regardless of mobility status. A problem with the prediction equation approach is that equations developed using data for one sample generally lose accuracy when applied to another, even if the populations are similar with regard to age, sex, ethnicity, and socioeconomic status. The application of certain statistical techniques, such as robust or ridge regression, and cross-validation analyses will reduce, but may not eliminate, this problem.

There is an additional problem in the development of a plethora of competing prediction equations, as has occurred for equations predicting body fat from skinfold thicknesses. The choice of the "best" equation may not be clear. Care should be taken to use the impedance equipment applied originally in developing an equation when utilizing the equation to estimate body composition. The use of a prediction equation requires that all the independent variables be measured. This adds to the cost and difficulty of application of prediction equations and may limit their popularity. Also, in selecting an equation, one should evaluate carefully whether bioelectric impedance adds significantly to the accuracy of the prediction over and above the anthropometric variables. Despite these limitations, this approach is recommended for population studies.

SEGMENT VOLUME RESISTIVITY METHODS. The use of segment *volume* resistivities has potential as a method of calculating body composition for the whole body or a body segment of an individual, but its present use is limited by the difficulty of establishing volume resistivities accurately, especially for the trunk [23, 24]. The use of "band" rather than spot electrodes and the accurate definition of internal as well as external geometry of the segments may help to overcome some of the problems inherent in this method. Band electrodes may provide a more uniform current density distribution for complex body segments such as the trunk [2]. Smith [111] has suggested the application of two currents, one on each side of the body, as another means of obtaining a more uniform current density distribution.

The measurement of *specific* resistivities in biological conductors is technically very difficult and most resistivities given in the literature are for composite volumes or mixtures of fluids, cells, or tissues and are therefore weighted averages of at least two or more *specific* resistivities. Anatomical and physiological variation among individuals in factors such as the size, location, structure, and hydration of organs and tissues will produce variable rather than constant volume resistivities. Certain types of conductors are anisotropic so that the current is passed more easily in one direction than in any other. Skeletal muscle is highly anisotropic and the volume resistivity for a body segment will be influenced by variation in the alignments of muscle fibers with regard to the direction of flow of the current. This problem may be minor in the arm and leg when impedance is measured longitudinally, but may result in large differences for the trunk [15].

Future Possibilities

IMPEDANCE IMAGING. Baker [2] describes an approach called the "finite element technique," presently used for analyses of physiologic changes such as the cardiac cycle, that is basic to impedance imaging. In this method, a body segment is partitioned into discrete volumes with defined anatomical locations. Each volume is assigned a resistivity presumed to be characteristic of the tissues present at each location. Changes in the size, shape, and orientation of the volumes can be calculated based on measured changes in impedance. This is essentially a dynamic refinement of the segment volume resistivity approach and is subject to the same limitations. The volume-elements must be homogenous and discrete in order for specific resistivities to be assigned. Because volume resistivities may vary over a range, the definition of boundaries between volumes can be a problem for elements that are similar in their electrical properties. "Edge detection" algorithms used commonly in CT and MRI imaging can be applied, but partial or overlapping volume effects may be more serious and anisotropy must be considered. Spatial resolution is presently poor in impedance imaging and may limit the usefulness of this approach for quantifying body composition [3].

MULTIFREQUENCY METHODS. The multifrequency approach may be most useful in the clinical setting where interest primarily concerns changes in the distribution of body fluids. The ratio of low (1–5 kHz) to high (>200 kHz) frequency resistances and reactance and phase angle at moderate (50 kHz) frequency may provide useful indices of the ratio of ECF/TBW or estimates of body cell mass [55, 74, 77, 115, 116]. More complex multifrequency techniques consisting of the analysis of impedance or admittance plots remain to be developed [1, 59]. Analysis of the components of impedance plots, such as characteristic frequency (f_c), β dispersion or relaxation time, and depression angle, is complex mathematically and requires numerical solutions on computers. Nonetheless, this approach may have considerable potential for monitoring changes in fluid distribution due to therapy (dialysis, diuretics), dehydration, or exercise [59]. The multifrequency approach may be useful in impedance imaging also [3].

CONCLUSION

Despite more than 100 years of research on bioelectric impedance, a great deal remains to be learned regarding factors influencing the conduction of electric currents in the living body. The application of bio-electric methods to the estimation of body composition is relatively recent. The present whole-body and segment prediction equation approaches are based on empirical and possibly fortuitous correlations. Nonetheless, these correlations have been demonstrated to be high across a range of samples with different sex, age, and ethnic compositions. Although the estimates obtained have been demonstrated generally to be accurate, this accuracy may be less for some types of individuals, especially patients with abnormal levels or distributions of body fluids. Thus, the present methods are most appropriate for epidemiologic and other field studies in which they will provide quick, easy, reliable, and accurate estimates of body composition in normal individuals. Several more complex approaches are being developed, including the analysis of complex impedance plots and impedance imaging, that have potential for body composition studies, but these will be useful mostly in clinical or laboratory settings and the implementation of these methods may be several years into the future.

ACKNOWLEDGMENTS

This work was supported by Grant HD-12252 from the National Institutes of Health, Bethesda, MD.

REFERENCES

1. Ackmann JJ, Seitz MA: Methods of complex impedance measurements in biologic tissue. *Crit Rev Biomed Eng* 11:281–311, 1984.
2. Baker LE: Principles of the impedance technique. *IEEE Eng Med Biol* 3:11–15, 1989.
3. Barber DC: A review of image reconstruction techniques for electrical impedance tomography. *Med Phys* 16:162–169, 1989.
4. Barillas-Mury C, Vettorazzi C, Molina S, Pineda O: Experience with bioelectrical impedance analysis in young children: sources of variability. In Ellis KJ, Yasumura S, Morgan WD (eds): *In Vivo Body Composition Studies.* Upton, Long Island, NY, The Institute of Physical Sciences in Medicine, Brookhaven National Laboratory, 1987, pp 87–90.
5. Barnett A: The basic factors in proposed electrical methods for measuring thyroid function. I. The effect of body size and shape. *West J Surg Obstet Gyn* 45:322–326, 1937a.
6. Barnett A: The basic factors in proposed electrical methods for measuring thyroid function. II. Resistance and Q factor in relation to sex and physical conformation. *West J Surg Obstet Gyn* 45:380–387, 1937b.
7. Barnett A: The basic factors in proposed electrical methods for measuring thyroid function. III. The phase angle and the impedance of the skin. *West J Surg Obstet Gyn* 45:540–554, 1937c.
8. Barnett A: The basic factors in proposed electrical methods for measuring thyroid function. IV. A combined study of the skin and deep tissues of the 2, 3, and 4-electrode techniques. *West J Surg Obstet Gyn* 45:612–623, 1937d.

9. Barnett A: The phase angle of normal human skin. *Am J Physiol* 93:349–366, 1938.
10. Barnett A: Electrical method for studying water metabolism and translocation in body segments. *Proc Soc Exp Biol Med* 44:142–147, 1940a.
11. Barnett A: Seasonal variations in the epidermal impedance of human skin. *Am J Physiol* 129:306–307, 1940b.
12. Barnett A, Bagno S: The physiological mechanisms involved in the clinical measure of phase angle. *Am J Physiol* 114:366–382, 1936.
13. Baumgartner RN, Chumlea WC, Roche AF: Associations between bioelectric impedance and anthropometric variables. *Hum Biol* 59:235–244, 1987.
14. Baumgartner RN, Chumlea WC, Roche AF: Bioelectric impedance phase angle and body composition. *Am J Clin Nutr* 48:16–23, 1988.
15. Baumgartner RN, Chumlea WC, Roche AF: Estimation of body composition from segment impedance. *Am J Clin Nutr* 50:221–226, 1989.
16. Bolot J-F, Fournier G, Bertoye A, Lenoir J, Jenin P, Thomasset A: Determination de la masse maigre chez l'adulte par la methode de l'impedance. *Nouv Press Med* 6:2249–2251, 1977.
17. Brazier MAB: The impedance angle test for thyrotoxicosis. *West J Surg Obstet Gyn* 43:514–527, 1935.
18. Burger HC, van Milaan JB: Measurements of the specific resistance of the human body to direct current. *Acta Med Scand* 114:584–607, 1943.
19. Burger HC, van Dongen R: Specific electric resistance of body tissues. *Physics Med Biol* 5: 431–447, 1960.
20. Caton JR, Mole PA, Adams WC, Heustis DS: Body composition analysis by bioelectrical impedance: effect of skin temperature. *Med Sci Sports Exerc* 20:489–491, 1988.
21. Chumlea WC, Baumgartner RN, Roche AF: Segmental bioelectric impedance measures of body composition. In Ellis KJ, Yasumura S, Morgan WD (eds): *In Vivo Body Composition Studies*. Upton, Long Island, New York, The Institute of Physical Sciences in Medicine, Brookhaven National Laboratory, 1987, pp 103–107.
22. Chumlea WC, Roche AF, Guo S, Woynarowska B: The influence of physiologic variables and oral contraceptives on bioelectric impedance. *Hum Biol* 59:257–270, 1987.
23. Chumlea WC, Baumgartner, RN, Roche AF: The use of specific resistivity to estimate fat-free mass from segmental body measures of bioelectric impedance. *Am J Clin Nutr* 48:7–15, 1988.
24. Chumlea WC, Baumgartner RN, Roche AF: Fat volumes and total body fat from impedance. *Med Sci Sports Exerc* 20:S82, 1988.
25. Cole KS, Curtis HJ: Bioelectricity: electric physiology. In Glasser O (ed): *Medical Physics*. Chicago, IL, Year Book, 1944, pp 82–90.
26. Cooley WL, Lehr JL: Electrical impedance fluctuation as an indicator of fluid volume changes in a living organism. *Biomed Eng* 8:313–315, 1972.
27. Colvin A, Pollock M, Graves J, Braith R: Validity and reliability of three different bioelectrical impedance analyzers. *Med Sci Sports Exerc* 20:S82, 1988.
28. Conway JM: Total body water (TBW) determined by bioelectric impedance analysis (BIA) in older women. *FASEB J* 2:1202, 1988.
29. Cordain L, Whicker RE, Johnson JE: Body composition determination in children using bioelectrical impedance. *Growth, Develop Aging* 52:37–40, 1988.
30. Davies PSW, Preece MA, Hicks CJ, Halliday D: The prediction of total body water using bioelectrical impedance in children and adolescents. *Ann Hum Biol* 15:237–240, 1988.
31. de Cossio TG, Diaz E, Delgado HL, Mendoza R, Gramajo L: Accuracy and precision of bioelectrical impedance and anthropometry for estimating body composition. In Ellis KJ, Yasumura S, Morgan WD (eds): *In Vivo Body Composition Studies*. Upton, Long Island, New York, The Institute of Physical Sciences in Medicine, Brookhaven National Laboratory, 1987, pp 195–200.

32. Delozier M, Gutin B, Wang J, Zybert P, Basch C, Rips J, Shea S, Contento I, Irigoyen M, Pierson R: Bioimpedance-derived estimates of body composition in 4–8 year olds. *Med Sci Sports Exerc* 20:S31, 1988.

33. Deurenberg P, Westrate JA, Hautvast JGAJ: Changes in fat-free mass during weight loss measured by bioelectrical impedance and by densitometry. *Am J Clin Nutr* 49:33–36, 1989.

34. Deurenberg P, Weststrate JA, van der Kooy, K: Body composition changes assessed by bioelectrical impedance measurements. *Am J Clin Nutr* 49: 401–403, 1989.

35. Ducrot H, Thomasset A, Joly R, Jungers F, Lenoir J, Eyraud C: Determination du volume des liquids extracellulaires chez l'homme par la mesure de l'impedance corporelle totale. *Presse Med* 78:2269–2272, 1970.

36. Elsen R, Siu M-L, Pineda O, Solomons NW: Sources of variability in bioelectrical impedance determinations in adults. In Ellis KJ, Yasumura S, Morgan WD (eds): *In Vivo Body Composition Studies*. Upton, Long Island, New York, The Institute of Physical Sciences in Medicine. Brookhaven National Laboratory, 1987, pp 184–188.

37. Fjeld CR, Freundt-Thurne J, Schoeller DA: Validation of bioelectrical impedance for predicting total body water in well and malnourished children. *FASEB J* 3:A1053, 1989.

38. Gambini D, Raggueneau JL, Spector M, Levante A, Thurel C: Détermination des volumes extracellulaire et intracellulaire par mesure de l'impédance corporelle totale. Comparison avec les techniques isotopiques. *Agressologie* 21:219–224, 1980.

39. Geddes LA, Baker LE: The specific resistance of biological material—a compendium of data for the biomedical engineer and physiologist. *Med Biol Eng Comput* 5:271–293, 1967.

40. Going SB, Lohman TG, Wilmore JH, Boileau RA, Van Loan M, Sinning W, Golding L, Carswell C: Segmental versus whole body bioelectrical impedance measurements for estimation of body composition. *Med Sci Sports Exerc* 19:S39, 1987.

41. Graves JE, Pollock ML, Colvin AB, Van Loan M, Lohman TG: Comparison of different bioelectrical impedance analyzers in the prediction of body composition. *Am J Hum Biol* 1:603–612, 1989.

42. Gray DS: Changes in bioelectrical impedance during fasting. *Am J Clin Nutr* 48:1184–1187, 1988.

43. Guo S, Roche AF, Chlimlea WC, Miles DS, Pohlman RL: Body composition predictions from bioelectric impedance. *Hum Biol* 59:221–233, 1987.

44. Guo S, Roche AF, Houtkooper L: Fat-free mass in children and young adults predicted from bioelectric impedance and anthropometric variables. *Am J Clin Nutr* 50:435–443, 1989.

45. Guzman MJ, Elsen R, Padilla A, Solomons NW, Whalen C, Siu M-L, Mazariegos M, Molina S, Neufeld L, Rosas A, Barillas-Mury C, Canales D, Vettorazzi C, Beltranena F, Pineda O: Body composition determinations by bioelectrical impedance in Olympic-Class Athletes at the Third Central American Games. In Ellis KJ, Yasumura S, Morgan, WD (eds): *In Vivo Body Composition Studies*. Upton, Long Island, NY, The Institute of Physical Sciences in Medicine, Brookhaven National Laboratory, 1987, pp 108–113.

46. Hartman C, Bowers RW, Liu NY: Relationships between bio-resistance body composition analyzer and hydrostatic methods for body composition. *Med Sci Sports Exerc* 20:S82, 1988.

47. Helenius MYT, Albanes D, Micozzi MS, Taylor PR, Heinonen OP: Studies of bioelectric resistance in overweight, middle-aged subjects. *Hum Biol* 59: 271–277, 1987.

48. Hodgdon JA, Fitzgerald PI: Validity of impedance predictions at various levels of fatness. *Hum Biol* 59:281–298, 1987.

49. Hoffer EC, Meador CK, Simpson DC: A relationship between whole body impedance and total body water volume. *Ann NY Acad Sci* 170:452–461, 1970.

50. Hoffer BC, Meador CK, Simpson DC: Correlation of whole-body impedance with total body water volume. *J Appl Physiol* 27:531–534, 1969.

51. Horton JW, Van Ravenswaay AC: Electrical impedance of the human body. *J Franklin Inst* 20:557–572, 1935.

52. Houtkooper LB, Lohman TG, Going SB, Hall MC, Harrison GG: Validity of whole-body bioelectrical impedance analysis for body composition assessment in children. *Med Sci Sports Exerc* 19:S39, 1987.

53. Hughes VA, Evans WJ: Assessment of fat-free mass in an older population using bioelectric impedance. *Fed Proc* 46:1186, 1987.

54. Jackson AS, Pollock ML, Graves JE, Mahar MT: Reliability and validity of bioelectrical impedance in determining body composition. *J Appl Physiol* 64:529–534, 1988.

55. Jenin P, Lenoir J, Roullet C, Thomasset AL, Bucrot H: Determination of body fluid compartments by electrical impedance measurements. *Aviat Space Environ Med* 46:152–155, 1975.

56. Johnson K, Rinke W, Burman K: Comparison of circumference, skinfold, bioelectrical impedance and hydrodensitometry to estimate percent body fat during weight loss. *Fed Proc* 46:575, 1987.

57. Joly R: *Signification de l'impedance globale du corps humain à 1 kHz.* Unpublished Thèses de Médecine, Université de Lyon, France, 1964.

58. Jones TE, Araujo J, Thomas TR, Aguiar CA: Predicting body density by electrical impedance. *Med Sci Sports Exerc* 20:S41, 1988.

59. Kanai H, Haeno M, Sakamoto K: Electrical measurement of fluid distribution in legs and arms. *Med Prog Technol* 12:459–470, 1987.

60. Katch FI, Keller B, Solomon R: Validity of BIA for estimating body fat in cardiac and pulmonary patients, and Black and White men and women matched for age and body fat. *Med Sci Sports Exerc (Suppl)* 18:S17, 1986.

61. Katch FI, Solomon RT, Shayevitz M, Shayevitz B: Validity of bioelectrical impedance to estimate body composition in cardiac and pulmonary patients. *Am J Clin Nutr* 43:972–973, 1986.

62. Keller B, Katch FI: Validity of bioelectrical resistive impedance for estimation of body fat in lean males. *Med Sci Sports Exerc* 17:272, 1985.

63. Keller B, Katch FI: Validity of BIA to predict body fat in underfat, normal and overfat males and females and comparison to sex-specific fatfold equations. *Med Sci Sports Exerc (Suppl)* 18:S17, 1986.

64. Khaled MA, McCutcheon MJ, Reddy S, Pearman PL, Hunter GR, Weinsier RL: Electrical impedance in assessing human body composition: the BIA method. *Am J Clin Nutr* 47:789–792, 1988.

65. Kushner RF, Kunigk A, Alspaugh M, Aodronis P, Lietch K, Schoeller DA: Validation of bioelectric 1 impedance analysis (BlA) as a measurement of change in body composition in obesity. *FASEB J* 3:A335, 1989.

66. Kushner RF, Schoeller DA, Bowman BB: Comparison of total body water (TBW) determination by bioelectrical impedance analysis (BIA), anthropometry, and D_2O dilution. *Am J Clin Nutr* 39:658, 1984.

67. Kushner RF, Schoeller DA: Estimation of total body water by bioelectrical impedance analysis. *Am J Clin Nutr* 44:417–424, 1986.

68. Lawlor MR, Crisman RP, Hodgdon JA: Bioelectrical impedance analysis as a method to assess body composition. *Med Sci Sports Exerc* 17:271, 1985.

69. Löfgren B: The electrical impedance of a complex tissue and its relation to change in volume and fluid distribution. A study of rat kidneys. *Acta Physiol Scand* 23 (Suppl 81):5–50, 1951.

70. Lohman TG: Skinfolds and body density and their relation to body fatness: a review. *Hum Biol* 53:181–225, 1981.

71. Lohman TG: Applicability of body composition techniques and constants for children and youths. In Pandolf KB (ed): *Exercise and Sport Sciences Reviews*. New York, MacMillan, 1986, pp 325–357.
72. Lohman TG, Going SB, Golding L, Wilmore JH, Sinning W, Boileau RA, Van Loan M: Interlaboratory bioelectric resistance comparisons. *Med Sci Sports Exerc* 19:S40, 1987.
73. Lohman TG, Roche AF, Martorell R (eds): *Anthropometric Standardization Reference Manual*. Champaign, IL, Human Kinetics, 1988.
74. Lukaski HC, Bolonchuk WW: Estimation of body fluid volumes using tetrapolar bioelectrical impedance measurements. *Aviat Space Environ Med* 59:1163–1169, 1988.
75. Lukaski H, Bolonchuk WW, Hall CB, Siders WA: Validation of tetrapolar bioelectrical impedance method to assess human body composition. *J Appl Physiol* 60:1327–1332, 1986.
76. Lukaski HC, Johnson PE, Bolonchuk WW, Lykken GI: Assessment of fatfree mass using bioelectric impedance measurements of the human body. *Am J Clin Nutr* 41:810–817, 1985.
77. McDougall D, Shizgal HM: Body composition measurements from whole body resistance and reactance. *Surg Forum* XXXVI: 42–44, 1986.
78. Marks C, Katch VL: Stature as body conductor length for whole-body resistance. *Am J Clin Nutr* 46:864–865, 1987.
79. Martorell R, Habicht J-P, Haas J: Predicting total body water from bioelectrical impedance in children. *Ann Hum Biol* 16:173–174, 1989.
80. Miles DS, Stevens AG: Body composition measured by bioelectrical impedance and hydrostatic weighing. *Med Sci Sports Exerc* 17:272–273, 1985.
81. Miranda E, Lombard VP, Troxel RK, Menon J: Percentage body fat estimation via bioelectrical impedance, hydrostatic weighing and skinfold assessment. *Med Sci Sports Exerc* 18:S31, 1986.
82. Mitchell C, Baumgartner RN, Chumlea WC: Estimation of body composition from segmental measures of bioelectric impedance in the elderly. In *Book of Abstracts, International Symposium on In Vivo Body Composition Studies, 1989*. Toronto, Canada, 1989.
83. Morgan P, Golden B, Bocage C, Golden M: Prediction of total body water and body composition from bioelectrical impedance measures in Jamaican infants during recovery from severe malnutrition. *FASEB J* 3:A1053, 1989.
84. Nyboer J: *Electrical Impedance Plethysmography*. Springfield, IL, Charles C Thomas, 1959.
85. Nyboer J: Electrorheometric properties of tissues and fluids. *Ann NY Acad Sci* 170:410–420, 1970.
86. Nyboer J: Percent body fat by four terminal bio-electrical impedance and body density in college freshmen. In *Proceedings of the Vth International Conference on Electrical Bio-Impedance*, August, 1981, Tokyo, 1981.
87. Nyboer J, Khalafalla AS: Workable volume and flow concepts of biosegments by electrical impedance plethesmography. *TIT J Life Sci.* 2:1–13, 1972.
88. Patterson R: Body fluid determinations using multiple impedance measurements. *IEEE Eng Med Biol*, 3: 16–18, 1989.
89. Patterson R, Ranganathan C, Engel R, Berkseth R: Measurement of body fluid volume change using multisite impedance measurements. *Med Biol Eng Comput* 26:33–37, 1988.
90. Rathbun E, Pace N: Studies on body composition. *J Biol Chem* 158:667–676, 1945.
91. Renk CM, Breitlow LV, Sander E: Body composition analysis: correlation between skinfold and bioelectrical impedance measurements in a normal population. *Med Sci Sports Exerc* 18:S31, 1986.

92. Roche AF, Chumlea WC, Guo S: *Identification and Validation of New Anthropometric Techniques for Quantifying Body Composition* (Technical Report No. TR-86-058). Natick, MA, U.S. Army Natick Research, Development and Engineering Center, 1986.
93. Roche AF, Guo S: Biased estimation of fat-free mass. *1988 Proceedings of the Biopharmaceutical Section,* Annual Meeting of the American Statistical Association, New Orleans, LA, August 22–25. 188–191, 1988.
94. Runge PJ, Eisenman PA, Johnson SC: Effects of exercise induced dehydration on bioelectrical impedance analyzation to determine body composition. *Med Sci Sports Exerc* 19:S38, 1987.
95. Rush S, Abildskov JA, McFee R: Resistivity of body tissues at low frequencies. *Circ Res* 12:40–50, 1963.
96. Salansky I, Utrata F: Electrical tissue impedance of the organism and its relation to body fluids. *Physiol Biochem* 21:295–304, 1972.
97. Schwan HP, Kay CF: Specific resistance of body tissues. *Circ Res* 4:664–670, 1956a.
98. Schwan HP, Kay CF: The conductivity of living tissues. *Ann NY Acad Sci* 65:1007–1013, 1956b.
99. Schwan HP, Li K: Capacity and conductivity of body tissues at ultrahigh frequencies. *Proceed IRE* 4:1735–1740, 1953.
100. Schwan HP: Electrical properties of body and impedance plethysmography. *IRE Trans Med Electron* PGME-3:32–45, 1955.
101. Schell B, Gross R: The reliability of bioelectrical impedance measurements in the assessment of body composition in healthy adults. *Nutr Rep Int* 36:449–459, 1987.
102. Segal KR, Kral IG, Wang J, Pierson RN, Van Itallie TB: Estimation of body water distribution by bioelectrical impedance. *Fed Proc* 46:1334, 1987.
103. Segal KR, Gutin B, Presta E, Wang J, Van Itallie TB: Estimation of human body composition by electrical impedance methods: a comparative study. *J Appl Physiol* 58:1565–1571, 1985.
104. Segal KR, Van Loan M, Fitzgerald PI, Hodgdon JA, Van Itallie TB: Estimation of lean body mass by bioelectrical impedance: a multicenter validation study. *Med Sci Sports Exerc (Suppl)* 19:S39, 1987.
105. Segal KR, Van Loan M, Fitzgerald PI, Hodgdon JA, Van Itallie TB: Lean body mass estimation by bioelectrical impedance analysis: a four-site cross-validation study. *Am J Clin Nutr* 47:7–14, 1988.
106. Settle RG, Foster KR, Epstein BR, Mullen JL: Nutritional assessment: whole body impedance and body fluid compartments. *Nutr Cancer* 2:72–80, 1980.
107. Sinning WE, Moore CE, Boileau RA, Going S, Lohman TG, Van Loan M, Wilmore JH: Variability of estimating body composition measures by skinfolds and bioresistance. *Med Sci Sports Exerc* 19:S39, 1987.
108. Siri WE: Body composition from fluid spaces and density, analysis of methods. In Brozek J, Henschel A (eds): *Techniques for Measuring Body Composition.* Washington, D.C., National Academy of Sciences, Natural Resources Council, 1961.
109. Siu M-L, Elsen R, Mazariegos M, Solomons NW, Pineda O: Evaluation through sequential determination of the stability of bioelectrical impedance measurements for body composition analysis. In Ellis KJ, Yasumura S, Morgan WD (eds): *In Vivo Body Composition Studies.* Upton, Long Island, NY, The Institute of Physical Sciences in Medicine, Brookhaven National Laboratory, 1987, pp 189–194.
110. Siu M-L, Mazariegos M, Pineda O, Solomons NV: Estimation of body composition of Guatemalan elderly by anthropometric indices and bioelectrical impedance analysis. *FASEB J* 2:1423, 1988.
111. Smith DN: Body composition by tetrapolar impedance measurements—correlation or con? In *Proceedings of the VIIth International Conference on Electrical Bio-Impedance,* May, 1987, Portschach, Austria, 1987.

112. Spence JA, Baliga R, Nyboer J, Seftick J, Fleischmann L: Changes during hemodialysis in total body water, cardiac output and chest fluid as detected by bioelectric impedance analysis. *Trans Am Soc Artif Intern Organs* 25:51–55, 1979.

113. Subramanyan R, Manchanda SC, Nyboer J, Bhatia ML: Total body water in congestive heart failure. A pre and post treatment study. *J Assoc Physicians India* 28:257–262, 1980.

114. Stump CS, Houtkooper LB, Hewitt MJ, Going SB, Lohman TG: Bioelectric impedance variability with dehydration and exercise. *Med Sci Sports Exerc* 20:S82, 1988.

115. Tedner B, Lins L-E, Asaba H, Wehle R: Evaluation of impedance technique for fluid-volume monitoring during hemodialysis. *Int J Clin Monitor Comput* 2:3–8, 1985.

116. Tedner B, Lins L-E: Fluid volume changes during hemodialysis monitored with the impedance technique. *Artif Organs* 9:416–427, 1985.

117. Thomasset A, Lenoir J, Jenin MP, Roullet C, Ducrot MH: Appreciation de la situation electrolytique tissulaire par le rapport des impedances globales du corps humain en base et haute frequence. *Rev Med Aer Spat* 46:312–315, 1973.

118. Thomasset A: Bio-electrical properties of tissues. *Lyon Med* 209:1325–1352, 1963.

119. Thomasset A: Mesure du volume des liquides extra-cellulaires par la methode electro-chimique signification biophysique de l'impedance a I kilocycle du corps humain. *Lyon Med* 214:131–143, 1965.

120. Thomasset A: Proprietes bio-electriques des tissus mesures de l'impedance en clinique signification des courbes obtenues. *Lyon Med* 207:107–118, 1962.

121. Tokunaga K, Matsuzawa Y, Ishikawa K, Tarui S: A novel technique for the determination of body fat by computed tomography. *Int J Obes* 7:437–445, 1988.

122. Van Loan M, Mayclin P: Bioelectrical impedance analysis: is it a reliable estimation of lean body mass and total body water? *Hum Biol* 59:299–309, 1987.

123. Vettorazzi C, Barillas C, Pineda O, Solomons NW: A model for assessing body composition in amputees using bioelectrical impedance analysis. *Fed Proc* 46:1186, 1987.

124. Zebatakis PM, Gleim GW, Vitting KE, Gardenswartz M, Agrawal M, Michelis MF, Nicholas JA: Volume changes effect electrical impedance measurement of body composition. *Med Sci Sports Exerc (Suppl)* 19:S40, 1987.

125. Zillikens MC, Conway JM: Estimation of lean body mass in black adults by total body impedance. *Fed Proc* 46:1335, 1987.

7
Human Body Segment Inertia Parameters: A Survey and Status Report

J. GAVIN REID, Ph.D
ROBERT K. JENSEN, Ph.D.

The researcher interested in studying the human body in dynamic situations has long been confronted with the problem of how to adequately describe body motion in quantitative terms. Unlike a rigid object where there is a relatively straightforward relationship between the forces producing motion and the translation and rotation of the object, the human body is more realistically represented by a system of linked segments that reposition during movement. The linear acceleration and, consequently, velocity and displacement of a segment are dependent on both the segment mass and the sum of all of the external forces, including muscle forces, acting on the segment. Angular acceleration, velocity, and displacement are dependent on both the segment principal moments of inertia and the external moments applied to the segment [70]. The researcher, then, must know the mass, location of the center of mass, and the inertia tensor of each body segment. These are the body segment inertia parameters. Without these parameters it is not possible to proceed with simulation or optimization of human movement, using the direct dynamics approach, nor to analyze human movement, using the inverse dynamics approach. Consideration of a movement would have to be restricted to a kinematic description without precise reference to the forces creating the movement.

The purpose of this paper is to review the literature concerning the segment inertia parameters and to draw conclusions as to the current state of our understanding of these parameters. Studies in this area can be classified conveniently into those conducted on cadavers and those in which living subjects were used. An alternative classification is by methodology, where the prospect of applying each method to cadavers and living subjects can be considered. The major methodologies for measuring or estimating segment inertia parameters can be classified into direct measurement, immersion, reaction change, photogrammetry, mathematical modelling, and radiation.

Unfortunately, to date there are no results from the studies of segment inertia parameters, which are universally accepted as indicating the protocol to be followed for estimating these parameters. It is evident from anthropometric surveys that a wide range of differences in inertia

225

parameters can be expected between and within various populations, such as males and females, different races, occupational groups, and sports groups [51]. Furthermore, considerable changes in parameters will occur across the life span as individuals grow, develop, and age. In order to become acceptable, a protocol will have to be judged across the expected range of inertial parameters.

CADAVER STUDIES

Attempts to provide data on segment inertia parameters began in the 19th century with the onset of cadaver studies. These studies consisted of sectioning cadavers into segments and measuring the parameters directly. One of the earliest studies was conducted by Harless [22] in Germany, who dismembered each of two male cadavers into 15 segments. Each of the segments had the soft tissue end-flaps sewn up to prevent tissue fluid loss. Each segment was weighed and the center of mass determined using a balance platform with the segment positioned in a state of equilibrium. The accuracy of the balance method is questionable, however, and the shift in tissue caused by the sewing of the end-flaps would have also affected the results. Furthermore, both of the cadavers were decapitated prisoners and thus had lost unknown quantities of fluid prior to segment dismemberment. The cadavers were then left unfrozen, thus making it certain that further fluid loss occurred. Such losses would have affected the estimation of segment mass.

In estimating the center of mass of the two trunk segments, Harless preceded by almost a century the modern method of modelling the body segments mathematically. He represented the upper torso as a truncated cone and the lower torso as an elliptical solid. Using anthropometric measurements from the cadaver and an assumed density of 1.066 g·cm^{-3} he was able to estimate the segment masses and the centers of mass. The accuracy of the assumed density would have affected his results.

Braune and Fischer [8, 9] collected data from three muscular male cadavers, thought to be representative of the average German soldier. Segment centers of mass were determined by the suspension method, where three thin metal rods were driven through the segment at right angles to the three cardinal planes. The segment was then suspended in turn from each rod and the intersection of the three vertical equilibrium planes was taken as the center of mass. Braune and Fischer also determined the moments of inertia about the longitudinal axis and a second axis perpendicular to the longitudinal axis by using a compound pendulum approach. Unlike the study by Harless, their cadavers were frozen to prevent tissue and fluid loss during dismemberment. Freezing, however, changes body fluid to ice, thereby increasing volume, decreasing density, and affecting the measured inertia parameters.

Dempster [15] using eight male cadavers, conducted the most extensive study on segment inertia parameters to that date. Primary joints of the limbs were frozen in a mid-flexed position and then transected through the apparent center of rotation. This midflexion position was thought to distribute the mass more equitably between segments. After weighing each segment, segment mass centers were determined using a balance plate. Segment moments of inertia were measured using the compound pendulum method and results were presented for parallel transverse axes through the mass center and proximal joint center. Dempster's study is regarded as one of the most comprehensive of the cadaver studies and the proportions reported for mass with respect to total mass and radius to the mass center and radius of gyration with respect to link length have been used extensively in biomechanics research. It must be remembered, however, that his data are from a small number of males aged 52–83 years, all of whom were emaciated to some extent.

Research on segment inertia parameters was also pursued in Japan by Mori and Yamamoto [47] and Fujikawa [19]. Both of these studies involved the dissection of six cadavers, three males and three females. Due to the incomplete reporting of techniques by Mori and Yamamoto and obvious inaccuracies found in Fujikawa's paper, little significance can be attached to their findings. However, their research was an attempt to determine racial and sex differences but, as has been pointed out by Miller and Nelson [46], these data should not be combined statistically with those for Caucasian cadavers.

Clauser et al. [14] dissected a sample of 13 male cadavers in order to facilitate the prediction of segment inertia parameters from anthropometric measures. Unlike previous studies, Clauser et al. used preserved cadavers, which permitted sampling over an extended time period and thus a larger sample. The density of the preservation solution was 1.0615 g·cm^{-3} [14], which was close to the average density of healthy young men (1.063 g·cm^{-3}). [6]. The effect of the preserving solution on total body density therefore was considered to be negligible.

Using techniques similar to those of their predecessors, Clauser et al. [14] measured the mass and the center of mass of each segment. Unfortunately, segment moments of inertia were not measured. Unlike the others, Clauser et al. also measured 73 anthropometric variables and used cine- and still-roentgenograms to more accurately locate the centers of rotation needed for segmentation. A stepwise regression computer program was then applied, which selected the best three predictor variables from the anthropometric variables, for segment weight and location of the center of mass.

Partial dissections have also been used to measure the inertias of selected segments. Liu et al. [42] measured the moments of inertia about three orthogonal axes through sections of the torso of eight cadavers. Becker [5] extended the procedure for determining the moments of inertia by measuring the ellipsoid of inertia and thus the principal moments and axes of the heads of nine cadavers. The studies of segment moments of inertia were reviewed by Chandler et al. [12] and found to be restricted to nonprincipal axes and/or too few segments. Reynolds [56], however, in a review for NASA concluded that the moments of inertia about the anatomical axes closely approximate the principal moments about the principal axes.

Chandler et al. [12] have produced the most comprehensive cadaver study of segment moments of inertia. Segment mass, center of mass, and anthropometric parameters were also measured. Six male embalmed cadavers, which had been stored for at least 1 year were dismembered using segmentation planes similar to those reported by Clauser et al. [14]. The mean age was 54.3 years with a standard deviation of 7.4 years. Principal moments of inertia and the directional angles of the principal moments were calculated for the three segments of the upper extremity and the lower extremity, the head, and the torso. Styrofoam specimen holders were used with six swing axes to determine the moments and products of inertia, a procedure that has been extended and further validated by Lephart [41]. Simple linear regression equations were derived to predict mass and the principal moments from body mass and segment volume. Although Chandler et al. cautioned that the data could not be construed to reflect population parameters due to the limited number of specimens, the study has been used to estimate segment principal moments. Hinrichs [27] used the anthropometric measures from Chandler et al. as predictor variables for the transverse and longitudinal principal moments. The computed multiple linear regressions were restricted to two predictor variables because of the small number of specimens. Forwood et al. [18] used a scaling procedure based on weight and segment length or stature in an attempt to improve the accuracy of the estimate of segment principal moments. Morlock and Yeadon [48] used single variable and multivariable regression to predict the principal moments and came to the conclusion that, although the use of equations based on Chandler's data is questionable, a curvilinear fit should be used because there is a theoretical basis for doing so and the equations are more appropriate outside the sample range.

Barter [4] attempted to increase the size of the sample of cadavers by combining results from different studies. The validity of Barter's regression equations is questionable, however, due to the different methodologies used in the studies. These equations were updated by Reynolds [56], Clauser et al. [14], and Chandler et al. [12] to those from Braune and Fischer [8], and Dempster [15].

Stereophotogrammetry is a technique that can be used to estimate the shape and volume of irregular objects, such as the body segments [16]. Pairs of cameras are used to record the front and back surfaces of the body, and body shape is then reconstructed from the coordinates. If density is specified, inertia parameters can be calculated. McConville and Clauser [45] have compared the inertia parameters from six cadavers [12] with estimates from stereophotographs of the intact specimens. Different densities were used in the calculations. The density assumption of $1 \text{ g} \cdot \text{cm}^{-3}$ produced a mean error in body weight estimation of 5%, the average segment density from Chandler et al. [12] gave a difference of 2.1% and the average segment density from Clauser et al. [14] produced a difference of 9.4%. Similar differences were found for the whole-body principal moments of inertia. These results may be misleading, however, as the stereophotogrammetric technique has been shown to overestimate body volume when applied to living subjects.

The mathematical modelling technique pioneered by Harless [22] can be extended to a representation of all segments by geometric shapes. The personalized model of the body developed by Hanavan [21] has been examined by Chandler et al. [12]. Using the anthropometry from the six cadavers and the Tieber and Lindemuth [65] modifications to the Hanavan model, Chandler et al. calculated the absolute difference between the measured and predicted segment principal moments of inertia. With the actual segment masses used to estimate density, the average errors ranged from 4.4 to 112.5%. The ellipsoidal head, the elliptical cylinder trunk, and the spherical hands were least acceptable. Further modifications with a longer trunk and spherical head produced some improvements but it was concluded that the shapes used to model the segments are not adequate.

In recent years it has been recognized that computed tomography (CT) can be used to estimate the distribution of segment mass. Successive scans are taken, which are transverse to the longitudinal axis of the segment, and the attenuation data are interpreted as CT numbers representative of the absorption characteristics of the object. The computerized system has the capacity to contrast absorption coefficient differences of about 1%, compared with 5% for conventional x-ray. The different tissues can be differentiated, but the images for bone are clearer than those for the soft tissues. A computerized image, using grey-scale gradients, is then produced. Through calibration, the physical density can be estimated and the mass within definable boundaries calculated. Calibration checks against unknown densities and masses produced mean errors of 0.8 and 2.16%, respectively, for test samples of woods and graphite [49]. Henson et al. [25] have measured soft tissue and bone densities using dual energy scans and shown that different calibration gradients are needed for the two types of tissue. Errors of less than 1.3% were reported for the phantoms, and the mean errors for cross-sectional samples from a cadaver leg were 1.33–2.9% with error due to noise of up to 3.8%. Small increments of volume and the tissue density estimated from the three-dimensional computer images are used to estimate the distribution of the mass [28]. This technique has been applied to cadaver segments. Rodrigue and Gagnon [57] used CT to estimate the segment densities of 20 forearms of six male and four female embalmed cadavers. The mean error for the estimation of segment density was 2.1% and the segment was represented as three density regions; the wrist, central, and elbow regions. They found that, when the segment was represented by 20 transverse elliptical zones [29, 67] and CT densities were used in place of assumed uniform densities, the difference in mass centroid was less than 1%. Ackland et al. [2] used dual energy scanning densities for the leg segment [25] and area measured from the scans and found errors of 3.5% for measured mass and 2.6% for measured transverse axis moment of inertia compared to estimates based on Dempster's [15] uniform density. Although the estimates were based on only six zones, the results suggest that shape representation may be a greater source of error than the uniform density assumption.

The most comprehensive study of cadavers using CT scans has been by Huang. He scanned several child cadavers but has reported in detail only one of the specimens, a 3-year-old female child [28]. A series of 99 transverse scans was taken and area, mass, center of mass, and inertia tensor calculated for each section. Mass, density, and sectional inertias, I_{xx}, I_{yy}, I_{zz}, were presented as profiles based on the body longitudinal axis. The estimated mass was also distributed within a 15-segment model.

Cadaver studies have the advantage of permitting direct measurement of segment inertia parameters. These direct measurements can then be used to check the accuracy of the parameter estimates determined from other techniques. Direct or indirect comparisons can be made. Direct comparisons involve both the estimation and measurement of a parameter on a cadaver, for example, a CT scan estimate and a direct measurement of the mass of a segment. Very little research has been directed to this mode of validation. The primary emphasis has been on proportions, using body mass and segment lengths, and predictions, using anthropometric parameters and statistical regression. It is rare for these predictions to be checked against independent measures, such as the procedure used by Morlock and Yeadon [48] where their estimates based on the data of Chandler et al. [12] were compared with the contralateral limb. Indirect comparisons can also be made. The estimated parameter can be compared to cadaver studies. For example, segment proportional radii of gyration estimated from a mathematical model could be compared to data from cadaver studies. The primary disadvantages of the cadaver studies are due to sampling and the adequacy of the measurements. Samples are small and not representative of the population under investigation. This is particularly so for females, children, adolescents and younger adults, and populations other than Caucasians and Japanese. The difficulties associated with conducting cadaver studies make it unlikely that larger and more representative samples of the various populations will be drawn in the near future. Inconsistency in the sectioning of segments and in measurement procedures make it difficult to compare the results of different studies. For principal moments, the work by Chandler et al. [12] is the most comprehensive to date but these researchers caution against generalizing from their sample. The remaining inertia parameters can also be judged from the work of Dempster [15] and Clauser et al. [14], with the latter study providing the largest sample of the three. These samples are of elderly, male Caucasians and the findings should be restricted to that population.

LIVE SUBJECT STUDIES

The use of living subjects offers the possibility of sampling populations more adequately by increasing the size of the sample and through purposive selection. For some of the techniques used to estimate inertia parameters, it is relatively easy to obtain subjects. Other techniques are potentially more hazardous and their application is restricted. However, the result has been that the samples reported are generally larger and more representative of a wider range of populations than the cadaver samples. In the absence of criterion measures for the inertia parameters, the question of the accuracy of the estimates has to be approached through a variety of validation procedures. The most common of these involves checking the estimates of whole body inertia parameters against the more readily obtainable whole body measures.

One of the most simple techniques for estimating segment inertia parameters is the immersion technique. Using the assumption that the segment is homogeneous and of known density, the mass, radius to the mass center, and the moment of inertia relative to the anterior-posterior or transverse axis can be estimated. Volume is determined from the volume of the displaced fluid and multiplied by density to give the mass. By reimmersion to half the original volume, the plane of the center of mass can be estimated. Moment of inertia is estimated by displacing successive small equal volumes of fluid and then measuring the distance from the reference axis to the center of each successive volume. Using the parallel axis theorem and treating each volume as a cylinder, the moment of inertia is calculated [46]. Plagenhoef et al. [54] performed the water immersion technique on 135 college-aged athletes, 100 females and 35 males, to estimate segment mass as a percentage of total mass. Center of gravity calculations based on volume proportions of Clauser et al. [14] were carried out on 16 subjects. Three trunk segments were defined and the estimated inertia parameters were compared to values from a dissected male. The major limitation of the water immersion technique is the difficulty with measuring precise volume on living subjects. Planes of segmentation are difficult to judge, the immersion tubes have to fit the segments as closely as possible, and it is difficult for the subject to hold a steady position during measurement. These problems are compounded when partial volumes are being estimated. The assumption of uniform average density also affects the accuracy of the estimate. It is evident that the different tissues have different densities, but the detailed effect of this distribution on the center of mass and the moments and products of inertia is not known at this time.

Segment mass has been estimated by reaction change [16, 69]. The subject is placed on a horizontal board, which is supported at both ends on knife edges. One end is supported by a sensitive scale and the other is the reference axis. It is assumed that the distance from the joint axis to the center of mass of the segment to be measured is known. The change in reaction moment, when the segment is moved from the horizontal to a vertical position with its center of mass above the joint axis, is used to estimate segment mass, based on the principle of moments. The reaction change technique is difficult to apply to many segments.

Segment moments of inertia have also been estimated using the quick-release method and oscillation techniques. Bouisset and Pertuzon [7] restrained the segment by using a fixed moment of force that was suddenly released, and the moment of inertia about the supporting joint axis was then calculated from the peak angular acceleration. Bouisset and Pertuzon measured the moment of inertia of the forearm and hand about the transverse elbow axis of 11 subjects. Hatze [23] estimated segment moments of inertia about a joint axis from damped oscillations of the lower extremity and the leg/foot segments of a single subject. Allum and Young [1] used forced sinusoidal oscillation to determine the moments of inertia of the forearm and hand about the elbow axis of four subjects. Peyton [52] has developed a-further oscillation technique with moment of inertia estimated from frequency. A comprehensive study of limb moments of inertia was conducted on 34 young adults by Stijnen et al. [63] using gravitational force in a modified quick-release method. Several segments were tested and their results compared to those of the Hatze [23] technique, Dempster [15], and the mathematical model of Hanavan [21]. A major limitation of these approaches is the inaccessibility of many of the body segments and axes.

Stereophotogrammetry has also been used to estimate the shape of segments of live subjects. Herron et al. [26] measured surface points on cross-sections at 2-inch intervals with the points ordered serially around the cross-section. Using triangles as the elemental area, mass, centers of mass, and moments and products of inertia were calculated for the cross-sectional slices and for the segments. Body density was assumed to be uniform. This technique was used with a sample of 37 children, males and females 3–7 years of age [13]. Volume and principal volume moments of inertia (cm^5) were calculated for 15 segments. However, the method was found to overestimate body volume substantially. A sample of 46 adult females [72] , age 21–45 years, with the body divided into 17 primary segments including a subdivision of the proximal thigh flap, was also evaluated using stereophotogrammetry. Density was assumed to be constant at 1 $g \cdot cm^{-3}$. Regression equations were developed to predict the segment inertias from anthropometric parameters. The method was found to overestimate body volume by approximately 10% compared to results of an immersion technique [40]. A further study was conducted on 31 male subjects [45] with similar results and overestimations. That sample was designed to represent the extreme ends of the stature/weight distribution as well as the mean. Stereophotogrammetry, then, has been applied to diverse populations and the results reported in detail. The technique is limited by the equipment costs for recording and analyzing surface shape, the time needed for analysis, and the accuracy of the volume estimates.

The mathematical modelling technique is based on the representation of a segment or its component parts by geometric shapes of known density. These geometric models have become increasingly complex. Whitsett [68] refined an earlier model by Simmons and Gardner [59] into a 14-segment collection of frustums of right circular cones, an elliptical cylinder, spheres, an ellipsoid and rectangular parallelepipeds with inertia parameters calculated for each geometric form. Segment densities were from Dempster [15]. A personalized mathematical model by Hanavan [21] consisted of 15 geometric shapes dependent on the anthropometry of an individual [57] with segment mass predicted using Barter's regression equations [4]. Segment lengths and diameters were based on 25 anthropometric measurements with the head represented by an ellipsoid of revolution, upper and lower torso by right elliptical cylinders, the hands by solid spheres, and the remaining segments by frustums of right circular cones. The body center of mass was within 1.8 cm of the measured value and whole-body estimated moments of inertia were checked against the experimental data on 66 subjects [57]. One-half of the predicted values for the x and y axes were within 10% and for the z axis within 20% of the experimental data. The Hanavan model is simple to use but is clearly an oversimplification of the shape of the segments and is not considered to be very accurate.

The geometric model can be refined by defining more appropriate geometric shapes for various parts of the body and deriving the equations for the inertia parameters. Hatze [24] constructed such a 17-segment model based on 242 anthropometric measures and reported its use on a 12-year-old boy and three adults including a female. The shoulders were treated as separate segments, and variations in tissue density within segments, based on profiles reported by Dempster [15] and skinfold measures, were allowed. Estimated segment volumes were compared with immersion volumes, while the mass centroid radius proportions and principal moments about the transverse centroidal axis were compared with cadaver values reported by Dempster [15] and, for four segments, values from the suspension method [23]. Most comparisons were favorable and, despite the time required to measure the anthropometric variables, the method appears to be effective for determining inertia parameters. Sprigings et al. [62] have used the Hatze, Dempster, and Clauser et al. methods to predict the location of the total body center of mass during an airborne movement performed by 10 university-aged males. The mean square error for acceleration due to gravity was least for Hatze, followed by Dempster and then Clauser et al.

A mathematical model that considers the body to be composed of 16 segments and transverse elliptical zones 2-cm wide has also been developed [29]. The elliptical zone approach was used originally by Weinbach [67] who constructed body profiles, such as for volume and the moment of inertia, about the soles of the feet. The mathematical model uses the major and minor axes measured from projected orthogonal photographic images of the body to calculate the inertial properties of the zone. Through summation across zones and summation across segments, the mass, mass centroid, and principal moments and axes of the segments and body can be estimated. Segment densities were from Clauser et al. [14].

A sample of 12 males, originally 4, 6, 9, and 12 years and of different body types, has been followed over 9 years using the elliptical zone model. With attrition, a total of 88 annual observations has been made. Changes in the segment mass proportions, mass centroid radius proportions, and transverse axis radius of gyration proportions over 3 years [33] and 9 years [32, 35] have been reported from this mixed longitudinal study. The results showed some changes with age and were consistent with the adult values reported by Zatsiorski and Seluyanov [73]. The growth of segment mass and volume [34, 37] is different between segments and consistent with the principles of cephalocaudad and distal to proximal development [64]. Intraindividual changes and interindividual differences in segment principal moments have been reported [38] and the results by the age of adulthood found to compare favorably with the results from Chandler et al. [12] and Zatsiorski and Seluyanov [73]. Changes have also been investigated for whole-body moments of inertia [30, 31].

Segment mass and principal moments of inertia, estimated from the elliptical zone model, have been predicted [39] using the curvilinear regression rationale presented by Morlock and Yeadon [48] and the anthropometric parameters reported by Hanavan [21]. With the exception of the head and foot, all parameters were predicted effectively with a common variance (R^2) of at least 0.8. These results suggest that extrapolation beyond the sample age range, 4–20 years, should be feasible.

The elliptical zone method has also been used in a study of 255 Japanese male and female children, 3–15 years of age [71]. The children were classified into 18 groups according to age, sex, and body type and the results presented as means and standard deviations for mass, mass centroid, and radius of gyration proportions for the frontal, sagittal, and longitudinal axes through the segment mass centroid. Finch [17] has applied the elliptical zone method to 15 females, 20–29 years of age and classified into endo-, meso-, and ectomorphs. Segment inertias were compared to the results for the adult female from Hatze's study [24] and the values reported by Plagenhoef [53] and Zatsiorski and Seluyanov [73] and found to be reasonable. Significant differences were found between the different body types. Ackland et al. [3] used anthropometric measures as predictor variables for the elliptical zone estimates of the trunk, thigh, and leg inertia parameters. The data were from a longitudinal study of 13 subjects at 6-month intervals over 2.5 years. The prediction equations accounted for 84–94% of the variance.

The mass of the body obtained from the sum of the segment masses can be compared to the measured mass. The error reported by Jensen [32, 35] is −0.82% (SD = 2.63%, n = 88), which is similar to the error of 1.65% reported by Yokoi et al. [71] and the 0.77% (SD = 0.29%) error in the study by Finch [17]. Yokoi et al. [71] also estimated the body center of mass for five postures using a reaction board. The standard errors for the estimated locations were 1.64–3.0% (n = 29). A similar elliptical zone technique has been developed by Tupling et al. [66] and they report high day-today and intra-/interobserver reliability. The elliptical zone results were similar to mass estimations based on immersion and to center of mass and moment of inertia estimations based on anthropometry where the segment is subdivided into five frustums of cones. The leg segment of a live subject has also been analyzed [2]. Compared to estimates based on density and area measured from six CT scans, the elliptical zone estimates of mass and transverse moment of inertia were different by 3 and 2.7%, respectively. The elliptical zone model has been applied to some of the largest samples of males and females, children and adults and different races using both cross-sectional and longitudinal methodologies. A number of different checks have been made on its accuracy including indirect comparisons with cadaver studies. Refinements are needed, however, and the effects of variations in density and shape within segments need further investigation.

Segment mass and its distribution can be measured using radiation techniques. Casper et al. [11] were the first investigators to use radiation techniques to estimate the mass, center of mass, and moment of inertia of an object. Their technique was based on the premise that the ability of an object to absorb or attenuate high energy γ rays is proportional to the density of the object and relatively independent of its composition. A computer controlled the scanning of the object and calculated the results. Parameters for wood, metal, and plastic test objects were within ±1% of criterion values. Volume, and thus density, is not estimated by the γ radiation technique. The γ mass scanning technique was applied to biological tissue by Brooks and Jacobs [10]. They compared scanner estimates for a leg of lamb to measurements based on weighing, reaction change, and pendulum techniques and found errors of 1, 2.1, and 4.8%, respectively. The procedure was developed further by Zatsiorski and Seluyanov [73] for tests on humans. Segment masses, mass centroids, and principal moments of inertia about anteroposterior, transverse, and longitudinal axes were measured for 100 adult male subjects. Three segments were specified for the upper extremity, lower extremity, and the torso, with the head the 16th segment. The sample had a mean age of 23.8 years (SD = 6.2). The inertia parameters estimated by the scanner technique were predicted using multiple linear regression models with weight and stature as predictor variables. These regressions were supplemented by a further set in which segment anthropometric measures were used as predictor variables with the accuracy of prediction improved by the use of the segment-specific variables [74]. Although direct comparisons between the segment inertia parameters estimated by the γ radiation technique and cadavers are not given in the two reports by Zatsiorski and Seluyanov [73, 74], comparisons with other techniques indicate that the results for most parameters are plausible. The size of their sample makes the application of their results to young adult male Caucasians reasonable. However, it is unlikely that approval would be given for the use of the γ radiation technique in most laboratories.

CT and magnetic resonance imaging (MRI) have also been used on living subjects. Reid [55] analyzed the trunk segment of two male and two female subjects, ranging in age from 46 to 68 years, using computed tomography scans at 1-cm intervals. The mean center of mass of the trunk segment was 49.35% of the distance from the line joining the greater trochanters across the superior surface of the pubic symphysis to the suprasternal notch. Also, the segmental mass of the trunk was found to be 52.58% of total body weight. The accuracy and precision of CT and MRI area measurements has been evaluated by Zhu et al. [75]. They concluded that for the phantoms and scanners tested, the errors were smaller for CT and the scan time is less. Mungiole and Martin [50] have demonstrated the feasibility of using magnetic resonance imaging for estimating segment inertia parameters of living subjects. They determined the mass, mass centroid, and transverse moments of inertia of the lower leg of 12 males and concluded that the values were within the range reported for the traditional cadaver studies. The cost and availability of facilities for CT and MRI measurements of segment inertia parameters are likely to restrict the use of these techniques, however.

CONCLUSIONS AND RECOMMENDATIONS

In selecting a method or set of prediction equations for segment inertia parameters, it is recommended that the age and sex of the sample be given primary consideration. Generally, because of individual differences, it is preferable to use a mathematical model [24, 29], rather than simple proportions, so as to account for body shape. For elderly males, the results of the cadaver studies are appropriate, although strongly biased toward Caucasians. The tables provided by Reynolds [56] combine the results of the different studies effectively. Prediction equations for the principal moments from Chandler et al. [12] or using Chandler's data should be employed, with the study by Morlock and Yeadon [48] providing the best rationale. Appropriate results for the population of elderly females are not available. Until cadaver and radiation studies become available, the use of mathematical models, which take into consideration the changes in segment volume with aging [24, 29], are recommended. Predictions from the radiation studies by Zatsiorski and Seluyanov [73, 74] appear to be the most appropriate for adult males. The anthropometry of their sample is similar to the results of surveys conducted in other countries [51]. If direct measurements are preferred it is recommended that a mathematical model [24, 29] be used. Proportions from the study by Finch [17] or the elliptical zone mathematical model [29] should be used for young adult females.

For male children and adolescents, the changes in parameters with growth are substantial and predictions based on the elliptical zone mathematical model [35, 39] should be used. The study by Yokoi et al. [71] shows that there are developmental patterns for young females distinct from those of young males. However, their results may not be appropriate for other races. It is recommended that a mathematical model [29] be used directly. Segment inertia parameters for male and female Japanese children and adolescents should be based on the research by Yokoi et al. [71]. For the elderly, the cadaver studies by Mori and Yamamoto [47] and Fujikawa [19] should be used.

Although mathematical models appear best suited to take into consideration changes and differences in segment volume, further improvements are needed. Shape sensing should be improved by using three-dimensional techniques [36, 43, 60, 61] and verified using phantoms and cadavers. Also, further research is needed to establish the density profiles of the various segments from MRI, CT scans [2] and cadaver studies.

ACKNOWLEDGMENTS

This research was supported by Grants A7154 and A3693 from the Natural Sciences and Engineering Research Council of Canada and the School of Graduate Studies and Research, Queen's University, Canada. In addition, the assistance of the Faculty of Physical Education, University of Otago, New Zealand, in the preparation of this manuscript is gratefully acknowledged.

REFERENCES

1. Allum JHJ, Young LR: The relaxed oscillation technique for the determination of the moment of inertia of limb segments. *J Biomech* 9:21–25, 1976.
2. Ackland TR, Henson PW, Bailey DA: The uniform density assumption: its effect upon the estimation of body segment inertial parameters. *Int J Sports Biomech* 4:146–155, 1988.
3. Ackland TR, Blanksby BA, Bloomfield J: Inertial characteristics of adolescent male body segments. *J Biomech* 21:319–328, 1988.
4. Barter JT: Estimation of the mass of body segments. Technical Report, TR-57–260, Wright-Patterson Air Force Base, OH, 1957.
5. Becker EB: Measurement of mass distribution parameters of anatomical segments. In *Proceedings of the Sixteenth Stapp Conference*. Society of Automotive Engineers Report, 720964, New York, 1972.
6. Behnke AR: Comment on the determination of whole body density and a résumé of body composition. In Brozck J. (ed): *Techniques for Measuring Body Compositions*. Washington D.C., National Research Council, 1961, pp 118–133.
7. Bouisset S, Pertuzon E: Experimental determination of the moments of inertia of limb segments. In Wartenweiler J (ed): *Biomechanics I* New York, S Karger, 1968, pp 106–109.
8. Braune W, Fischer O: Uber den Schwerpunkt des menschlichen Korpers, mit Rucksicht auf die Austrustung des deutschen Infanteristen. *Abhandlugen der mathematische-physichen classe der Konigl, Sashsischen Gesellschaften der Wissenschaften* 26:561–672, 1889.
9. Braune W, Fischer O: Bestimung der tragheitsmomente des mensch lichen korpers and seiner glieder. *Abh d Math Phys 1C d K Sachs Gessel d Wiss* 18:409–492, 1892.
10. Brooks CB, Jacobs AM: The gamma mass scanning technique for inertial anthropometric measurement. *Med Sci Sports* 7:290–294, 1975.
11. Casper RM, Jacobs AM, Kennedy ES, McMaster IB: On the use of gamma ray images for determination of body segment parameters. Paper, presented at Quantitative Imagery in Biomedical Sciences, Houston, TX, 1971.
12. Chandler RF, Clauser CE, McConville JT, Reynolds HM, Young JW: Investigation of inertial properties of the human body. Technical Report, AMRL-TR-74-137, Wright-Patterson Air Force Base, OH, 1975.
13. Chandler RF, Snow CC, Young JW: Computation of mass distribution characteristics of children. In Coblentz AM, Herron RE (eds.): *Proc Soc Phot-Optic Instruments Eng* 166:158–161, 1978.
14. Clauser CE, McConville JT, Young JW: Weight, volume and center of mass of segments of the human body. AMRL Technical Report, TR-69-70, Wright-Patterson Air Force Base, OH, 1969.
15. Dempster WT: Space requirements of the seated operator. WADC Technical Report, 55-159, Wright-Patterson Air Force Base, OH, 1955.

16. Drillis R, Contini R, Bluestein M: Body segment parameters. *Artif Limbs* 8:44–66, 1964.
17. Finch CA: Estimation of body segment parameters of college age females using a mathematical model. Unpublished Masters Thesis, University of Windsor, 1985.
18. Forwood MR, Neal RJ, Wilson B: Scaling segmental moments of inertia for individual subjects. *J Biomech* 18:755–761, 1985.
19. Fujikawa K: The center of gravity in the parts of the human body. *Okajimas Folia Anat Jpn* 39:117–125, 1963.
20. Gagnon M, Rodrigue D: Determination of the forearm parameters by anthropometry, immersion and photography methods. *Res Q* 50:188–198, 1979.
21. Hanavan EP: A mathematical model of the human body. Technical Report, Aerospace Medical Research Laboratory TR64-102, Wright-Patterson Air Force Base, OH, 1964.
22. Harless E: Die statischen momente der menschlichen gliedmassen. *Abhandlugen der Mathemat.-Physickalichen Classe der Koeniglichen Bayerischen Akademie der Wissenschaften,* 8:69–96, 257–294, 1860.
23. Hatze H: A new method for the simultaneous measurement of the moment of inertia, the damping coefficient and the location of the centre of mass of a body segment. *Eur J Appl Physiol* 34:217–226, 1975.
24. Hatze, H: A mathematical model for the computational determination of parameter values of anthropomorphic segments. *J Biomech* 13:833–843, 1980.
25. Henson PW, Ackland T, Fox RA: Tissue density measurement using CT scanning. *Australas Phys Eng Sci Med* 10:162–166, 1987.
26. Herron RE, Cuzzi JR, Goulet DV, Hugg JE: Experimental determination of mechanical features of adults and children. DOT-HS-231-2-397, Washington D.C., U.S. Department of Transportation, 1974.
27. Hinrichs RN: Regression equations to predict segmental moments of inertia from anthropometric measurements: an extension of the data of Chandler *et al. J Biomech* 18:621–624, 1985.
28. Huang HK, Suarez FR: Evaluation of cross-sectional geometry and mass density distributions of humans and laboratory animals using computerized tomography. *J Biomech* 16:821–832, 1983.
29. Jensen RK: Estimation of the biomechanical properties of three body types using a photogrammetric method. *J Biomech* 11:349–358, 1978.
30. Jensen RK: The effect of a 12-month growth period on the body moments of inertia of children. *Med Sci Sports Exerc* 13:238–242, 1981.
31. Jensen RK: The growth of children's moment of inertia. *Med Sci Sports Exerc* 18:440–445, 1986.
32. Jensen RK: Changes in segment mass, radius and radius of gyration, four years to adulthood. In Allard P, Gagnon M (eds.): *Proceedings of the North American Congress on Biomechanics.* Montreal, Canada Society for Biomechanics, 1986, pp 227–228.
33. Jensen RK: Body segment mass, radius and radius of gyration proportions of children. *J Biomech* 19:359–368, 1986.
34. Jensen RK: Growth of estimated segment masses between four and sixteen years. *Hum Biol* 59:173–189, 1987.
35. Jensen RK: Changes in segment inertia proportions between four and twenty years. *J Biomech* 22:529–536, 1989.
36. Jensen RK, Marshall RN: Object surface coordinates from a single camera and two mirrors. In Baumann JU, Herron RE (eds): *Biostereometrics '88* SPIE Volume 1030, Bellingham, WA, International Society for Optical Engineering, 1989, pp 325–329.
37. Jensen RK, Nassas G: A mixed longitudinal description of body shape growth. In Coblentz AM, Herron RE (eds): *Biostereometrics '85* SPIE Volume 602, Bellingham, WA, International Society for Optical Engineering, 1986, pp 130–135.
38. Jensen RK, Nassas G: Growth of segment principal moments of inertia between four and twenty years. *Med Sci Sports Exerc* 20:5, 1988.

39. Jensen RK, Wilson BD: Prediction of segment inertias using curvilinear regression. In Cotton CE, Lamontagne M, Robinson DGE, Stothart JP (eds): *Proceedings of the Fifth Biennial Conference of the Canadian Society for Biomechanics*. Spodym, London, Ontario, 1988.

40. Kaleps I, Clauser CE, Young JW, Chandler RF, Zehner GF, McConville JT: Investigation into the mass distribution properties of the human body and its segments. *Ergonomics* 27:1225–1237, 1984.

41. Lephart SA: Measuring the inertial properties of cadaver segments. *J Biomech* 17:537–543, 1984.

42. Liu YK, Laborde JM, Van Buskirk WC: Inertial properties of a segmented cadaver trunk: their implications in acceleration injuries. *Aero Med* 42:650–657, 1971.

43. Magnant D: Three dimensional measurement on the human body using a scanning laser beam. In Coblentz AM, Herron RE (eds): *Biostereometrics '85* SPIE Volume 602, Bellingham, WA, International Society for Optical Engineering, 1986, pp 130–135.

44. McConville JT, Churchill TD, Kaleps I, Clauser CE, Cuzzi J: Anthropometric relationships of body and body segments moments of inertia. Aerospace Medical Research Laboratory Report, AFAMRL-TR-80-119, Wright-Patterson Air Force Base, OH, 1980.

45. McConville JT, Clauser CE: Anthropometric assessment of the mass distribution characteristics of the living human body. *Proceedings 6th Congress International Ergonomics Association*, College Park, MD, Human Factors Society, 1976, pp 379–383.

46. Miller DI, Nelson RC: *Biomechanics of Sport*. Philadelphia, Lea & Febiger, 1973.

47. Mori M, Yamamoto T: Die Massenanteile der einzelnen Korperabschnitte der Japaner. *Acta Anat (Basel)* 37:385–388, 1959.

48. Morlock M, Yeadon MR: Regression equations for segment inertia parameters. In Allard P, Gagnon M (eds): *Human Locomotion IV*. Montreal, Canadian Society for Biomechanics, 1986, pp 231–232.

49. Mull RT: Mass estimates by computed tomography: physical density from CT number. *Am J Roent* 143:1101–1104, 1984.

50. Mungiole M, Martin PE: Estimating segmental inertial properties: magnetic resonance imaging versus existing methods. In Allard P, Gagnon M (eds): *Human Locomotion IV*. Montreal, Canadian Society for Biomechanics, 1986, pp 229–230.

51. NASA Staff: *Anthropometry Source Book: Volume II, A Handbook of Anthropometric Data*. Houston, TX, National Aeronautics and Space Administration, 1978.

52. Peyton AJ: Determination of the moment of inertia of limb segments by a simple method. *J Biomech* 19:405–410, 1986.

53. Plagenhoef S: *Patterns of Human Motion*. Englewood Cliffs, NJ, Prentice-Hall, 1971.

54. Plagenhoef S, Evans FG, Abdelnour T: Anatomical data for analyzing human motion. *Res Q Exerc Sport* 54:169–178, 1983.

55. Reid JG: Physical properties of the human trunk as determined by computed tomography. *Arch Phys Med Rehabil* 65:246–250, 1984.

56. Reynolds HM: The inertial properties of the body and its segments. In *Anthropometric Source Book: Volume II, A Handbook of Anthropometric Data*. Houston, TX, National Aeronautics and Space Administration, 1978.

57. Rodrigue D, Gagnon M: Validation of Weinbach's and Hanavan's models for computation of physical properties of the forearm. *Res Q Exerc Sports* 55:272–277, 1984.

58. Santschi WR, DuBois J, Omoto C: Moments of inertia and centers of gravity of the living human body. Technical Report TDR-63-36, Wright-Patterson Air Force Base, OH, 1963.

59. Simmons JC, Gardner MS: Self-maneuvering for the orbital worker. Technical Report TR-60-748, Wright-Patterson Air Force Base, OH, 1960.

60. Schmitt F, Maitre H, Clainchard A, Lopez-Krahe J: Acquisition and representation of object surface data. In Coblentz AM, Herron RE (eds): *Biostereometrics '85* SPIE Volume 602, Bellingham, WA, International Society for Optical Engineering, 1986, pp 130–135.

61. Sheffer D, Schaer A, Baumann J: Stereophotogrammetric mass distribution parameter determination of the lower body segments for use in gait analysis. In Baumann JU, Herron RE (eds): *Biostereometrics '88* SPIE Volume 1030, Bellingham, WA, International Society for Optical Engineering, 1989, pp 361–368.

62. Sprigings EJ, Burko DB, Watson LG, Laverty WH: An evaluation of three segmental methods used to predict the location of the total body CG for human airborne movements. *J Hum Mov Stud* 13:57–68, 1987.

63. Stijnen VV, Willems EJ, Spaepen AJ, Peeraer L, Van Leemputte M: A modified release method for measuring the moment of inertia of the limbs. In Matsui H, Kobayashi K (eds): *Biomechanics VIII-B*. Champaign, IL, Human Kinetics, 1983, pp 1138–1143.

64. Tanner JM: *Growth at Adolescence*, ed 2. Oxford, Blackwell, 1962.

65. Tieber JA, Lindemuth RW: An analysis of the inertial properties and performance of the astronaut maneuvering system. Unpublished Masters Thesis, U.S. Air Force Institute of Technology, Wright-Patterson Air Force Base, OH, 1965.

66. Tupling SJ, Pierrynowski MR, Forsyth RD: Anthropometric estimates of the human body using photogrammetry. In Thornton-Trump AB (ed): *Human Locomotion III*. Winnipeg, Canadian Society for Biomechanics, 1984.

67. Weinbach AP: Contour maps, center of gravity, moment of inertia and surface area of the human body. *Hum Biol* 10:356–371, 1938.

68. Whitsett CE: Some dynamic response characteristics of weightless man. Unpublished Masters Thesis, U.S. Air Force Institute of Technology, Wright-Patterson Air Force Base, OH, 1962.

69. Williams M, Lissner HR: *Biomechanics of Human Motion*. Philadelphia, WB Saunders, 1962.

70. Winter DA: *Biomechanics of Human Movement*. New York, John Wiley & Sons, 1979.

71. Yokoi T, Shibukawa K, Ae M: Body segment parameters of Japanese children. *Jpn J Phys Ed* 31:53–66, 1986.

72. Young JW, Chandler RF, Snow CC, Robinette KM, Zehner GF, Lofberg MS: Anthropometric and mass distribution characteristics of the adult female. Technical Report, Oklahoma City, OK, FAA Civil Aeromedical Institute, 1983.

73. Zatsiorski V, Seluyanov V: The mass and inertial characteristics of the main segments of the human body. In Matsui H, Kobayashi K (eds): *Biomechanics VIII-B*. Champaign, IL, Human Kinetics, 1983, pp 1152–1159.

74. Zatsiorski V, Seluyanov V: Estimation of the mass and inertia characteristics of the human body by means of the best predictive regression equations. In Winter DA, Norman RW, Wells RP, Hayes KC, Patla AE (eds): *Biomechanics IX-B*. Champaign, IL, Human Kinetics, 1985, pp 233–239.

75. Zhu XP, Checkley DR, Hickey DS, Isherwood I: Accuracy of area measurements made from MR images compared with computed tomography. *J Comp Assist Tomogr* 10:96–102, 1986.

8

Physical Activity and Coronary Heart Disease Risk Factors during Childhood and Adolescence

JEAN-PIERRE DESPRÉS, Ph.D
CLAUDE BOUCHARD, Ph.D.
ROBERT M. MALINA, Ph.D.

INTRODUCTION

Coronary heart disease (CHD) is the major cause of death in North America [58]. Understanding the biological mechanisms that underlie its development is thus of paramount importance. Epidemiological studies have identified several important risk factors for CHD, including plasma lipoprotein levels, blood pressure, smoking, diabetes, obesity, sedentary life-style, and familial history of cardiovascular disease [15]. Many of the risk factors are apparent during childhood and adolescence as is evidence for the early stages of atherosclerosis, the main factor responsible for CHD. Atherosclerosis and the risk factors are related, so it may be possible, at least theoretically, to prevent or slow down the progression of atherosclerosis through modification of an individual's risk factor profile. In adult populations, for example, a substantial amount of scientific evidence suggests that regular aerobic exercise, through its favorable effects on risk factors such as plasma lipoprotein levels [39, 40, 90, 91], blood pressure [50, 73], and glucose homeostasis [7, 86], may have beneficial effects on the progression of atherosclerosis.

Because lipid deposition in the intima-media of blood vessels begins in childhood [60, 61, 92], it is important to study the potential effects of the level of habitual physical activity or regular exercise on cardiovascular risk factors during growth. However, interpretation of available data is often difficult, as growth processes may interact with the effects of regular exercise. On the other hand, it appears that very high risk children tend to remain categorized as such from the growing years into adulthood [69]. Modification of life-style, including increased regular physical activity, may, therefore, contribute to an improved metabolic condition of these children and, perhaps, slow lipid accumulation in the arteries.

This paper briefly reviews the main risk factors for CHD and their evolution during growth. Evidence for the beneficial effects of regular physical activity on risk factors is also discussed.

ATHEROSCLEROSIS IN CHILDREN

Atherosclerosis, which involves the deposition of cholesterol esters in the intima-media of the arteries, is the main cause of CHD [75]. Further, there is impressive epidemiological, experimental, and clinical evidence that plasma lipid and lipoprotein levels are important correlates of atherosclerosis and cardiovascular disease. Indeed, high levels of plasma cholesterol and low density lipoprotein (LDL) cholesterol are correlated with atherosclerosis and thus with CHD [43, 44]. On the other hand, the amount of cholesterol transported by high density lipoprotein (HDL) seems to play a protective role against the progression of atherosclerosis. High plasma HDL levels are generally associated with a low incidence of cardiovascular disease [35, 63]. Further, results from the Framingham Study suggest that the ratio of cholesterol transported by LDL to HDL is the best predictor of CHD and related death [15].

Although it is clear that the measurement of plasma levels of lipoproteins is useful in the prediction of CHD, a major question is whether changes in plasma lipoprotein levels will have beneficial effects on the progression of atherosclerosis and related mortality. Results of the Lipid Research Clinics Coronary Primary Prevention Trial [57] clearly indicate that a decrease in plasma LDL-cholesterol levels is associated with a reduction in the incidence of CHD and that the reduction in CHD is directly proportional to the decrease in LDL-cholesterol levels. A recent longitudinal study from Finland [29] also provides further support for a role of HDL in the protection against CHD. An increase in plasma HDL-cholesterol levels was associated with a reduction in the incidence of CHD. It thus appears that measures aimed at lowering LDL-cholesterol levels and increasing HDL-cholesterol levels should be encouraged.

Two related questions must be addressed. First, when should such measures be implemented, and second, on which individuals should they be implemented? To answer these questions, the evidence for the presence of atherosclerosis early in life must be evaluated. Enos et al. [24] provided evidence for the early development of atherosclerosis in an analysis of autopsies of 300 United States soldiers killed in the Korean War. Although the mean age of the soldiers was 22.1 years, there was gross evidence of coronary arteriosclerosis in 77% of the soldiers. Similar results were reported by McNamara et al. [62], who noted evidence of atherosclerosis in 45% of 105 United States soldiers killed in Vietnam. Results from the International Atherosclerosis Project [60, 61] confirmed these observations and further documented the presence of fatty streaks by 3 years of age in the aortas of many children. Fatty streaks were frequently observed in the coronary arteries by 10 years of age, and the presence of such lipid deposition in the coronary arteries was associated with adult arteriosclerosis [61]. There is, therefore, little doubt that lipid deposition in the arteries is a process that begins early in life.

The most striking example of early atherosclerosis comes from homozygous familial hypercholesterolemia, a disease of lipoprotein metabolism. This condition is associated with very high plasma LDL-cholesterol levels [34] that are caused by a deficiency of the apo-B,E receptor. This disease was characterized by Nobel prize winners Michael Brown and Joseph Goldstein [12]. The apo-B,E receptor is responsible for the binding of apo-B- and apo-E-containing lipoproteins and thus is responsible for the clearance of LDL from the plasma. Malfunction of the receptor is, therefore, associated with a low plasma clearance of LDL, leading to high plasma LDL-cholesterol levels. Although this may be the only metabolic defect observed in apo-B,E receptor-deficient children, they show severe coronary arteriosclerosis early in childhood and often die from myocardial infarction during the teens and sometimes earlier [34]. Although this example is extreme, it clearly indicates that arteriosclerosis can begin early in life if high plasma LDL-cholesterol levels or other important cardiovascular risk factors are present.

CARDIOVASCULAR RISK FACTORS IN ADULTS

The study of risk factors for cardiovascular disease in adult populations has been the subject of extensive research, and a comprehensive review of the topic is beyond the scope of this paper. The ratio of LDL-cholesterol to HDL-cholesterol provides the best estimate of the risk of CHD [15]. Other risk factors, however, have been identified. Hypertension and smoking are the two most important after the LDL-cholesterol/HDL-cholesterol ratio. In the Framingham Study, a hypertensive hypercholesterolemic smoker has a much greater risk of experiencing a heart attack than a normotensive nonsmoker with normal cholesterol levels [15]. Other risk factors for CHD include hyperinsulinemia [21] and diabetes mellitus [15], a high proportion of abdominal fat [53, 54], a sedentary life-style [55], a familial history of cardiovascular disease [4], and a high consumption of fat [44]. It is also important to note that the risk factors are not only additive, but that there is a significant interaction among them [15]. Therefore, the clustering of certain risk factors may substantially increase the risk of CHD in an individual. An example is provided by abdominal obesity. The regional distribution of body fat is more closely associated with CHD and its risk factors than obesity per se [17, 47, 51, 53, 54]. Indeed, individuals (men or women) with a high proportion of abdominal fat are more frequently glucose intolerant [47, 51], which potentially leads to diabetes [38], hypertension [9] and a low HDL-cholesterol/LDL-cholesterol ratio [2, 17, 36], whereas individuals with a gluteal-femoral accumulation of fat show less alterations in metabolic profiles and are generally comparable to lean subjects. Therefore, it appears that abdominally obese subjects are clearly at greater risk for cardiovascular disease than obese individuals in general. This high risk obese subgroup should be treated with more attention. The effect on the health of children of variation in the regional distribution of body fat has thus far received little attention.

Several risk factors can be modified, e.g., changes in the caloric content and lipid composition of the diet, and changes in the level of habitual physical activity. Thus, favorable changes in life-style may potentially reduce the progression of arteriosclerosis in adults [71]. It is important to indicate that it has not yet been possible to document the regression of atherosclerosis following changes in diet or exercise level in adults and that the regression of atherosclerosis has been observed only in animals [49]. However, favorable changes in cardiovascular risk factors have been associated with a reduced progression of atherosclerosis in humans [3]. Further, Newman et al. [66] have analyzed the relationship of risk factors for cardiovascular disease to atherosclerotic lesions in 35 individuals with a mean age of 18 years. Aortic fatty streaks were positively correlated with antemortem levels of LDL-cholesterol and negatively correlated to the HDL-cholesterol/LDL-cholesterol ratio. Given these results, it appears reasonable to suggest that favorable changes in lifestyle habits and in cardiovascular risk factors may have beneficial effects on the progression of atherosclerosis and that they should be implemented during childhood. In this regard, a National Institutes of Health Consensus Conference [58] has recommended that, because patterns of life-style are acquired in childhood, prevention should begin in this period and the moderate fat and moderate cholesterol diet that has been recommended for the entire population should be encouraged for all family members older than 2 years. The panel also recommended closer supervision of high risk children as well as measures aimed at reducing their LDL-cholesterol levels as in adults. There is, therefore, some consensus for the pediatric primary prevention of atherosclerosis [33].

RISK FACTORS FOR CARDIOVASCULAR DISEASE DURING CHILDHOOD AND ADOLESCENCE

Cardiovascular risk factors, i.e., high plasma LDL-cholesterol/HDL-cholesterol ratio, hypertension, smoking, abdominal obesity, physical inactivity, and high fat intake, will not have the same effect on the morbidity and mortality of children and youth as in adults. However, the presence of these risk factors, especially when clustered as in the obese child [74], could lead, over a period of many years, to the development of coronary arteriosclerosis. Such concern would appear especially relevant if cardiovascular risk factors track reasonably well during childhood and adolescence.

Plasma Lipoprotein and Lipid Levels

At birth, plasma total cholesterol, LDL-cholesterol, and triglyceride levels are very low and a sharp increase occurs during the first year of life [52]. After infancy, LDL-cholesterol and triglyceride levels are relatively stable until adulthood [77]. Values of HDL-cholesterol are relatively stable before puberty [77]. During sexual maturation, however, a marked sex difference is observed. Boys show a reduction in plasma HDL-cholesterol levels during puberty that is not observed in girls.

During the preschool years, year-to-year correlations for plasma cholesterol, triglycerides, and blood pressure are generally low [88]. Berenson et al. [5] reported little association between morphological variables and blood lipids during the preschool years. However, tracking improves with age during the school years, and year-to-year correlations increase after puberty [88]. Because plasma lipids increase with age [81], it seems that tracking is better during and after puberty than during childhood. In 2236 children 2–14 years of age who were examined three times over a 5-year period, Webber et al. [88] observed acceptable tracking of total cholesterol and β-lipoprotein (LDL)-cholesterol, but lower tracking of triglycerides and α-lipoprotein (HDL)-cholesterol. However, extreme plasma lipid values track better and very high lipid values tend to remain high throughout childhood [69, 88]. Even at these young ages, implementation of measures aimed at reducing high plasma lipid levels appears warranted. Kunze [52] has suggested that early identification of children at risk for cardiovascular disease by measurements of plasma cholesterol and LDL-cholesterol is possible, especially during puberty when plasma lipids track reasonably well.

Glucose and Insulin Metabolism

Berenson et al. [6] have reported increasing levels of fasting plasma insulin from 5 to 17 years of age. Accordingly, Orchard et al. [68] have shown that 5–10-year-old children display higher tissue insulin sensitivity than adolescents and adults. Young children have a lower insulin response to a glucose tolerance test than older children and adolescents. At puberty, a decrease in insulin sensitivity occurs in both girls and boys [1, 10].

Insulin sensitivity is negatively correlated to the proportion of free testosterone in the plasma in adults [26]. Such an association may explain the reduced insulin sensitivity in male adolescents but not in females. Further, males accumulate proportionally more subcutaneous fat on the trunk, including the abdomen, during adolescence. However, in contrast to boys, overall adiposity of girls increases significantly at puberty [59] and, because body fatness is negatively correlated with insulin sensitivity [11], increased fat deposition during puberty in girls may contribute to the reduced insulin sensitivity of girls. In adulthood, however, the abdominal accumulation of fat observed in obese men places them at greater risk for glucose intolerance and diabetes than obese women with peripheral accumulation of fat [8].

Tracking of plasma glucose levels appears to be moderate over a 3-year period in children aged 5–17 years [14]. Plasma insulin levels track well only in older children (ages 9–14 years at first examination) [14]. Because hyperinsulinemia is a significant risk factor for cardiovascular disease [21], these results suggest that high fasting plasma insulin levels measured after about 10 years of age could be a useful marker of cardiovascular risk. Further, fasting insulin levels are positively related to body fatness, blood pressure, plasma triglyceride, and cholesterol and are negatively correlated to α-lipoprotein (HDL)-cholesterol in 5–17-year-old children [14]. These results emphasize the importance of insulin sensitivity as a determinant of plasma lipoprotein levels and, therefore, in the cardiovascular disease risk profile of children. In addition, because relative insulin resistance is apparently associated with normal puberty, it is important, perhaps, to control variables that may further contribute to a poor metabolic profile and glucose intolerance, i.e., excess adiposity that is associated with insulin hypersecretion and insulin resistance [11].

Blood Pressure

Substantial variation in blood pressure is common in children. Blood pressure does not track very well (less than plasma cholesterol) during childhood [16]. In the Bogalusa Heart Study, systolic and diastolic blood pressures increase, respectively, by 2 and 1 mm Hg/year, except in 2–4-year-olds [88]. In the Muscatine Study of 5–18-year-old children followed over a 6-year period, changes in percentile rank order were large and the distribution of diastolic blood pressure quintiles after 6 years of follow-up could not be predicted by the initial quintiles [16]. Similarly, the tracking of blood pressure in children over a 5-year period in the Bogalusa Heart Study was not as good as tracking for plasma cholesterol levels [88]. However, a certain proportion of children with high systolic blood pressure tended to remain in that category during childhood and adolescence [88]. Because plasma insulin levels and obesity are significant correlates of systolic and diastolic blood pressure in children [16], it appears important to identify and treat children potentially at greater risk for atherosclerosis given the interactive effects of many risk factors.

Obesity and Regional Adipose Tissue Distribution

Several longitudinal studies have shown that obese children display higher blood pressure, plasma glucose and insulin, and lipid levels than the nonobese [46, 74]. Indeed, obesity is considered a major factor responsible for the clustering of other risk factors during growth [74]. It thus appears that excess adiposity should be thoroughly treated during childhood. In adults, on the other hand, regional adipose tissue distribution is apparently more important than obesity per se as a cardiovascular risk factor [2, 9, 17, 36, 38, 47, 51, 53, 54].

The relationship of body fat distribution to metabolic complications has been less studied in children than in adults. During childhood, absolute and relative adiposity increase gradually in both sexes. At about 8–9 years, fatness increases at a faster rate in girls until adulthood [59]. In boys, the increase in absolute and relative fatness after 8–9 years is less marked and, at puberty, there is a decrease in relative fatness in boys due to the marked increase in fat-free mass at this time [59]. The lowest relative fatness values in boys generally occur in late adolescence and then increase progressively into adulthood.

The proportion of central (trunk) fat is not substantially different between boys and girls until puberty, when boys experience a greater relative accumulation of fat on the trunk due in part to a reduction of subcutaneous fat on the upper and lower extremities. Puberty is associated, on the other hand, with a substantial deposition of fat in the femoral gluteal area of girls [59]. These sex differences in the amount of central atherogenic fat have been suggested as being involved in the sex difference observed later in life in the prevalence of cardiovascular disease in men and women [8, 20, 48, 82]. Whether a high proportion of abdominal fat in childhood is associated with metabolic complications has not been extensively studied but, from the results obtained in adults, there is high probability that abdominal obesity may be involved in the clustering of CHD factors in children.

PHYSICAL ACTIVITY AND CARDIOVASCULAR RISK FACTORS DURING GROWTH

It is generally believed that physically active children are leaner and healthier than sedentary children. However, before such a statement can be accepted, one must consider the fact that healthy and lean children may be more inclined to participate in physical activities than obese children and/or children prone to various diseases. Therefore, the important role of selection in studies of physical activity and risk factors must be considered. Comparisons of young athletes to sedentary children also suffer from this bias. It is, therefore, important to examine the consistency of cross-sectional and longitudinal data for the potential beneficial effects of physical activity on CHD risk factors. A related issue that deserves discussion is the effects of physical activity versus physical fitness. This question has not yet been completely resolved in adults.

Physical Activity and Plasma Lipoproteins and Lipids during Growth

Relatively few papers have addressed the issue of the effect of regular physical activity on plasma lipid and lipoprotein levels in children.

Viikari et al. [84] reported cross-sectional comparisons of sedentary and active children and found no evidence for a significant effect of physical activity among 3-year-old children, but noted a significant positive correlation between the HDL-cholesterol/cholesterol ratio and participation in school sport clubs in older children. Durant et al. [22] did not observe an association between level of participation in sport activities and lipoprotein levels in 7–11-year-old black children, but noted a significant negative association with the cholesterol/HDL-cholesterol ratio among 12–15-year-old black adolescents. In 6–7-year-old children, Gilliam et al. [32] found little association between the amount of cumulative work performed on a bicycle ergometer and plasma lipid and lipoprotein levels, with the exception of total cholesterol, which showed a small but significant negative correlation (7% of the variance) with the amount of work performed during the exercise test. Välimäki et al. [83] reported no difference in plasma cholesterol levels among sedentary and trained 11–13-year-old boys and girls, but observed higher triglyceride levels in sedentary compared to trained girls. In both sexes, HDL-cholesterol levels were higher in trained than in sedentary boys and girls [83]. Among boys aged 8–11 years, Thorland and Gilliam [78] found lower plasma triglyceride levels and a higher HDL-cholesterol/cholesterol ratio in active individuals than in children displaying low levels of physical activity. In a sample of 14–16-year-old adolescents, Wanne et al. [87] observed higher triglyceride levels in inactive boys than in active boys, but found no difference in girls. These authors also found higher HDL-cholesterol levels in boys involved 8 hr or more per week in sport activities compared to boys not involved in school sports, but no difference in HDL-cholesterol was observed between active and sedentary girls [87].

Although the activity levels of trained children undoubtedly differ among studies, the available data suggest that fit and active children tend to have lower triglyceride and higher HDL-cholesterol levels. This association appears to be stronger in boys at puberty when a decrease in HDL-cholesterol and an increase in plasma lipids is generally observed. The association between the training status and plasma lipids and lipoprotein appears to be weaker in girls, especially after puberty, when the plasma level of HDL-cholesterol tends to increase in all girls. Finally, the low lipid levels observed in young children make it difficult to evaluate and/or detect possible significant relationships between habitual physical activity and lipid levels. The problem is further confounded by difficulties in assessing habitual activity in young children.

An additional limitation of cross-sectional studies that compare trained and sedentary children is the problem of selection. This also applies to comparisons of adult athletes and nonathletes. For obvious reasons related to selection processes, it is possible that skilled and physiologically fit children enroll in school teams because of their partly inherited high level of fitness, whereas poorly fit children are seldom able to support the strain of rigorous training. Therefore, it is important that longitudinal studies are performed in children in order to sort out the potential effects of exercise (dependent upon the level of physical activity) and physical fitness (determined by both the level of physical activity and inherited characteristics).

Unfortunately, the literature on the effect of exercise training programs on plasma lipid and lipoprotein levels is limited and has yielded mixed results, which can be explained in part by variation in age of subjects, initial levels of lipids, and characteristics of the exercise training programs. Gilliam and Burke [30], for example, studied 14 girls, 8–10 years of age, who exercised 6 days/week, 40 min/day for a period of 6 weeks. No change in plasma cholesterol levels was observed but a significant increase in plasma HDL-cholesterol levels occurred. Gilliam and Freedson [31] exercised-trained 7–9-year-old boys and girls 25 min/day, 4 days/week over 12 weeks and found no significant change in plasma cholesterol and triglyceride levels. However, one hypertriglyceridemic child involved in the training program showed normal triglyceride levels after training, which suggests that if plasma lipid levels are normal or low at the start (as it is often the case in children) there may be less chance of detecting a statistically significant exercise-training effect.

Savage et al. [72] did not find evidence for an exercise-training effect in two groups of 8–9-year-old boys exposed to 10 weeks of low (40% Vo_2max) or high (75% Vo_2max) intensity training (walking, jogging, and running). It is of interest that significant decreases in HDL-cholesterol levels occurred in both groups after training. In 7th grade children, Fisher and Brown [27] observed that 30 min of physical activity, 5 days/week over 12 weeks produced a significant decrease in serum cholesterol levels and an increase in HDL-cholesterol levels. On the other hand, Linder et al. [56] randomly assigned 50 boys, 11–17 years of age, to a physical conditioning program or a control group. The exercise group participated in an 8-week aerobic exercise program that included four 30-min sessions/week. No changes in plasma lipid and lipoprotein levels were observed at the end of the exercise program. Finally, Hunt and White [41] reported no effect of 10-week, moderate and high intensity exercise training programs on the plasma lipoprotein and lipid levels in late adolescents.

The literature on the effects of exercise training in children is thus equivocal. Further research is clearly warranted. One possible explanation for the discordant results is the heterogeneity of the children studied relative to age and initial physiological and metabolic characteristics. As previously indicated, plasma lipid levels progressively increase with age during childhood and adolescence. Low levels are generally observed in younger children. However, individual variation is considerable and some children even have plasma lipid levels that require dietary and/or pharmacological intervention. In this regard, it is well known that

CHD risk factors cluster in children and that obesity is a condition frequently associated with the simultaneous observation of metabolic disturbances, such as high lipid and glucose levels and high blood pressure. It would, therefore, appear important to further investigate the effects of exercise-training in obese children. This issue is discussed subsequently in the section on obesity.

Physical Activity and Glucose and Insulin Metabolism during Growth

Glucose intolerance and hyperinsulinemia are risk factors for diabetes and CHD. In normal children, physical fitness and glucose tolerance are apparently not related [65], but reported levels of physical activity are negatively related to the product of 1-hr plasma glucose × insulin levels during an oral glucose tolerance test in the Bogalusa Heart Study [85]. The heart rate response to a step test had a low ($r = 0.1–0.2$) but significant correlation with blood glucose levels in children and adolescents, 10–19 years of age, in the Tecumseh Study [64], and this effect was largely independent of the effect of fatness. In contrast, obese children had a higher insulin response to a glucose tolerance test than did lean, fit children [93]. Further, after exercise-training, obese children who significantly lost weight had lower fasting plasma insulin levels compared to obese children who did not lose weight in response to training.

Exercise-training in adults improves insulin sensitivity and consequently produces a reduction in the insulin response to a glucose challenge [7, 86]. However, in lean nondiabetic adults with normal glucose tolerance, exercise-training does not further improve glucose tolerance [7, 19, 80]. Therefore, it appears that obese, hyperinsulinemic children may potentially benefit from an increase in daily energy expenditure in physical activity. Further, there is substantial data that indicate significant associations between glucose and insulin metabolism and plasma lipid and lipoprotein levels in both adults [18, 67] and children [14]. The improvement in insulin sensitivity in the obese child subjected to an exercise training program may thus contribute to improved plasma lipid transport. The effect of exercise training on glucose and insulin metabolism and the relationship with plasma lipid transport in children and adolescents is an important area that warrants further research.

Physical Activity and Blood Pressure during Growth

Very few studies have addressed the effect of exercise-training on blood pressure in children and adolescents. Further, as blood pressure measurements often vary from day-to-day during growth, it is difficult to obtain conclusive results. Cross-sectional analyses of the correlates of blood pressure in children and adolescents have indicated an independent association between physical fitness, as measured by the PWC_{170}, and systolic blood pressure in preadolescent boys and in adolescents of both sexes [28]. However, some data indicate no significant correlation between maximal aerobic power and blood pressure in 8–12-year-old boys [89].

Exercise-training studies on children generally show little change in blood pressure following training. For example, no changes were observed in blood pressure of 11–17-year-old boys after an 8-week aerobic exercise program [56] and in the resting or exercise blood pressure of 11–13-year-old children after 4 months of training [25]. On the other hand, diastolic blood pressure declined in 7th grade children after a 12-week exercise program that included five weekly sessions of 30 min for a period of 12 weeks [27]. Ylitalo [93] studied, in obese children, the effects of an intervention that included reduced energy intake and increased physical activity, and he reported that children who lost a significant amount of weight showed a reduction in systolic blood pressure. Among 25 exercised-trained hypertensive adolescents over a period of 6 months, significant reductions in systolic and diastolic blood pressure occurred although body weight and subcutaneous skinfolds were not altered [37]. Thus, results in obese and hypertensive children suggest that those in the high percentile for fatness and blood pressure can benefit the most from an increase in physical activity. There is little evidence that exercise-training can decrease blood pressure in normotensive children.

Physical Activity, Obesity, and Regional Body Fat Distribution during Growth

Regular physical activity can potentially have a substantial effect on body fatness if exercise sessions of sufficient intensity and duration are performed [79]. In addition, a negative energy balance induced by an exercise-training program preserves fat-free mass so that the composition of weight loss includes a very high proportion of fat in contrast to low calorie diets, which induce a loss of both fat mass and fat-free mass [79]. However, during growth, it is difficult to dissociate training effects from age- and maturity-associated gains in fat-free mass, especially in adolescent boys. Nonetheless, because obesity is partly responsible for the clustering of cardiovascular risk factors in children and adolescents, increased physical activity is important in the management of the obese child. However, it is important to remember that a substantial amount of exercise is essential to substantially alter energy balance and that the duration of the prescribed exercise sessions must be high. The form of exercise is especially important as the feasibility of prescribing 40 min of jogging or bicycling for an 8-year-old child is questionable. Many cross-sectional studies have shown that physically active children are leaner than sedentary children [42, 76], and longitudinal training studies have generally shown that an increase in physical activity can result in a reduction in fatness [13, 23, 70]. In adults, reduction in fatness induced by exercise-training is associated with significant metabolic improvements, and this generally appears to be the case in children. One study has observed a reduction in atherogenic abdominal-trunk fat after training in adults and it was associated with a reduction in plasma insulin levels and in plasma cholesterol and LDL-cholesterol [19]. It is not known whether a preferential loss of abdominal-central fat occurs in children in response to negative energy balance induced by exercise-training.

PHYSICAL ACTIVITY AND CARDIOVASCULAR RISK FACTORS DURING GROWTH: FURTHER CONSIDERATIONS AND CONCLUSIONS

Although the exercise literature for adults generally indicates that regular physical activity is associated with a healthy metabolic profile, such as low plasma lipid levels, a high HDL-cholesterol/total cholesterol ratio, high insulin sensitivity, and low blood pressure, results for children are not conclusive and may reflect difficulties in further improving the "normal" metabolic profile of most children. An exception to this notion is the obese child who often displays high triglyceride and low HDL-cholesterol levels, hyperinsulinemia, and increased blood pressure.

An additional issue is whether an increase in habitual physical activity during growth will slow the atherosclerosis process. Direct experimental evidence for a beneficial effect of exercise-training on the progression of atherosclerosis in children is lacking. From the results of Newman et al. [66], which show an association between cardiovascular risk factors and the extent of atherosclerotic lesions in late adolescents, it is reasonable to speculate that the beneficial effects of exercise training on cardiovascular risk factors may well slow the progression of coronary lipid accumulation, at least in some high risk children. Because other life-style variables are associated with the development of atherosclerosis, i.e., percentage of lipids and of saturated fat in the diet, smoking, positive energy balance, and so on, a multifactorial approach including increased habitual physical activity or training is essential, especially for high risk children.

Another aspect of the effects of exercise-training on cardiovascular risk factors that deserves further discussion is individual variation in the magnitude of metabolic responses to aerobic exercise-training. Experiments performed on young adult males clearly indicate a significant role for genetic variation in the adaptation to physical training. For example, six pairs of young adult male monozygotic twins exercised-trained on bicycle ergometers at 58% of their $\dot{V}O_2max$ for 22 consecutive days [19, 80]. The exercise duration, 116 min/day, was calculated to induce a net daily energy deficit of 4.2 MJ (1000 kcal). Baseline energy needs were evaluated before the training program and were rigorously controlled (subjects lived in a metabolic ward during the protocol) during the training experiment in order to ensure that the energy deficit was the same for all subjects and that the deficit was due solely to the daily exercise. Following the exercise-training program, the subjects lost weight and, as expected, insulin response during an oral glucose tolerance test was markedly reduced [80]. Plasma triglyceride levels were significantly reduced and the HDL-cholesterol/total cholesterol ratio was significantly increased [19]. All these metabolic adaptations to exercise training in young adult males are well documented and are consistent with the notion that exercise-training improves the metabolic profile. However, substantial variation in changes in the insulin area/glucose area and in plasma lipid and lipoprotein levels was apparent. Some subjects showed very little improvement, whereas others experienced marked alterations in cardiovascular disease risk factors, although the exercise-training protocol was rigorously the same for all subjects. However, changes in the insulin area/glucose area and in plasma cholesterol, apolipoprotein B, LDL-cholesterol, HDL-cholesterol, and the HDL-cholesterol/LDL-cholesterol ratio were quite similar within monozygotic twin pairs. The most likely explanation for these observations is that the genotype is a significant determinant of the sensitivity of some cardiovascular risk factors to exercise-training. Current studies of the DNA polymorphism for the genes related to glucose, insulin, and lipoprotein metabolism may permit the identification of individuals who are sensitive or resistant to exercise-training in terms of alterations in the metabolic profile. Such information would be especially helpful in childhood and adolescence to discriminate especially among high risk children, those who will benefit the most from regular exercise and those who would require more rigorous multifactorial intervention. The presence of low and high responders to exercise-training among children and adolescents is clearly an area that deserves further investigation.

Finally, the issue of physical fitness versus physical activity merits consideration. It is obvious that children who are actively involved in school sport activities (and therefore who have a high level of physical activity) may also be the fittest due to genotypic characteristics and, of course, the selection process in youth sports. Cross-sectional comparisons of sedentary and active children, therefore, include the effects of both fitness and physical activity. This may explain why more convincing evidence for a beneficial effect of regular physical activity on cardiovascular risk factors is apparent in cross-sectional studies than in generally short-term longitudinal experiments.

However, results of a 100-day exercise-training study with moderately obese young men are encouraging. After the measurement of baseline energy needs, the subjects were involved in an exercise-training program during which they exercised on bicycle ergometers (two 53-min sessions/day) 6 days/week at an intensity below 60% $\dot{V}o_2$max (Després

JP, Tremblay A, Moorjani S, Lupien PJ, Thériault G, Nadeau A, Bouchard A, unpublished observations). At the end of the training period, the subjects lost a substantial amount of body weight (reduction of about 9%) and their metabolic profile was markedly improved, i.e., reduced insulin response to glucose and increased HDL-cholesterol/total cholesterol ratio, but due to the low intensity of exercise, no significant increase in maximal aerobic power occurred. These results indicate that an increase in V̇o₂max is not a prerequisite for exercise training to induce some beneficial metabolic effects as long as the program is of proper duration and substantially affects energy balance. There is, therefore, hope for the sedentary unfit and/or obese child or adolescent who is frequently not involved in sport activities. Low intensity, but prolonged aerobic exercise appears to have the potential to reduce body fatness and improve the metabolic profile even if no substantial increase in maximal aerobic power occurs. This concept, however, requires experimental testing in children.

ACKNOWLEDGMENTS

This work was supported by the Quebec Heart Foundation, the Fonds de la Recherche en Santé du Québec (FRSQ), Merck Frosst Canada, the Medical Research Council of Canada, and the United States National Institutes of Health.

REFERENCES

1. Amiel SA, Sherwin RS, Simonson DC, Lauritano AA, Tamborlane WV: Impaired insulin action in puberty. A contributing factor to poor glycemic control in adolescent with diabetes. *N Engl J Med* 315:215–219, 1986.
2. Anderson AJ, Sobocinski KA, Freedman DS, Barboriak JJ, Rimm AA, Gruchow HW: Body fat distribution, plasma lipids and lipoproteins. *Arteriosclerosis* 8:88–94, 1988.
3. Arntzenius AC, Kromhout D, Barth JD, Reiber JHC, Bruschke AVG, Buis B, van Gent CM, Kempen-Voogd N, Strikwerda S, van der Velde EA: Diet, lipoproteins, and the progression of coronary atherosclerosis. The Leiden Trial. *N Engl J Med* 312:805–811, 1985.
4. Barrett-Connor E, Khaw K: Family history of heart attack as an independent predictor of death due to cardiovascular disease. *Circulation* 59:1065–1069, 1984.
5. Berenson GS, Foster TA, Frank GC, Frerichs RR, Srinivasan SR, Voors AW, Webber LS: Cardiovascular disease risk factor variables at the preschool age. The Bogalusa Heart Study. *Circulation* 57:603–612, 1978.
6. Berenson GS, Radhakrishnamurthy B, Srinivasan SR, Voors AW, Foster TA, Dalferes ER Jr, Webber LS: Plasma glucose and insulin levels in relation to cardiovascular risk factors in children from a biracial population. The Bogalusa Heart Study. *J Chronic Dis* 34:379–391, 1981.
7. Björntorp P: The effects of exercise on plasma insulin. *Int J Sports Med* 2:125–129, 1981.

8. Björntorp P: Morphological classifications of obesity: what they tell us, what they don't. *Int J Obes* 8:525–533, 1984.

9. Blair D, Habicht JP, Sims EAH, Sylwester D, Abraham S: Evidence for an increased risk for hypertension with centrally located body fat and the effect of race and sex on this risk. *Am J Epidemiol* 119:526–540, 1984.

10. Bloch CA, Clemons P, Sperling NA: Puberty decreases insulin sensitivity. *J Pediatr* 110:481–487, 1987.

11. Bogardus C, Lillioja S, Mott DM, Hollenbeck C, Reaven G: Relationship between degree of obesity and in vivo insulin action in man. *Am J Physiol* 248:E286-E291, 1985.

12. Brown MS, Goldstein JL: A receptor-mediated pathway for cholesterol homeostasis. *Science* 232:34–47, 1986.

13. Brownell KD, Kaye FS: A school-based behavior modification, nutrition education, and physical activity program for obese children. *Am J Clin Nutr* 35:277–283, 1982.

14. Burke GL, Webber LS, Srinivasan SR, Radhakrishnamurthy B, Freedman DS, Berenson GS: Fasting plasma glucose and insulin levels and their relationship to cardiovascular risk factors in children: Bogalusa Heart Study. *Metabolism* 35:441–446, 1986.

15. Castelli WP: Epidemiology of coronary heart disease. The Framingham Study. *Am J Med* 76:4–12, 1984.

16. Clarke WR, Schrott HG, Leaverton PE, Connor WE, Lauer RM: Tracking of blood lipids and blood pressures in school age children: The Muscatine Study. *Circulation* 58:626–634, 1978.

17. Després JP, Allard C, Tremblay A, Talbot J, Bouchard C: Evidence for a regional component of body fatness in the association with serum lipids in men and women. *Metabolism* 33:967–973, 1985.

18. Després JP, Poehlman ET, Tremblay A, Lupien PJ, Moorjani S, Nadeau A, Pérusse L, Bouchard C: Genotype-influenced changes in serum HDL cholesterol after short-term overfeeding in man: association with plasma insulin and triglyceride levels. *Metabolism* 36:363–368, 1987.

19. Després JP, Moorjani S, Tremblay A, Poehlman ET, Lupien PJ, Nadeau A, Bouchard C: Heredity and changes in plasma lipids and lipoproteins after short-term exercise training in men. *Arteriosclerosis* 8:402–409, 1988.

20. Després JP, Tremblay A, Bouchard C: Regional adipose tissue distribution and plasma lipoproteins. In Bouchard C, Johnston FE (eds): *Fat Distribution during Growth and Later Health Outcomes*. New York, Alan R. Liss, 1988, pp 221–241.

21. Ducimetière P, Eschwege E, Papoz L, Richard JL, Claude JR, Rosselin GE: Relationship of plasma insulin levels to the incidence of myocardial infarction and coronary heart disease in a middle-aged population. *Diabetologia* 19:205–210, 1980.

22. Durant RH, Linder CW, Harkess JW, Gray RG: The relationship between physical activity and serum lipids and lipoproteins in Black children and adolescents. *J Adolesc Health Care* 4:55–60, 1983.

23. Dwyer T, Coonan WE, Leitch DR, Hetzel BS, Baghurst RA: An investigation of the effects of daily physical activity on the health of primary school students in South Australia. *Int J Epidemiol* 12:308–313, 1983.

24. Enos WF, Holmes RH, Beyer J: Coronary disease among United States soldiers killed in action in Korea. *JAMA* 152:1090–1093, 1953.

25. Eriksson RO, Koch G: Effect of physical training on hemodynamic response during submaximal and maximal exercise. *Acta Physiol Scand* 87:27–39, 1973.

26. Evans DJ, Hoffman RG, Kalkhoff RK, Kissebah AH: Relationship of body fat topography to insulin sensitivity and metabolic profiles in premenopausal women. *Metabolism* 33:68–75, 1984.

27. Fisher AG, Brown M: The effects of diet and exercise on selected coronary risk factors in children (Abstract). *Med Sci Sports Exerc* 14:171, 1982.

28. Fraser GE, Phillips RL, Harris LR: Physical fitness and blood pressure in schoolchildren. *Circulation* 67:405–412, 1983.

29. Frick MH, Elo O, Haapa K, Heinonen OP, Heinsalmi P, Helo P, Huttunen JK, Kaita-
niemi P, Koskinen P, Manninen V, Mäenpää H, Mälkönen M, Mänttari M, Norola S,
Pasternack A, Pikkarainen J, Romo M, Sjösblom T, Nikkila EA: Helsinki Heart Study:
Primary prevention trial with gemfibrozil in middle-aged men with dyslipidemia. *N
Engl J Med* 317:1237–1245, 1987.
30. Gilliam TB, Burke MB: Effects of exercise on serum lipids and lipoproteins in girls,
ages 8 to 10 years. *Artery* 4:203–213, 1978.
31. Gilliam TB, Freedson PS: Effects of a 12-week school physical fitness program on peak
V̇o₂, body composition and blood lipids in 7- to 9-year-old children. *Int J Sports Med*
1:73–78, 1980.
32. Gilliam TB, Freedson PS, MacConnie SE, Geenen DL, Pels AE III: Comparison of
blood lipids, lipoproteins, anthropometric measures, and resting and exercise cardiovascular responses in children, 6–7 years old. *Prev Med* 10:754–764, 1981.
33. Glueck CJ: Pediatric primary prevention of atherosclerosis. *N Engl J Med* 314:175–
177, 1986.
34. Goldstein JL, Brown MS: Familial hypercholesterolemia. In Stanbury JB, Wyngaar-
den JB, Fredrickson DS, Goldstein JL, Brown MS (eds): *The Metabolic Basis of Inherited
Disease.* ed 5. New York, McGraw-Hill, 1983, pp 672–712.
35. Gordon T, Castelli WP, Hortland MC, Kannel WB, Dawber TR: HDL as a protective
factor against CHD. The Framingham study. *Am J Med* 62:707–714, 1977.
36. Haffner SM, Stern MP, Hazuda HP, Pugh J, Patterson JK: Do upper-body and centralized adiposity measure different aspects of regional body-fat distribution? Relationship to non-insulin-dependent diabetes mellitus, lipids, and lipoproteins. *Diabetes*
36:43–51, 1987.
37. Hagberg JM, Goldring D, Ehsani AA, Heath GW, Hernandez A, Schechtman K,
Holloszy JO: Effect of exercise training on the blood pressure and hemodynamic
features of hypertensive adolescents. *Am J Cardiol* 52:763–768, 1983.
38. Hartz AJ, Rupley DC, Kalkhoff RD, Rimm AA: Relationship of obesity to diabetes:
influence of obesity and body fat distribution. *Prev Med* 12:351–357, 1983.
39. Haskell WL: Exercise-induced changes in plasma lipids and lipoproteins. *Prev Med*
13:23–36, 1984.
40. Haskell WL: The influence of exercise training on plasma lipids and lipoproteins in
health and disease. *Acta Med Scand Suppl* 711:25–37, 1986.
41. Hunt JF, White JR: Effects of ten weeks of vigorous daily exercise on serum lipids and
lipoproteins in teenage males (Abstract). *Med Sci Sports Exerc* 12:93, 1980.
42. Johnson ML, Burke BS, Mayer J: Relative importance of inactivity and overeating in
the energy balance of obese high school girls. *Am J Clin Nutr* 4:37–44, 1956.
43. Kannel WE, Dawber TR, Friedman GD, Glennan WE, McNamara PM: Risk factors in
coronary heart disease: an evaluation of several serum lipids as predictors of coronary
heart disease. *Ann Intern Med* 61:888–899, 1964.
44. Keys A, Anderson JT, Grande F: Prediction of serum cholesterol responses of man to
changes in fats in the diet. *Lancet* 2:959–966, 1957.
45. Keys A: Coronary heart disease in seven countries. *Circulation* (Suppl)41:I1–I211,
1980.
46. Khoury P, Morrison JA, Kelly K, Mellies M, Horvitz R, Glueck CJ: Clustering and
interrelationships of coronary heart disease risk factors in schoolchildren, ages 6–19.
Am J Epidemiol 112:524–538, 1980.
47. Kissebah AH, Vydelingum N, Murray R, Evans DJ, Hartz AJ, Kalkhoff RK, Adams
PW: Relation of body fat distribution to metabolic complications of obesity. *J Clin
Endocrinol Metab* 54:254–260, 1982.
48. Kissebah AH, Peiris A, Evans DJ: Mechanisms associating body fat distribution to
glucose intolerance and diabetes mellitus. In Bouchard C, Johnston FE (eds): *Fat
Distribution during Growth and Later Health Outcomes.* New York, Alan R. Liss, 1988,
pp 203–220.

49. Kramsch DM, Aspen AJ, Abramowitz BM, Kreimendahl T, Hood WB: Reduction of coronary atherosclerosis by moderate exercise in monkeys on an atherogenic diet. *N Engl J Med* 305:1483–1489, 1981.
50. Krotkiewski M, Mandroukas K, Sjöström L, Sullivan L, Wetterquist H, Björntorp P: Effects of long-term physical training on body fat, metabolism, and blood pressure in obesity. *Metabolism* 28:650–658, 1979.
51. Krotkiewski M, Björntorp P, Sjöström L, Smith U: Impact of obesity on metabolism in men and women: importance of regional adipose tissue distribution. *J Clin Invest* 72:1150–1162, 1983.
52. Kunze D: Reference values and tracking of blood lipid levels in childhood. *Prev Med* 12:806–809, 1983.
53. Lapidus L, Bengtsson C, Larsson B, Pennert K, Rybo E, Sjöström L: Distribution of adipose tissue and risk of cardiovascular disease and death: a 12-year follow-up of participants in the population study of women in Gothenburg, Sweden. *Br Med J* 289:1261–1263, 1984.
54. Larsson B, Svardsudd K, Welin L, Wilhemsen L, Björntorp P, Tibblin G: Abdominal adipose tissue distribution, obesity, and risk of cardiovascular disease and death: 13-year follow-up of participants in the study of men born in 1913. *Br Med J* 288:1401–1404, 1984.
55. Leon AS, Connett J, Jacobs DR, Rauramaa R: Leisure-time physical activity levels and risk of coronary heart disease and death. The Multiple Risk Factor Intervention Trial. *JAMA* 258:2388–2395, 1987.
56. Linder CW, Durant RH, Mahoney OM: The effect of physical conditioning on serum lipids and lipoproteins in white male adolescents. *Med Sci Sports Exerc* 15:232–236, 1983.
57. Lipid Research Clinics Program. The Lipid Research Clinics Coronary Primary Prevention Trial Results. II: The relationship of reduction in incidence of coronary heart disease to cholesterol lowering. *JAMA* 251:365–374, 1984.
58. Lowering cholesterol to prevent heart disease. *JAMA* 253:2080–2086, 1985.
59. Malina RM, Bouchard C: Subcutaneous fat distribution during growth. In Bouchard C, Johnston FE (eds): *Fat Distribution during Growth and Later Health Outcomes.* New York, Alan R. Liss, 1988, pp 63–84.
60. McGill HC Jr, Arias-Stellen J, Carbonnell LM, Correa P, de Veyra EA, Donoso S, Eggen DA, Galindo L, Guzman MA, Lichtenberger E, Loken AC, McGarry PA, McMahan CA, Montenegro MR, Mossy J, Perez-Iamayo R, Restrepo C, Robertson WB, Salas J, Solberg LA, Strong JP, Tejada C, Wainwright J: General findings of the international atherosclerosis project. *Lab Invest* 18:466–502, 1968.
61. McGill HC Jr: Morphologic development of the atherosclerotic plaque. In Lauer RM, Shekelle RR (eds): *Childhood Prevention of Atherosclerosis and Hypertension.* New York, Raven Press, 1980, pp 41–49.
62. McNamara JJ, Molot, MA, Stremple JF, Cutting RT: Coronary artery disease in combat casualties in Vietnam. *JAMA* 216:1185–1187, 1971.
63. Miller NE, Thelle DS, Forde OH, Mjos OD: The Tromso heart study—high-density lipoprotein and coronary heart disease, a prospective case-control study. *Lancet* 1:965–967, 1977.
64. Montoye HJ, Block W, Keller JB, Willis PW: Glucose tolerance and physical fitness: an epidemiologic study in an entire community. *Eur J Appl Physiol* 37:237–242, 1977.
65. Montoye HJ, Mikkelsen WM, Block WD, Gayle R: Relationship of oxygen uptake capacity, serum uric acid and glucose tolerance in males and females, age 10–69. *Am J Epidemiol* 108:274–282, 1978.
66. Newman WP III, Freedman DS, Voors AW, Gard PD, Srinivasan SR, Cresanta JL, Williamson GD, Webber LS, Berenson GS: Relation of serum lipoprotein levels and systolic blood pressure to early atherosclerosis. The Bogalusa Heart Study. *N Engl J Med* 314:138–144, 1986.

67. Olefsky JM, Farquhar JW, Reaven GM: A reappraisal of the role of insulin in hypertriglyceridemia. *Am J Med* 57:551–560, 1974.
68. Orchard TJ, Becker DJ, Kuller LH, Wagener DK, LaPorte RE, Drash AL: Age and sex variations in glucose tolerance and insulin responses: parallels with cardiovascular risk. *J Chron Dis* 35:123–132, 1982.
69. Orchard TJ, Donahue RP, Kuller LH, Hodge PN, Drash AL: Cholesterol screening in childhood: Does it predict adult hypercholesterolemia? The Beaver County experience. *J Pediatr* 103:687–691, 1983.
70. Parizkova J: Physical training in weight reduction of obese adolescents. *Ann Clin Res* 34:63–68, 1982.
71. Rationale of the diet-heart statement of the American Heart Association. Report of the AHA Nutrition Committee. *Arteriosclerosis* 4:177–191, 1982.
72. Savage MP, Petratis MM, Thompson WH, Berg K, Smith JL, Sady SP: Exercise training effects on serum lipids of prepubescent boys and adult men. *Med Sci Sports Exerc* 18:197–204, 1986.
73. Seals DR, Hagberg JM: The effect of exercise training on human hypertension: a review. *Med Sci Sports Exerc* 16:207–215, 1984.
74. Smoak CG, Burke GL, Webber LS, Harsha DW, Srinivasan SR, Berenson GS: Relation of obesity to clustering of cardiovascular disease risk factors in children and young adults. The Bogalusa Heart Study. *Am J Epidemiol* 125:364–372, 1987.
75. Solberg LA, Strong JP: Risk factors and atherosclerosis lesions. A review of autopsy studies. *Arteriosclerosis* 3:187–198, 1983.
76. Stefanick PA, Heald FP, Mayer J: Caloric intake in relation to energy output in obese and non-obese adolescent boys. *Am J Clin Nutr* 7:55–62, 1959.
77. Tamir I, Heiss G, Glueck CJ, Christensen B, Kwiterovich P, Rifkind BM: Lipid and lipoprotein distribution in white children ages 6–19 yr. The Lipid Research Clinics Program Prevalence Study. *J Chronic Dis* 34:27–39, 1981.
78. Thorland WG, Gilliam TB: Comparison of serum lipids between habitually high and low active pre-adolescent males. *Med Sci Sports Exerc* 13:316–321, 1985.
79. Tremblay A, Després JP, Bouchard C: The effects of exercise-training on energy balance and adipose tissue morphology and metabolism. *Sports Med* 2:223–233, 1985.
80. Tremblay A, Poehlman E, Nadeau A, Pérusse L, Bouchard C: Is the response of plasma glucose and insulin to short-term exercise-training genetically determined? *Horm Metab Res* 19:65–67, 1987.
81. Tyroler HA: Cholesterol and cardiovascular disease. An overview of Lipid Research Clinics (LRC) epidemiologic studies as background for the LRC Coronary Primary Prevention Trial. *Am J Cardiol* 54:14C–19C, 1984.
82. Vague J, Vague P, Jubelin J, Barré A: Fat distribution, obesities and health: Evolution of concepts. In Bouchard C, Johnston FE (eds): *Fat Distribution during Growth and Later Health Outcomes*. New York, Alan R. Liss, 1988, pp 9–41.
83. Välimäki I, Hursti ML, Pihlaskoski L, Viikari J: Exercise performance and serum lipids in relation to physical activity in school children. *Int J Sports Med* 1:132–136, 1980.
84. Viikari J, Välimäki I, Telama R, Siren-Tiusanen HK, Anderblom HK, Dahl M, Lahde PL, Personen M, Pietikainen M, Sudninen P, Uhari N: Atherosclerosis precursors in Finnish children: physical activity and plasma lipids in 3- and 12-year-old children. In Ilmarinen J, Välimäki I (eds): *Children and Sports*. Berlin, Springer-Verlag, 1984, pp 231–240.
85. Voors AW, Harsha DW, Webber LS, Radhakrishnamurthy B, Srinivasan SR, Berenson GS: Clustering of anthropometric parameters, glucose tolerance, and serum lipids in children with high and low B- and pre-B-lipoproteins: Bogalusa Heart Study *Arteriosclerosis* 2:346–355, 1982.
86. Vranic N, Berger M: Exercise and diabetes mellitus. *Diabetes* 28:147–167, 1979.

87. Wanne O, Viikari J, Välimäki I: Physical performance and serum lipids in 14–16-year-old trained, normally active, and inactive children. In Ilmarinen J, Välimäki I (eds): *Children and Sport.* Berlin, Springer-Verlag, 1984, pp 241–246.
88. Webber LS, Cresanta JL, Voors AW, Berenson CS: Tracking of cardiovascular disease risk factor variables in school-age children. *J Chronic Dis* 36:647–660, 1983.
89. Wilmore JH, McNamara JJ: Prevalence of coronary heart disease risk factors in boys, 8 to 12 years of age. *J Pediatr* 84:527–533, 1974.
90. Wood PD: Physical activity and high-density lipoproteins. In Miller NE, Miller GJ (eds): *Clinical and Metabolic Aspects of High-Density Lipoproteins.* Amsterdam, Elsevier, 1984, pp 133–165.
91. Wood PD, Stefanick ML, Dreon DS, Frey-Hewitt B, Garay SC, Williams PT, Superko HR, Fortman SP, Albers JJ, Vranizan KM, Ellsworth NM, Terry RB, Haskell WL: Changes in plasma lipids and lipoproteins in overweight men during weight loss through dieting as compared with exercise. *N Engl J Med* 319:1173–1179, 1988.
92. Ylä-Herttuala S: Development of atherosclerotic plaques. *Acta Med Scand (Suppl)* 701:7–14, 1985.
93. Ylitalo V: Treatment of obese schoolchildren. *Acta Paediatr Scand Suppl* 290:1–108, 1981.

9
Measuring the Cardiovascular Endurance of Persons with Mental Retardation: A Critical Review

BARRY LAVAY, Ph.D.
GREG REID, Ph.D.
MARSHA CRESSLER-CHAVIZ, M.S.

Engaging in proper physical fitness activities contributes to a person's healthy life-style for work and leisure [23, 68]. However, there is a lack of a universally accepted group of fitness components and a consensus of how these components can be most effectively measured. Most experts agree that the single best indicator of aerobic fitness is the measurement of an individual's cardiovascular capacity or maximum oxygen uptake consumption [68].

A healthy life-style is no less important for persons with mental retardation. For this reason, recent attention has focused on programs of physical fitness that enhance the cardiovascular endurance of this population (e.g., see Refs. 27, 29, 53, and 54). The focus of this chapter will be the measurement of cardiovascular fitness of persons with mental retardation.

The importance of physical fitness for persons with mental retardation is not only justified from the standpoint of promoting a healthy life-style, but also from a vocational perspective [9, 40]. The trend toward deinstitutionalization and the passage of the Education for All Handicapped Children's Act (Public Law 94–142) have increased the number of persons with mental retardation joining the work force. Coleman et al. [18] stated that programs of physical fitness are essential if this population is to qualify, maintain, and compete for employment of most manual occupational tasks. Employers concerned with optimal productivity prefer workers who can sustain a light to moderate work output over a long period of time without undue physical and/or mental fatigue. A study conducted by Beasley [9] demonstrated that an 8-week jogging program for persons with mental retardation not only improved their cardiovascular endurance level but also increased their work performance on piece-goods production.

Although the benefits of physical fitness improvement for individuals with mental retardation are well argued and supposedly documented [12, 16, 54], the difficulties of measuring their fitness casts doubt on

263

some of the supporting research. Too often, tests of cardiovascular endurance that have been validated with the general population are used indiscriminately with persons who are mentally retarded with little regard to their limited mental ability, movement proficiency, or prior learning experiences [67]. Bundschuh and Cureton [13] have questioned whether instruments used to assess the cardiovascular endurance of persons with normal intelligence can be used with this specific population.

This situation leaves professionals and scientists interested in the physical well being of this population with the dilemma of choosing appropriate measures and procedures of cardiovascular assessment. Without valid, reliable, and administratively feasible measurement instruments, proper assessment procedures and, consequently, appropriate programs of physical fitness improvement can not be fully realized. This review will begin by highlighting the pertinent intellectual, psychological, and physical characteristics of persons with mental retardation as they relate to cardiovascular fitness testing. Each mode of testing (step tests, bicycle ergometry, treadmill, and run/walk field tests) and corresponding empirical studies in the mental retardation literature will then be described as follows: (*a*) technical concerns, including preparing subjects for testing, reliability, validity, and underlying assumptions and (*b*) test performance, including availability of specific test protocols, norms, test score results, age, and gender differences.

PERSONS WITH MENTAL RETARDATION

Mental retardation is a common label for individuals who function at a significantly subaverage intellectual level and demonstrate deficits in adapted behavior during the developmental period [36]. Intellectual levels refer to performance on an IQ test, whereas adapted behavior refers to maturation and social responsibility. The first 18 years of life constitute the developmental period.

While the definition of mental retardation is relatively clear, it does not convey the enormous differences existing among persons so labeled. This variance has lead to a number of classifications in the field of mental retardation. A common system used by psychologists distinguishes among mild, moderate, severe, and profound retardation. The contents of Table 9.1 attest to the vast heterogeneity of the population. Those who are mildly handicapped may be totally integrated into society at adulthood because, for example, they work, drive a car, and marry. At the other extreme are some profoundly retarded individuals who have significant difficulties with rudimentary personal care and language. Clearly, the physical fitness appraiser is faced with a difficult task; one test or protocol is unlikely to be satisfactory for all levels of retardation.

TABLE 9.1
Characteristics of Persons with Mental Retardation

Level of Retardation	Characteristics
Mild	Retardation often not apparent until school difficulties arise
	Minimal delay in motor development and motor skill acquisition
	May learn academic skills up to grade 6 level
	Will learn social and vocational skills for self-support
	May require assistance in difficult economic times
Moderate	Can learn to talk and communicate but at delayed rate
	Motor deficits and coordination problems are common
	May learn academic skills up to g'ade 2 level
	Require specific training in social ɛ.ɪd vocational skills
	Often will require some supervision in adult living but may succeed in unskilled or semi-skilled work
Severe	Speech is minimal and delayed
	Significant delay in motor development
	Can be taught basic self-care skills
	Will require supervision and support in most vocational pursuits and adult living
Profound	Speech may be absent
	Significant delays in motor development physical abnormalities are common
	Will require assistance in self-care skills
	May require nursing-type care

In fact, Bar-Or et al. [7] noted that the appropriate test may be related to IQ or even place of residence. Therefore, it is likely that the optimal technique of cardiovascular assessment may interact with degree of retardation.

Levels of motor development and performance are also widely variable among those with mental retardation. Many persons with mild mental retardation are capable of behavior that matches or exceeds nonhandicapped peers. Perusal of Special Olympian records supports this assertion. More commonly, however, it is repeatedly noted that Special Olympians perform jumping, catching, throwing, balance, and general coordination of body management tasks with considerably less proficiency than would be expected for their age (e.g., see Refs. 32, 39, 60, and 75). Poor coordination has been noted as a reason for subject failure to complete a maximal graded treadmill walking regime [7]. There is also evidence indicating that motor performance generally declines as the severity of retardation increases (e.g., see Ref. 47), although there are significant numbers of individuals who perform contrary to this generalization. Finally, measurement issues notwithstanding, the physical fitness-related data indicate that children, youth, and adults with mental retardation are in poor physical condition [27, 54, 67].

Thus, the person with mental retardation may come to a cardiovascular testing situation with limited coordination and low physical fitness. Protocols for highly trained individuals (e.g., see Ref. 48) are obviously not appropriate and it is conceivable that even the initial workloads of standard protocols (e.g., see Refs. 6, 11, and 46) will be too demanding for the majority of these subjects. This could make the prediction of maximum oxygen uptake difficult if the prediction is based on a heart rate-work load relationship. There exists a linear relationship between heart rate and low to moderate work rates, whereas at high work rates the work output may increase without a corresponding increase in heart rate due to anaerobic energy contribution. If testing begins at a high work load for that person but the experimenter assumes it is a low or moderate level, then the maximum oxygen uptake is likely to be overestimated [5, 23].

Persons with mental retardation are unique not only intellectually and with regard to motor coordination but also they are often physically distinct. There is a tendency for this population to be shorter than age peers, with this difference increasing with the degree of retardation [34, 44]. In the large clinical subgroup of persons with Down syndrome they are not only shorter than nonhandicapped peers but are disproportionately short. Individuals with Down syndrome have unusually stunted limbs, whereas their trunks more closely approximate typical expectations [55, 71]. In addition, health specialists are concerned with the prevalence of obesity in persons with Down syndrome and mental retardation [31, 42]. Oxygen cost of activities with substantial body movement is influenced by body weight. When body size differences between mildly mentally retarded and nonretarded children are statistically removed, there are fewer motor performance tasks that differentiate between the two groups [24]. Therefore, physical characteristics must be considered when administering cardiovascular tests and interpreting the results.

It is also important to identify medical conditions that may affect test selection, administration, and/or interpretation, particularly in the moderate, severe, and profound retardation levels, where such problems are frequent. For example, persons with Down syndrome may have congenital heart disorders or respiratory problems. Atlantoaxial instability also occurs in approximately 15% of persons with Down syndrome and thus excessive flexion or extension of the neck is contraindicated [19]. Epilepsy is also common in mental retardation. Thus, cardiovascular fitness appraisers must be aware of the pathological correlates that will influence the testing protocol.

Finally, some additional observations have been noted that affect the efficacy of cardiovascular testing of these persons. Difficulties in maintaining the cadence of the protocol have been commonly cited [54, 62, 74]. Also, it is likely that the physiological efficiency of persons with mental retardation is less than nonhandicapped peers, due probably to poor coordination and less practice at the mode of exercise [66]. This is likely to lead to underestimations of maximum oxygen uptake. Also, cardiovascular fitness tests require a certain degree of motivation, either to complete two or three work loads in a submaximal protocol or to push oneself to near exhaustion in a maximal protocol. Researchers have often suggested that persons with mental retardation lack such motivation on tests of cardiovascular endurance [13, 54, 62, 74] and consequently stop before achieving true target heart rates or work loads.

This brief overview of persons with mental retardation highlights the extreme heterogeneity of the population and the need to adjust the assessment process in light of the competencies of the individual being tested. Additional considerations specific to the mode of exercise testing will be discussed next.

TESTS OF MAXIMAL AND SUBMAXIMAL OXYGEN UPTAKE

In a laboratory environment, primarily three types of cardiovascular endurance tests exist: bench stepping, treadmill, and bicycle ergometer exercise. Shephard [69] stated that each mode of exercise has "merit in certain specific situations" (p. 14). When selecting the protocol, a choice must be made with respect to direct or indirect measurement of oxygen consumption ($\dot{V}o_2$) and maximal or submaximal intensity of work. Field tests also have been used to estimate cardiovascular fitness including the 12-min run/walk [20] and runs ranging from 300 yards (274 meters) to 2000 meters [1, 35] or 9–12 min [2].

In all cardiovascular testing regardless of the intellectual characteristics of the subjects, it is important to prepare them for optimal performance by maintaining a cool room temperature (20–22°C), restricting eating (2 hr) and smoking (4 hr) prior to testing, having subjects comfortably dressed, avoiding vigorous exercise for several hours prior to testing, providing the subjects with appropriate warm-up and cool-down and being aware of any medication being taken by the individual [3].

Another important concept is familiarization with the mode of exercise. Persons with mental retardation may be apprehensive to attempt new test procedures and/or to use a certain piece of exercise equipment. Therefore, every effort must be made to familiarize, accommodate, and make the person feel comfortable and secure during the procedure [45]. Technical concerns and test performance will be specifically addressed in the following sections: step tests, bicycle ergometry, treadmill, and field tests of running walking.

Step Tests

TECHNICAL CONCERNS. The step test is an attractive method of exercise testing because of its simplicity and because most North Americans have extensive experience climbing stairs. For persons with limited mental ability this will likely minimize anxiety and habituate the individual to the experimental situation very quickly.

Familiarity with stepping is important to the validity of the step test. However, there is both concentric and eccentric work, with the latter requiring 25–33% less energy. As Heyward [38] pointed out, the issue of eccentric work coupled with adjusting the height and rate of stepping for differences in body weight make the standardization of work very difficult. Because oxygen uptake is predicted from work rate, any protocol in which it is difficult to maintain a consistent work rate will prove problematic. Thus, step testing was considered to be the least desirable mode of stress testing by Heyward [38].

Another consideration when using the step test is the assumption of 16% stepping efficiency, which is used in the prediction formula for maximum oxygen uptake in submaximal protocols. Recently, Seidl et al. [66] have shown that women with mental retardation are significantly less efficient than nonhandicapped peers (15.7 versus 17.1%), but the efficiency of the former group did not differ significantly from the assumed 16%. Although these data support additional research on the efficiency assumption for all persons, they do not invalidate the step test for persons with mental retardation.

A valid step test protocol requires the subject to maintain the required cadence of stepping, a problem noted when administering this test to persons with mental retardation [21, 30, 58, 62]. As noted in the next section, subjects are commonly eliminated for failing to maintain or increase cadence on a step test. Although needed, no study currently exists that directly addresses the issue of validity. The reliability (r) of the Canadian Home Fitness Test, a stepping protocol, has been assessed for adults with mental retardation at .84 [62] and .95 [21]. However, these results must be interpreted with caution, as the Canadian Home Fitness test stepping protocol has not been specifically validated for persons with mental retardation.

TEST PERFORMANCE. Few investigators have administered a bench-stepping test protocol to measure the cardiovascular endurance of persons with mental retardation (see Table 9.2). Also the few studies conducted have not used similar bench-stepping test procedures. The Ohio State University submaximal step test (Callan modification) was used by Peries [58], to ascertain the submaximal cardiovascular capacity of 129 children and adolescents (7–19 years of age) who were trainable (similar to moderate) mentally retarded. Apparatus included a split-level bench with 15- and 20-inch steps and handbars that could be adjusted to each individual's height. The test included 18 exercise innings with each divided into a 30-s work period and a 20-s rest period. During the testing, assistance was provided to the children by either one or more of the following methods: (*a*) stepping on the bench with an assistant, (*b*) playing a tape recording of the stepping sequence, and (*c*) providing visual

TABLE 9.2
Summary of Step Test Studies

Study	Subjects	Protocol	Exercise Program	Results
Fox et al. (1984)	42 adults	Ohio State Step Test	No program	Inferior fitness scores compared to general population
Peries (1973)	129 children	Ohio State Step Test (Callan Modification)	No program	Inferior fitness scores compared to general population
Reid et al. (1985)	220 adults, sheltered workshop	Modified Canadian Home Fitness Test	No program	Inferior fitness scores compared to general population
Seidl et al. (1989)	30 women	Modified Canadian Home Fitness Test	No program	Women with mental retardation were less efficient than nonhandicapped peers

and tactile cues. The test was stopped when either the subjects could not keep the proper stepping cadence, reached a heart rate of 174 bpm (Callan modification), or successfully completed all 18 innings. The obtained score was the number of innings completed. During the administration of the test, 85 of the students (66%) were able to successfully perform the test procedures. The remaining 44 students (34%) were unable to perform the test protocol correctly and were excluded from testing. The results of the investigation for those individuals who successfully completed the protocol revealed a score of 9.7 innings completed. Peries then compared the results to the scores of a group of nonhandicapped children and adolescents (similar age and same protocol). Results for the nonhandicapped population yielded a group mean score of 13.42 innings completed. Comparison of mean values between the two groups revealed that the group of children and adolescents with mental retardation produced significantly lower scores.

The Ohio State submaximal step test was also used in an investigation conducted by Fox et al. [30] to measure the submaximal cardiovascular endurance capacity of 42 adults employed in a sheltered workshop for persons with mental retardation. The adults were identified as obese ($n = 22$) or nonobese ($n = 20$) through a skinfold thickness measure. The protocol and apparatus was similar to that used in the investigation by Peries [58]. However, the investigators terminated testing when the subjects reached 150 bpm rather than 174 bpm. The step test was completed by 26 of the adults (62%) whereas the remaining 16 persons (37%) were eliminated because they failed to keep pace with the prescribed cadence. Interestingly, this success rate of 62% is similar to the 66% success rate reported in the 1973 study by Peries, although it should be noted that the adults in the Fox et al. [31] study were made to stop at a lower heart rate count of 150 bpm. The investigators summarized their findings by reporting that the obese adult scores were inferior to those of the nonobese adults. Also as a group, the mentally retarded persons were in a poorer fitness category when compared to normative data taken from a study using the same stepping protocol [50].

The Canadian Standard Test of Fitness [35] was administered to a total of 220 adults who were employed in a sheltered workshop setting for persons with mental retardation [62]. The test item selected to measure the cardiovascular endurance of the adults was a step test modified from the Canadian Home Fitness Test. This test required the individuals to complete three successive 3-min work bouts, although subjects were stopped if their heart rates exceeded predetermined rates. The individual ascended and descended two steps at a preestablished tempo set to a music tape. The beginning tempo was set according to the age of each subject. However, a pilot study of 20 adults who were mentally retarded determined that they could not maintain the stepping rate on the tape. Therefore, the regression equation to predict the maximum oxygen uptake was modified to account for the actual number of steps completed rather than the desired tempo of stepping during the last 3 min work bout. When the adults stepped at a rate slower than recommended, the oxygen uptake scores were interpolated from values provided by Jetté et al. [41]. In order to decrease the participant's level of anxiety, verbal encouragement, modelling, physical guidance, and prompting procedures were provided by trained instructors throughout the test protocol. Results of this study demonstrated poor fitness scores by the majority of the adults. However, the authors cautioned that the actual values may have been an underestimation, because 45% of the adults tested were stopped prior to reaching their target heart rate because they had not increased their tempo of stepping. Also, 2% refused to continue to the next level, whereas the remaining 53% were stopped because their heart rates equalled or exceeded the target heart rates prescribed in the protocol.

SUMMARY OF STEP TESTING. The simplicity and familiarity of stepping remains the step test's most attractive point. The assumption of 16% efficiency does not seem to be violated by mentally retarded subjects [66]. The step test has been reported to be reliable [21, 62] when administering a prediction equation developed by Jetté et al. [41] and modified by Reid et al. [62]. The difficulty for subjects to maintain the appropriate cadence and the problem of standardizing work output because of the down phase of stepping remain serious concerns to validity. Modifications that need to be considered are the following: (*a*) a nonhandicapped partner stepping with the person and giving physical prompts and verbal encouragement to maintain cadence; and (*b*) regression equations [62] designed to measure the actual steps completed rather than adhering to the actual tempo of the stepping cadence.

The three studies noted [31, 58, 62] all "lost" subjects for a variety of reasons. Thus, if a step protocol was subsequently demonstrated to be valid, the statement of validity would have to be considered in terms such as "under the following conditions . . ." and "for persons with a range of retardation from _____ to _____," etc. This is in keeping with the notion that a given mode and/or protocol may be useful for only a certain classification of the mentally retarded population. Studies to validate step test protocols with this population are clearly needed.

Bicycle Ergometry Tests

TECHNICAL CONCERNS. Bicycle ergometry testing is often conducted in laboratory settings adhering to specific equipment, test protocols, and procedures that are usually unfamiliar to persons with mental retardation. Although some persons with mental retardation may have recreational experience riding a bicycle, it is likely that they are unfamiliar with maintaining a steady speed in order to successfully adhere to a specific test protocol [45]. Also, riding a bicycle ergometer may quickly tire weak quadriceps, thus inducing local muscle fatigue and a desire to stop. To date, few investigations have conducted orientation and extensive practice sessions prior to actual test administration [21, 45, 49].

Research conducted with the general population has indicated that $\dot{V}o_2$max on the bicycle ergometer is 5–12% lower than that obtained on the treadmill [51]. Also, submaximal tests tend to overestimate the physical work capacity in well-trained individuals and to underestimate the physical work capacity in poorly trained individuals [5, 27]. Certainly, the majority of persons with mental retardation would be in the untrained category (Table 9.3). This should be an important consideration during the selection of submaximal exercise test protocols.

If subjects are to successfully adhere to the prescribed bicycle ergometry test protocol, they must maintain the indicated work load by following a steady and consistent speed. The majority of the investigations conducted in this area have reported difficulties in subjects following the prescribed work bout [13, 21, 45, 57]. Difficulties encountered by subjects have included: (*a*) inability to cycle the proper number of revolutions per minute in order to maintain the proper work rate; (*b*) performing quick bursts of pedalling while riding and not maintaining a steady and constant speed; (*c*) successfully completing only one work rate, which makes extrapolation difficult; and (*d*) experiencing general fatigue and specific tiredness in the legs following increased work rates, which deteriorates pedalling performance. The use of an electronically braked bicycle ergometer may solve some of these problems; however, to date, few investigators have used this piece of equipment [10, 49, 57].

No studies have addressed the issue of validity for persons with mental retardation. The test-retest reliability of the bicycle ergometry physical working capacity (PWC) test for the general population has been shown to have a correlation of $\tau = 0.88$ [23] for adults with mental retardation; the reliability for the PWC has been documented at $\tau = 0.84$ [13] and $\tau = 0.64$ [21]. A limitation to the interpretation of these latter reliability studies is that they did not use the same PWC protocol as was used with the general population.

Another technical concern is that the majority of the studies conducted with persons who are mentally retarded have used a variety of bicycle ergometry test protocols and procedures (Table 9.3) that are standardized with the general population. Few studies have taken into consideration the subject's age, mental classification, or training level. Investigations have included subjects who range in age from children to adults and encompass various mental classifications. The test protocols used were the Åstrand Submaximal Test [10, 45, 70], the Physical Work Capacity Test [13, 21, 22], and the Sjostrand Modification Technique [18]. Only a few investigators have incorporated procedural modifica-

TABLE 9.3
A Summary of Bicycle Ergometer Test Studies

Study	Subjects	Protocol	Exercise Program	Results
Bennett et al. (1989)	3 Down syndrome adults	Åstrand Submaximal Protocol	Token economy contingency program	Decreased heart rate after exercise program
Bundschuh and Cureton (1982)	14 adolescents	PWC_{170} Test	16-week bicycle program	No significant increase compared to control group
Coleman et al. (1976)	37 male adults	Sjostrand Modification	No program	20–30% below general population in fitness capacity
Maksud and Hamilton (1974)	62 EMR children	50 and 75 watts	No program	Low cardiovascular fitness levels
Nordgren (1970)	63 young adults	Various work loads	No program	16 of the subjects were unable to perform protocol
Skrobak-Kaczynski and Vavik (1980)	20 male adolescents and adults	Åstrand Submaximal Protocol	5-Circuit fitness program	Significant improvement of adult age group

tions in the test protocol [18, 22, 49]. The use of different bicycle ergometry protocols makes comparison of various investigations difficult. Few studies have incorporated $\dot{V}o_2$max procedures [10, 18, 49].

There has been minimal work comparing bicycle ergometry tests to other forms of cardiovascular fitness testing (Table 9.4). One study compared subjects in the Physical Working Capacity Bicycle Ergometer Test to the 12-Min/1.5-Mile Run Test [22]. The protocol was administered to nine adolescents with mild to moderate mental retardation. A comparison during testing revealed that subjects participating in the 12-Min Run/Walk Test elicited a greater fluctuation in heart rate. At various times, pulse rates exceeded 85% of an individual's predicted maximum heart rate. This was not the case during the administration of the bicycle ergometer test and the investigators concluded that this was a safer and more accurate method to determine cardiovascular fitness levels for adults with mental retardation who exhibit low levels of fitness. These results must be interpreted with caution, as the validation of either test protocol specific to persons with mental retardation was never conducted.

TEST PERFORMANCE. As noted, the majority of the investigations conducted in this area have encountered a number of difficulties with this population adhering to the prescribed test protocol and work bouts. For example, 16 of 63 (25%) individuals tested in an investigation by Nordgren [56] were unable to successfully complete the physical work ergometry test protocol. To overcome these difficulties, few investigators have included the following test modifications: (a) an electric metronome or tape recording of the prescribed work load to monitor pedal frequency, (b) a visual cue in the form of a piece of tape placed on the speedometer at the prescribed work load, (c) physical prompting by an assistant in order to assure the subject maintains the proper pedal frequency, and/or (d) verbal encouragement [18, 21, 22, 45]. These modifications are also often used with the general population. Whether these modifications improve performance in persons with mental retardation needs to be further investigated. The application of test modifications may vary among age groups and classifications of mental retardation.

All but one study [70] has reported subjects to display inferior maximum oxygen uptake scores compared to those of the general population. In this investigation the mean group scores of the adults in group one as measured by the Åstrand Bicycle Ergometry Test improved from 36 to 49 ml/kg/min after subjects participated in a 12-week exercise circuit program. Interestingly, the mean maximum oxygen uptake test scores after training were 2 ml/kg/min above the mean score of healthy Norwegian males of the same age. The authors noted that this group of men with mental retardation was more familiar with physical training, less time was needed for motivation or instruction, and consequently more time was devoted to an intensive 12-week training session. How-

TABLE 9.4
A Comparison of Different Cardiovascular Test Protocols

Study	Subjects	Protocols Compared	Results
Cressler et al. (1988)	17 adults employed in a workshop	1. Cooper 12-min run 2. Balke Ware Treadmill 3. PWC Bicycle Ergometer Test 4. Canadian Home Fitness Step Test	Reliability scores of the protocols varied
DePauw et al. (1985)	9 adolescents	1. 12-min run/walk 2. PWC Bicycle Ergometer Protocol	Bicycle ergometer PWC is a more accurate and safer measure
Fernhall and Tymeson (1988)	15 adults employed in a workshop	1. 300-yard and 1.5-mile runs 2. $\dot{V}O_2$max protocol	1.5-mile run a valid indicator of fitness with populations studied
Lavay et al. (1987)	6 adults employed in a workshop	1. Cooper 12-min run 2. Modified Balke Ware Treadmill 3. Åstrand Bicycle Ergometer	With modifications the individuals could engage in all tests

ever, the majority of the studies using bicycle ergometry test protocols have reported inferior scores when compared to the general population [13, 18, 48]. For example, one investigation reported 37 male adult subjects with mental retardation to display fitness scores 20–30% inferior to their nonhandicapped counterparts [18]. The likely reasons for the lower $\dot{V}o_2max$ values for persons with mental retardation may be lack of both physical condition and an understanding of the exercise test procedures.

SUMMARY OF BICYCLE ERGOMETRY TESTING. The administration of bicycle ergometry testing is a widely accepted procedure used with the general population to measure cardiovascular fitness. However, the majority of the studies conducted of persons with mental retardation have encountered a number of difficulties. Before actual test administration, it is important to familiarize subjects with the test environment (i.e., laboratory setting), the equipment used, and the prescribed test protocol. Orientation and sufficient practice sessions are imperative.

Another major concern is that the studies have used bicycle ergometry test protocols (e.g., Physical Work Capacity Test) standardized for the general population. Studies have not taken into consideration the specific ages, training levels, and different mental classifications of the mentally retarded population. This can be a major reason why the majority of the reported studies have found these persons to display difficulties in successfully following the prescribed work bouts and protocols while engaged in bicycle ergometry testing. In general these subjects displayed difficulty cycling the required number of pedal revolutions per minute. Although a few investigators have made some test modifications, to date no study has been conducted that validates bicycle ergometry test procedures for persons with mental retardation.

Treadmill Tests

TECHNICAL CONCERNS. In laboratory settings, the assessment of oxygen consumption on a treadmill is a widely accepted means of measuring cardiovascular endurance capacity [23]. However, using a treadmill is limited to one person at a time and requires expensive equipment and laboratory facilities [26].

Treadmill tests follow specific procedures and test protocols using either maximal or submaximal measures of oxygen consumption. Treadmill studies conducted of persons with mental retardation have used a variety of protocols (Table 9.5). While walking is a familiar activity for this population, walking on a moving belt is a new experience for the majority.

Before testing can begin, it is important to familiarize subjects with the equipment that will be used such as the actual treadmill, headgear, electrodes, mouthpiece, etc. [61]. An early investigation did not discuss in

TABLE 9.5
A Summary of Treadmill Test Studies

Study	Subjects	Protocol	Exercise Program	Results
Andrew et al. (1979)	20 adults	Modified Balke Protocol	12-week exercise program	Exercise group increased duration of treadmill
Bar-Or (1971)	161 children	3 different all-out walking tests	No program	85% of the group could complete the protocol
Burkett (1984)	5 TMR adolescents	Bruce Multistage Protocol	No program	Max $\dot{V}o_2$ scores inferior to general population
Campbell and Shannon (1970)	6 institutionalized adolescents	Balke Maximum Work Capacity Protocol	No program	Reliable method of measuring fitness levels
Fernhall and Tymeson (1987)	21 EMR adults	Graded exercise $\dot{V}o_2$max protocol	No program	Successfully completed protocol with proper modification
Millar (1988)	14 Down syndrome adolescents and adults	Balke Ware Protocol	10-week walk/jog program	No significant difference in scores
Schurrer et al. (1985)	5 adults	Based on individual fitness levels	23-week walk/jog program	Improved fitness scores over 23-week program
Tomporowski and Ellis (1984)	65 institutionalized adults	Balke Ware Protocol	11-month aerobic exercise program	Increased group duration on the treadmill
Tomporowski and Jameson (1985)	19 adults	Treadmill walk/run was part of the exercise program	18-week aerobic exercise program	Increased group duration on the treadmill

detail the actual orientation and practice sessions conducted to familiarize mentally retarded subjects with the test equipment [7]. The lack of a pretest orientation may have been a contributing factor to subject dropout during testing. In this investigation, 24 of 161 individuals (15%) did not participate in testing for the following reasons: refusal to get on the treadmill, refusal to complete the walk, refusal to wear the mouthpiece, and difficulty breathing [7].

Later investigations conducted orientation and practice sessions with subjects (e.g., see Refs. 21, 25, 45, 64, and 73). The actual time spent and procedures used to familiarize subjects with specific equipment and test procedures have varied greatly. Some studies have conducted minimal orientation period(s): two separate 10-min sessions [15] or one 10-min session for each subject [73]. Other studies have described in detail the orientation and practice sessions conducted: a 2-week period [21], a 3-week period [14], six of eight visits to the laboratory [4], a two-phase orientation program [25], and sufficient practice sessions with spotters until each subject felt comfortable on the treadmill and could walk with a steady gait [45]. To date, the Fernhall and Tymeson study [25] is the only investigation to chronicle familiarization procedures and identify specific criteria that will denote functional familiarization specific to this population while on the treadmill.

The majority of the studies conducted in this area have used a variety of treadmill test protocols and procedures standardized with the general population. As with step tests and bicycle ergometer tests, the majority of investigations have selected test protocols with little regard to age, mental ability, or training level of the subjects. Investigators have administered a variety of standardized test protocols, such as the Balke Treadmill Test [16], Modified Balke Treadmill Test [4], Balke Ware Treadmill Test [21, 52, 73], Modified Balke Ware Treadmill Test [25, 26, 45], and the Bruce Multistage Protocol [14]. Some investigations have based protocol selection on the individual fitness levels of subjects tested [64] and pilot study data [21].

To date, only one study has used oxygen uptake results from a treadmill protocol to validate another protocol [26]. Adults with mild mental retardation walked on an exercise treadmill maintained at a constant speed of 3 mph (1.34 m/s) throughout the test. During the first 2 min, subjects exercise at a 0% grade, followed by a 2.5% grade for an additional 2 min. Following these initial stages the grade was raised 2.5% every minute until exhaustion. Results demonstrated that the 1.5-mile run/walk test was a valid indicator of cardiovascular fitness with this population (Table 9.4).

Reliability coefficient scores on maximum oxygen uptake treadmill tests for the general population usually range from $\tau = 0.97$ to 0.99 [5]. A reliability score of $\tau = 0.93$ has been reported using the Balke Ware Treadmill Test protocol for adults with mild to moderate mental retardation [21]. Also the Balke Maximum Work Capacity Treadmill Test protocol has been reported to demonstrate high reliable scores when measuring cardiovascular fitness for children with mental retardation [15].

As stated earlier in this section, a variety of studies have been conducted that provide subjects with sufficient orientation and practice sessions to adequately prepare for treadmill testing. Spotters have been used to physically guide subjects onto the treadmill and to help them walk with a steady gait [45]. For some subjects, walking with a steady and comfortable gait on the treadmill is difficult without holding on to the handrails and looking down on the belt. These factors can seriously alter test scores and the validity of the protocol [5]. Strategies used to alleviate these problems include: spotters positioned to the side and back of the subject, and motivating posters placed on the wall directly in front of the treadmill, which help to keep the subject's head erect [45].

TEST PERFORMANCE. Studies indicate that subjects with mental retardation display lower maximum oxygen uptake scores for their age when compared to their nonhandicapped counterparts [14, 25, 52]. These test results have been reported with different age groups and classifications of mental retardation such as: adults with mild to moderate mental retardation [4, 25, 64], adolescents with moderate mental retardation [14], and adolescents and young adults with Down syndrome [52]. For example, in the Burkett et al. study [14], variations in $\dot{V}O_2max$ among five adolescents with moderate mental retardation varied from 20 to 38 $ml \cdot kg^{-1} \cdot min^{-1}$. Millar et al. [52] reported pretraining $\dot{V}O_2max$ mean scores of 26.9 and 26.2 $ml \cdot kg^{-1} \cdot min^{-1}$ for adolescents and young adults with Down syndrome. Fernhall and Tymeson [25] reported an overall mean $\dot{V}O_2max$ score of 26.3 $ml \cdot kg^{-1} \cdot min^{-1}$ for 17 young adults (mean age = 29 years) with mental retardation. These authors [25] noted that the nonhandicapped adult population below the age of 30 years will exhibit an average $\dot{V}O_2max$ score between 40 and 50 $ml \cdot kg^{-1} \cdot min^{-1}$.

Some investigators have reported the treadmill to be advantageous compared to other means of exercise testing such as the bicycle ergometer, steps, and run/walks [25, 72–74]. One advantage to treadmill testing is that the pace of the exercise is externally controlled. Whereas maintaining the desirable cadence on a step test or bicycle has proven problematic for subjects with mental retardation, the treadmill minimizes the possibility of subjects accelerating and decelerating during testing. The treadmill moves at a set speed, allowing for precise control of each subject's pace during testing. This may explain why the treadmill has been used successfully with persons with severe mental retardation (e.g., see Ref. 74).

SUMMARY OF TREADMILL TESTING. Research has demonstrated that the treadmill is a desirable means of cardiovascular fitness testing and training for persons with mental retardation. However, it is important for future investigators to consider that initially many persons with mental retardation may perceive the laboratory setting as frightening and will be apprehensive to run and/or walk on the treadmill, wear headgear and electrodes, and breath though a respiratory collection system. There are unique challenges and strategies necessary to test this particular population with the treadmill. In order to determine a true measure of cardiovascular fitness, investigators must conduct sufficient orientation and practice sessions in a nonthreatening atmosphere if these subjects are to adapt to equipment and feel comfortable with test procedures.

Recent studies have taken into consideration modifications and sufficient practice sessions to familiarize subjects with the necessary equipment and test procedures. One study has compared the treadmill $\dot{V}o_2max$ for adults with mental retardation to predict $\dot{V}o_2max$ from walk/run field tests [26]. More validation studies of this nature need to be conducted in laboratory settings with different age groups and with individuals of various classifications of mental retardation. These validation studies would assist practitioners in field settings, such as the school or community, in selecting the best test(s) for the particular population.

Run/Walk Field Tests

TECHNICAL CONCERNS. Run/walk field tests are attractive because they are simple to administer and require little equipment. Tests of this nature have ranged from 300 yards (274 meters) to 2000 meters and from 6 to 12 min (Table 9.6). It is assumed that the subjects are familiar with walking and running.

Although run/walk field tests may be simple to administer, they are always indirect measures of aerobic capacity [27]. Fernhall and Tymeson [26] have examined the issue of validity of such field tests specific to persons with mental retardation. The investigators reported the 1.5-mile run/walk component of the AAHPERD Health Related Fitness Test to be a valid measure of cardiovascular fitness of mildly mentally retarded adults. The reported correlation between $\dot{V}o_2max$ and the 1.5-mile run/walk component was $\tau = 0.88$. In this particular investigation it should be noted that the number of mentally retarded adults tested was limited to 15. Another important finding of this study was that the 300-yard (274-meter) run/walk test was not a significant predictor of $\dot{V}o_2max$. These results are important because this field test is commonly used with this population to measure cardiovascular fitness.

Koh and Watkinson [43] studied the heart rate responses of moderately retarded youngsters as they performed the endurance run of the Canada Fitness Awards, Adapted Format. A telemetry chest belt was used to record heart rate. A 10–12-year-old group ($N = 9$) was required to run 1200 meters whereas a 13-year and older group ($N = 7$) ran 2000

TABLE 9.6
A Summary of Run/Walk Field Test Studies

Study	Subjects	Protocol	Exercise Program	Results
Beasley (1982)	30 adults in sheltered workshop	Cooper 12-min run/walk	8 weeks, 5 days/week	Experimental group significant reduction in mean run/walk time
Findlay (1981)	644 TMR (children)	Endurance run of Canada Fitness Test	No program	Youngsters had difficulty completing distance
Halle et al. (1983)	9 TMR children	600-yard run/walk	7 months, 5 days/week	Group significant gain in distance completed
Jansma et al. (1986)	71 institutionalized adults	300-yard run/walk	14 weeks, 4 days/week Fitness/hygiene	Modified from 600 yard, based on pilot study
Koh and Watkinson (1988)	16 children and adolescents, moderate retardation	1200-m and 2000-m runs of Canada Fitness Awards	No program	Participants helped by pacer
Londeree and Johnson (1974)	1005 TMR children and adolescents	300-yard run/walk	No program	Modified from 600-yard AAHPER Youth Fitness Test
Pizarro (1982)	126 EMR/TMR	880-yard run/walk	No program	Modified from 9-min AAHPERD HRPFT, based on pilot study
Rarick et al. (1970)	4235 EMR	300-yard run/walk	No program	Modified from 600-yard AAHPER Youth Fitness Test
Tomporowski and Jameson (1985)	19 severe/profound institutionalized adults	No protocol	18 weeks, 5 days/week	Group increase in miles completed and decrease in time each week
Watkinson and Koh (1988)	16 EMR children	1200–2000 m	No program	High heart rate responses for a relatively long duration

meters. The mean completion times for the groups without the aid of a pacer were 8:26 and 14:14 (min:s), respectively. A vigorous intensity level was defined as a heart rate above 160 bpm. More than 80% of the recorded heart rate responses of the younger group fell into this category. Sixty-five percent of responses of the older group were considered as vigorous although this increased to 74% when the subjects were paced during the run. Such high heart rates for a relatively long duration suggest that this field test is assessing the cardiovascular systems of the subjects. Thus, the data from Fernhall and Tymeson [26] and Watkinson and Koh [76] support the validity of the field tests, at least for the small number of subjects studied.

Run/walk field tests do present unique issues and concerns when administered to persons with mental retardation. The successful administration of run/walk field tests can be difficult, especially for persons exhibiting moderate to severe mental retardation. The majority of these individuals are limited in their mental ability and may lack the necessary motivation required to complete such a task. Despite the success of the limited number of subjects in the Watkinson and Koh [76] study, Findlay [28] reported the drop-out rates of trainable mentally handicapped children and youth on the endurance runs of the Canadian Fitness Awards. In general there was a greater than 50% drop out of subjects at half the required distance. For example 8-year-old children were required to run 800 meters, yet 57% of the girls and 64% of the boys stopped at 400 meters. The situation deteriorated with older youths. For example, 15-year-old adolescents were required to run 2400 meters. However, 71% of the girls and 83% of the boys did not run beyond 1200 meters. Other concerns with walk/run testing include: (*a*) completing a prescribed time, such as 12 min, which is an abstract concept [26], (*b*) the inability to cope with breathlessness and fatigue, (*c*) lack of knowledge of pace or concept of distance [8, 59], and (*d*) the perseverence needed to complete the required distance in an "all out effort" to determine true cardiovascular fitness [22].

Modifications have been made by reducing the distance of the run/walk in order to accommodate this populations' unique needs. The early work of Rarick et al. [60] established fitness norms for children with mild mental retardation. The AAHPER Youth Fitness Test item of the 600-yard run/walk was reduced to 300 yards (274 meters). The investigators felt the shorter distance would be long enough to determine the individual's endurance level. Similar modifications were made by Londeree and Johnson [47] in establishing physical fitness standards for individuals with moderate mental retardation. Jansma et al. [40] in their physical fitness and hygiene study with mentally retarded adults residing in an institution reduced the distance of the fitness run/walk from 600 (549 meters) to 300 (274 meters) yards. This was based on the results of an earlier pilot study in which a high percentage of adults could not successfully complete the longer distance. Pizarro [59] substituted the 9-min run on the Health Related Fitness Test with an 800-yard (712-meter) run when over 70% of the participants in a pilot study either quit or completed less than 1100 yards (1005 meters). In the actual investigation, the majority of children with mild and moderate mental retardation spent a greater amount of time walking than running, whereas some stopped before finishing.

However, it should be noted that the shortening of the distance to 300 yards (274 meters), although often used, has never been validated for children with mental retardation and has been found to be an invalid measure of cardiovascular fitness for adults with mental retardation [26]. Administrators of these field tests with this population are faced with a serious dilemma. By reducing the distance and/or duration of the run/walk test, an adequate measure of cardiovascular fitness is questionable [8, 26, 27]. However, if they do not limit the distance and/or duration, the majority of this population will be unable to successfully complete the test. Before this population can successfully complete such a field test they need to be properly prepared with systematic, individualized, self-paced, and highly motivated training techniques.

The majority of these field tests with the general population have reported high reliability scores $r = 0.92$ [20]. For persons with mild and moderate mental retardation the research is limited. The reliability of the Cooper 12-min run/walk in one study was reported to be $r = 0.81$ for adults with mild mental retardation [21].

TEST PERFORMANCE. For children with mental retardation, Koh and Watkinson [43] have investigated the effect of pacers on the time to complete the endurance runs of the Canada Fitness Award, Adapted Format. Based upon the youngsters' pretest performance the pacers were able to individualize the pace on three subsequent tests. The pacers ran slightly in front of the children, providing verbal encouragement and instructions. The authors concluded that not only do more children complete the distance with a pacer but also the time to complete improves. In addition, a few studies that implement a systematic run/walk program with this population have been conducted in order to prepare this population for testing [9, 37, 74]. Training modifications to prepare a person with mental retardation for testing have included: meeting weekly running standards [37], systematic distance increase [9], and running with a pacer [43, 47].

SUMMARY OF FIELD TESTING. Although run/walk field tests are attractive because they are simple to administer and require little equipment, they present unique issues and considerations when administered to persons with mental retardation. The limited research reveals that systematic training programs are needed to prepare these subjects for run/walk field tests. Without consideration for motivational factors, it is unlikely that persons with mental retardation will perform well on run/walk field tests, which in turn will contribute to inaccurate estimates of cardio-vascular fitness [27, 67]. Conversely, Koh and Watkinson [43, 76] have demonstrated that some moderately retarded youngsters are capable of expending considerable energy during endurance runs and that their timed performance can be enhanced with the help of pacers. Such results favor the continued use of field tests. However, an attempt should be made to replicate these findings to determine if the subjects in Koh and Watkinson's research are representative of other persons with mental retardation.

Studies of training programs to prepare this population for testing have reported individual as well as group improvement in the distance or the time the subjects needed to complete the run/walk. Typically the subjects were afforded the opportunity to run/walk consistently 4–5 days a week over a period of 2–7 months. All of the studies established individualized standards based on personal performance and ability, an important training as well as motivational consideration with this population. Few studies have paired subjects with a partner while participating in a run/walk testing or training program [43, 74], which is a modification that should be given serious consideration because these subjects lack the necessary knowledge and ability regarding proper pacing techniques [43, 59].

CONCLUSIONS AND FUTURE DIRECTIONS

The heterogeneity of persons with mental retardation makes cross-study comparisons almost impossible unless authors provide detailed descriptions of the subjects. Simply listing IQs or the range of retardation (e.g., moderate, severe, etc.) is not sufficient. Among the many relevant characteristics that might impinge upon cardiovascular test performance include: (*a*) recreation patterns, (*b*) sport involvement, (*c*) body size and weight, (*d*) living conditions, and (*e*) prominent behavioral characteristics such as abnormal fears, hyperactivity, etc. Knowledge of each subject's present level of performance will help reconcile apparent contradictions such as the vigorous energy expenditure of subjects in the Watkinson and Koh [76] study and the more frequent observation that motivating persons with mental retardation to perform on standardized tests is a problem (e.g., see Ref. 62). It is quite possible that the subjects are vastly different in studies with results that appear to be at odds with each other. Detailed descriptions of subjects will also promote the ultimate emergence of clusters of individuals who share common characteristics. It is conceivable that different protocols or modes of cardiovascular assessment will become matched to the various clusters. As previously noted, one procedure is not going to be sufficient for accurate assessment of all persons with mental retardation.

The validation of testing modes of cardiovascular endurance within this population is in its infancy and much more research is needed. Poor mechanical efficiency will lead to underestimation of maximum oxygen uptake as will submaximal protocols with untrained persons. Because persons with mental retardation may be inefficient movers [66] and they are no doubt generally in poor physical condition, it is possible that current estimates of their cardiovascular fitness are actually underestimations of their true aerobic fitness. More studies devoted to questions of validity are required. Reliability studies are beginning to emerge (e.g. see Ref. 21) and researchers should not be allowed to publish their work without providing such information.

Future research must also address the relative merits of the various means of assessment. Some comparative research of this type has begun (Table 9.4). It is usually demonstrated with nonhandicapped subjects that the highest oxygen uptake values are elicited by graded treadmill protocols, whereas cycle ergometry yields lower scores [51]. However, Reid [61] described a pilot study of persons with mental retardation indicating that bench-stepping and cycle ergometry protocols produced higher Vo_2max scores compared to those of a graded treadmill protocol. Similarly, Lavay et al. [45] found a significant difference in favor of cycle ergometry over a treadmill procedure. More research of this nature is required to determine if the Reid [61] and Lavay et al. [45] results are robust and, if so, why do they differ from those of nonhandicapped persons. DePauw et al. [22] concluded that a PWC bicycle ergometry test was more accurate than a 12-min run/walk. These results must be interpreted with caution as neither test was validated specifically for persons with mental retardation. Other researchers have found such endurance runs to be quite satisfactory (e.g., see Refs. 26 and 76). Again, these findings must be couched in terms of subject characteristics, that is, protocol X is appropriate and reliable for persons with mental retardation who display characteristics A, B, and C.

It is critical that persons with mental retardation be familiar with the testing protocol. Reid et al. [63] have provided a number of suggestions for pretest familiarization including: using testers who are known to the subjects, explaining why a procedure is used and not assuming that the person is unable to understand, allowing for refamiliarization with mouthpieces, etc. if multiple testing occurs, and teaching subjects to use hand signals to indicate discomfort if breathing apparatus is used. In addition, Tomporowski and Ellis [72] have demonstrated that, with structured physical assistance, some severely and profoundly retarded individuals can perform desired exercises. However, their study was not one of cardiovascular endurance, so future studies should address the specific means by which subjects can be accommodated in endurance tests.

Large intraindividual variability plagues researchers who use a pretest-posttest design to evaluate the effectiveness of exercise programs. A posttest result that differs from the pretest could be the result of functional cardiovascular improvement or normal variation within subjects. One could posit further that posttest scores would systematically increase, given the greater familiarity at posttest with the testing procedures, facilities, and personnel. Therefore, it would be desirable to adopt multiple measures at both pre- and posttest phases of the research [67]. Repeating a test two or three times should yield a realistic baseline or pretest performance. Similarly, having subjects repeat the test several times at the conclusion of a program should produce a clearer picture of typical performance. Of course, future research is required to determine the optimal number of repeated tests and whether or not there is a systematic trend across the multiple tests. Perhaps most importantly, studies must be conducted that validate appropriate familiarization procedures for different age groups and classifications of persons with mental retardation [26].

There is a need to adopt and evaluate novel measurement and training techniques for some persons with severe or profound retardation who are unable to learn typical standardized procedures. Such techniques may evaluate exercise programs without established estimates of $\dot{V}O_2$max. Sechrest [65] used a simple behavioral measure of number of pedal turns as a dependent variable in a study designed to assess the influence of visual stimulation, candy, and trinkets as reinforcers of youngsters with mental retardation on a stationary bicycle. Likewise, Caouette and Reid [17] used a time-series design to compare visual and auditory stimulation as potential reinforcers of severely retarded adults on a bicycle ergometer. The ergometer was the exercise medium rather than a testing vehicle, work output over 15 min being the dependent measure. Heart rate responses can also be used to assess program effectiveness. In some settings it is not feasible for standard protocols of maximum oxygen uptake to be used. However, alternative behavioral measures exist (e.g., work output, number of pedal turns, total time cycling), which can provide researchers with a rigorous means to evaluate the exercise program of persons with mental retardation. In this manner, we can promote and objectively assess the influence of exercise testing protocols for all persons with mental retardation.

It is obvious from the many measurement and administrative issues presented in this review that research and study in this area needs to continue. It is a false assumption that tests that are appropriate with the general population are valid and can be effectively administered to persons with mental retardation, especially when one considers the heterogeneity of this population. Case managers and professionals in the areas of special physical education, exercise physiology, and rehabilitation must collaborate in an effort to develop true measures of cardiovascular endurance that are appropriate with this population. Most importantly, quality research will lead to effective cardiovascular fitness testing that will enhance program application, which in turn will lead to healthy lifestyle changes in persons with mental retardation [21].

ACKNOWLEDGMENTS

This paper was supported in part by the financial assistance provided to Dr. Reid from Fitness Canada and the Canadian Fitness Lifestyle and Research Institute. The authors wish to acknowledge the helpful comments of the reviewers on an earlier draft of this chapter.

REFERENCES

1. American Alliance for Health, Physical Education and Recreation. *Youth Fitness Test Manual*. Reston, VA, 1976.
2. American Alliance for Health, Physical Education, Recreation and Dance. *Health-Related Physical Fitness Test Manual*. Reston, VA, 1980.
3. American College of Sports Medicine. *Guidelines for Exercise Testing and Prescription*. Philadelphia: Lea & Febiger, 1986.
4. Andrew GM, Reid JG, Beck S, McDonald W: Training of the developmentally handicapped young adult. *Can J Appl Sport Sci* 4:289–293, 1979.
5. Åstrand PO, Rodahl K: *Textbook of Work Physiology*. New York, McGraw-Hill, 1977.
6. Balke B, Ware R: An experimental study of physical fitness of Air Force personnel. *US Armed Forces Med J* 10:675–688, 1959.
7. Bar-Or O, Skinner JS, Bergsteinova V, Shearburn C, Royer D, Bell W, Haas J, Buskirk ER: Maximal aerobic capacity of 6–15-year-old girls and boys with subnormal intelligence quotients. *Acta Paediatr Scand (Suppl)* 217:108–113, 1971.
8. Baumgartner TA, Horvat MA: Problems in measuring the physical and motor performance of the handicapped. *J Phys Ed Rec Dance* 59:48–52, 1988.
9. Beasley CR: Effects of jogging program on cardiovascular fitness and work performance of mentally retarded adults. *Am J Ment Defic* 86:609–613, 1982.
10. Bennett F, Eiseman P, French R, Henderson H, Shulz B: The effect of a token economy on cardiorespiratory fitness exercise behavior of individuals with Down's syndrome. *Adapt Phys Activity Q* 6:230–246, 1989.
11. Bruce RA, Kusumi F, Hosmer D: Maximal oxygen intake and homographic assessment of functional aerobic impairment in cardiovascular disease. *Am Heart J* 85:546–562, 1973.
12. Bruininks RH: Physical and motor development of retarded persons. In Ellis NR (ed): *International Review of Research in Mental Retardation*, New York, Academic Press, 1974, pp 209–261.
13. Bundschuh EL, Cureton KJ: Effect of bicycle ergometer conditioning on the physical work capacity of mentally retarded adolescents. *Am Correct Ther J* 36:159–163, 1982.
14. Burkett LN: Max $\dot{V}O_2$ uptake on five trainable mentally retarded high school students. In Kroll W (ed): *AAHPERD Abstracts*, Reston, VA, 1984, pp 73.

15. Campbell DE, Shannon CH: Reliability of cardiovascular evaluation of mentally retarded subjects. Abstracts of Research Papers. AAHPER Convention, Washington, D.C., American Alliance of Health, Physical Education and Recreation, 1970.
16. Campbell J: Physical fitness and the mentally retarded: a review of research. *Ment Retard* 11:26–29, 1973.
17. Caouette M, Reid G: Increasing the work output of severely retarded adults on a bicycle ergometer. *Ed Training Ment Retard* 20:296–304, 1985.
18. Coleman AE, Ayoub MM, Friedrich DW: Assessment of the physical work capacity of institutionalized mentally retarded males. *Am J Ment Defic* 80:629–635, 1976.
19. Cooke RE: Atlantoaxial instability in individuals with Down's syndrome. *Adapt Phys Activity Q* 1:194–196, 1984.
20. Cooper K: *Aerobics.* New York, M. Evans, 1968.
21. Cressler M, Lavay B, Giesse M: The reliability of four measures of cardiovascular fitness with mentally retarded adults. *Adapt Phys Activity Q* 5:285–292, 1988.
22. DePauw KP, Hiles M, Mowatt M, Goc-Karp G: Cardiovascular endurance of mentally retarded adolescents as assessed by the 12-minute run and cycle ergometry. Paper presented at the 5th International Symposium on Adapted Physical Activity, Toronto, Canada, October, 1985.
23. DeVries HA: *Physiology of Exercise for Physical Education and Athletes.* ed 4. Dubuque, IA, WC Brown, 1986.
24. Dobbins DA, Garron R, Rarick GL: The motor performance of educable mentally retarded and intellectually normal boys after covariate control for difference in body size. *Res Q Exerc Sport* 52:1–8, 1981.
25. Fernhall B, Tymeson GT: Graded exercise testing of mentally retarded adults: a study of feasibility. *Arch Phys Med Rehab* 68:363–365, 1987.
26. Fernhall B, Tymeson GT: Validation of cardiovascular fitness field tests for adults with mental retardation. *Adapt Phys Activity Q* 5:49–59, 1988.
27. Fernhall B, Tymeson GT, Webster GE: Cardiovascular fitness of mentally retarded individuals. *Adapt Phys Activity Q* 5:12–28, 1988.
28. Findlay HI: Adaptation of Canada Fitness Award for the trainable mentally handicapped. *Can Assoc Health, Phys Ed Rec J* 48:5–12, 1981.
29. Folkins CH, Sime WE: Physical fitness training and mental health. *Am Psychol* 36:373–389, 1981.
30. Fox R, Burkett JE, Rotatori AF: Physical fitness and personality characteristics of obese and nonobese retarded adults. *Int J Obes* 8:61–67, 1984.
31. Fox R, Rotatori A: Prevalence of obesity among mentally retarded adults. *Am J Ment Defic* 87:228–230, 1982.
32. Francis RJ, Rarick GL: Motor characteristics of the mentally retarded. *Am J Ment Defic* 63:292–311, 1959.
33. Glassford RG, Baycroft GHY, Sedwick AW, McNab RBJ: Comparison of maximal oxygen uptake values determined by predicted and actual methods. *J Appl Physiol* 20:509–513, 1965.
34. Goddard HH: The height and weight of feeble-minded children in American institutions. *J Nerv Ment Dis* 39:217–235, 1912.
35. Government of Canada: *Standardized Test of Fitness Operations Manual.* ed 2, Ottawa, Fitness and Amateur Sport, 1981.
36. Grossman HJ (ed): *Manual or Terminology and Classification in Mental Retardation.* Washington D.C., American Association on Mental Deficiency, 1984.
37. Halle JW, Silverman NA, Regan L: The effects of a data-based exercise program on physical fitness of retarded children. *Ed Training Ment Retard* 18:221–225, 1983.
38. Heyward VH: Designs for Fitness. Minneapolis, Burgess Publishing, 1984.
39. Holland BV: Fundamental motor skill performance of nonhandicapped and educably mentally impaired students. *Ed Train Ment Retard* 22:197–204, 1987.

40. Jansma P, Ersing WF, McCubbin JA: *The effects of physical fitness and personal hygiene training on the preparation for community placement of institutionalized mentally retarded adults.* (Final Report, Project No. G008300001), Washington D.C.: U.S. Department of Eduction, Office of Special Education and Rehabilitation Services, 1986.

41. Jetté M, Campbell J, Mongeon J, Routhier R: The Canadian Home Fitness Test as predictor of aerobic capacity. *Can Med Assoc J* 114:680–682, 1976.

42. Kelly LE, Rimmer JH, Ness RA: Obesity levels in institutionalized mentally retarded adults. *Adapt Phys Activity Q* 2:167–176, 1986.

43. Koh MS, Watkinson EJ: Endurance run pacing of moderately mentally handicapped children. *Can Assoc Health Phys Ed Rec J* 54:12–15, 1988.

44. Kugel RB, Mohr J: Mental retardation and physical growth. *Am J Ment Defic* 68:41–48, 1963.

45. Lavay B, Giese M, Bussen M, Dart S: Comparison of three measures of predictor $\dot{V}O_2$ maximum protocols with mentally retarded adults: a pilot study. *Ment Retard* 25:39–42, 1987.

46. Léger LA, Lambert JA: A maximal multistage 20-m shuttle run test to predict $\dot{V}O_2$max. *Eur J Appl Physiol* 49:1–12, 1982.

47. Londeree BR, Johnson LE: Motor fitness of TMR vs. EMR and normal children. *Med Sci Sport* 6:247–252, 1974.

48. Maksud MG, Coutts KD: Comparison of a continuous and discontinuous graded treadmill test for maximal oxygen uptake. *Med Sci Sports* 3:63–65, 1971.

49. Maksud MG, Hamilton LH: Physiological responses of EMR children to strenuous exercise. *Am J Ment Defic* 79:32–38, 1974.

50. Matthews DK: *Measurement of Physical Education.* Philadelphia, WB Saunders, 1968.

51. McArdle WD, Katch FI, Pechar GS: Comparison of continuous and discontinuous treadmill and bicycle test for max $\dot{V}O_2$. *Med Sci Sports* 5:156–160, 1973.

52. Millar AL, Fernhall B, Burkett LN, Tymeson, G: Effects of training on maximal oxygen uptake of mentally retarded adolescents and adults. *Med Sci Sports Exerc* 20 (Suppl):S28, 1988.

53. Montgomery DL, Reid G, Seidl C: The effects of two physical fitness programs designed for mentally retarded adults. *Can J Sport Sci* 13:73–78, 1988.

54. Moon MS, Renzaglia A: Physical fitness and the mentally retarded: a critical review of the literature. *J Spec Ed* 16:268–287, 1982.

55. Mosier HD, Grossman HJ, Dingman HF: Physical growth in mental defectives. *Pediatrics* 36:465–519, 1965.

56. Nordgren B: Physical capabilities in a group of mentally retarded adults. *Scand J Rehab Med* 2:125–132, 1970.

57. Nordgren B: Physical capacity and training in a group of young adult mentally retarded persons. *Acta Paediatr Scand (Suppl)* 217:119–121, 1971.

58. Peries VP: Sub-maximal cardiovascular endurance of trainable mentally retarded boys. Unpublished doctoral dissertation, Ohio State University, 1973.

59. Pizarro D: Health related fitness of mainstreamed emr/tmr children. *Unpublished doctoral dissertation.* University of Georgia, 1982.

60. Rarick GL, Widdop JH, Broadhead GD: The physical fitness and motor performance of educable mentally retarded children. *Except Child* 6:509–519, 1970.

61. Reid G: Preparing mentally retarded adults for physical fitness tests. Paper presented at the meeting of the American Alliance for Health, Physical Education, Recreation and Dance, Las Vegas, 1987.

62. Reid G, Montgomery D, Seidl C: Performance of mentally retarded adults on the Canadian Standardized Tests of Fitness. *Can J Public Health* 76:187–190, 1985.

63. Reid G, Seidl C, Montgomery DL: Preparing mentally retarded adults for cardiovascular fitness tests. *J Phys Ed Rec Dance* 60:76–78, 1989.

64. Schurrer R, Brammell H, Weltman A: Efforts of physical training on cardiovascular fitness and behaviour patterns of mentally retarded adults. *Am J Ment Defic* 90:167–169, 1985.

65. Sechrest L: Exercise as an operant response for retarded children. *Spec Ed* 2:311–317, 1968.

66. Seidl C, Montgomery DL, Reid G: Stair stepping efficiency of mentally handicapped and non-handicapped adult females. *Ergonomics* 32:519–526, 1989.

67. Seidl C, Reid G, Montgomery DL: A critique of cardiovascular fitness testing with mentally retarded persons. *Adapt Phys Activity* 4:106–116, 1987.

68. Sharkey BJ: *Physiology of Fitness: Prescribing Exercise for Fitness, Weight Control and Health.* ed 2. Champaign, IL, Human Kinetics, 1984.

69. Shephard RJ: Exercise test methodology. In Fox SA, (ed): *Coronary Disease—Learning System: Prevention, Detection, and Rehabilitation with Emphasis on Exercise Tests.* Denver, Department of Professional Education, 1974, pp 1–23.

70. Skrobak-Kaczynski J, Vavik T: Children and exercise IX. In Berg K, Erikson B (eds): *Physical Fitness and Trainability of Young Male Patients with Down's Syndrome.* Baltimore, University Park Press, 1980, pp 300–316.

71. Thelander HE, Pryor HB: Abnormal patterns of growth and development in mongolism. *Clin Pediatr* 5:493–501, 1966.

72. Tomporowski PD, Ellis NR: Preparing severely and profoundly mentally retarded adults for tests of motor fitness. *Adapt Phys Activity Q* 1:158–163, 1984.

73. Tomporowski PD, Ellis NR: Effects of exercise on the physical fitness, intelligence and adaptive behavior of institutionalized mentally retarded adults. *Appl Res Ment Retard* 5:329–337, 1984.

74. Tomporowski PD, Jameson LD: Effects of a physical fitness training program on the exercise behaviour of institutionalized mentally retarded adults. *Adapt Phys Activity Q* 2:197–205, 1985.

75. Ulrich D: A comparison of qualitative motor performance of normal, educable, and trainable mentally retarded. In Eason RL, Smith TL, Caron F (eds): *Adapted Physical Activity.* Champaign, IL, Human Kinetics, 1983, pp 219–225.

76. Watkinson EJ, Koh SM: Heart rate response of moderately mentally handicapped children and youth on the Canada Fitness Award adapted endurance run. *Adapt Phys Activity Q* 5:203–211, 1988.

10
Prevention of Ligament Injuries to the Knee

BRUCE E. BAKER, M.D.

Disruption of the ligamentous structures of the knee occurs commonly in sports such as American football and lacrosse [12, 37, 38, 42, 56]. Controversy exists not only as to the mechanism of injury and subsequent treatment but also regarding the efficacy of prophylactic bracing prior to injury, as a means of preventing ligamentous disruption, and the use of functional braces following an injury or surgery. In an effort to minimize the potential for further injury, many amateur and professional teams currently use extensive prophylactic bracing on previously uninjured players and functional braces on players who have sustained previous injuries [1–5, 8, 9, 11, 15, 19, 21, 23, 26, 39, 40, 41, 45, 46, 57]. The 1984 American Academy of Orthopaedic Surgeons' seminar report [11] on knee braces indicates that no conclusive evidence was obtained concerning the efficacy of either prophylactic or functional bracing and that significant research is required to document beneficial effects from the use of bracing. Garrick and Requa [15] reviewed the epidemiologic studies available and concluded that none of the studies could be used to support the contention that braces are effective in preventing injury.

High visibility of braces in the media, e.g., through TV and magazine sports coverage, and the available market allowed numerous manufacturers of prophylactic braces to advertise the devices inaccurately. Extensive basic science evaluation prior to marketing was not done by the manufacturers so that the advertised benefits of bracing were unrealistic. Subsequent basic science research has been conducted primarily by nonaffiliated laboratories [2, 3, 15, 33, 34]. Currently, public pressure is exerted on coaches and athletic administrators, particularly at the high school and college levels, to use the braces, with the assumption that they reduce the potential for injury. However, a *variety* of methods may be used to prevent ligamentous injuries in sports. These include strengthening and conditioning, attention to technique, and using protective equipment. Discussion of the mechanism of injury, factors affecting injury, and the evidence concerning the use of prophylactic and functional bracing will be presented in this chapter.

ANATOMY

The *medial collateral ligament* (MCL) is composed of two layers, the superficial and the deep [16, 32]. The origination of the superficial portion is well above the joint line on the medial femoral condyle with insertion on the medial aspect of the tibia, distal to the joint line and the pes anserine mechanism, composed of the sartorius, gracilis, and semitendinosus. The deep portion is primarily a reinforcement of the capsular structures of the medial aspect of the knee, and it also contributes to the stabilization of the medial meniscus. The medial collateral ligament structures control the static stability of the knee when valgus forces are applied to the knee, and they assist in controlling rotational stresses.

The *lateral collateral ligament* (LCL) originates on the lateral femoral condyle above the joint line and inserts on the fibula [16, 32]. The lateral collateral ligament assists in primarily controlling varus stresses on the knee, with a limited capacity to affect rotational stresses.

The iliotibial band originates on the pelvis and inserts distally just below the joint line on Gerdy's tubercle [16, 32]. This structure is important in terms of controlling varus stresses as well as rotational instabilities about the knee.

The *anterior cruciate ligament* (ACL) originates in the intercondylar notch from the medial aspect of the lateral femoral condyle posteriorly and inserts anteriorly on the tibia. The primary function of the anterior cruciate ligament is to control anterior translation of the tibia on the femur and also to control rotational stresses [50].

The *posterior cruciate ligament* (PCL) originates from the lateral aspect of the medial femoral condyle anteriorly and inserts posteriorly on the tibia [16, 32]. The PCL primarily controls posterior translation of the tibia on the femur and additionally assists in controlling some rotational stresses.

Additional stabilization of the knee is produced by the contour of the femoral condyles and articulation with the menisci. The menisci also produce a wedge-type configuration that increases the potential for stabilization of the femoral condyles on the tibial plateau.

The structures previously mentioned are involved in producing a static-type stabilization. Dynamic stability is created primarily by the quadriceps and hamstrings. For example, Solomonow et al. [44] demonstrated that there is a secondary reflex arc from the anterior cruciate ligament to the hamstrings that causes the hamstrings to contract, protecting the knee from anterior translation. This produces joint stabilization. Additionally, these authors have demonstrated that there is a reflex arc from the joint capsule and/or muscle to the hamstrings with an ACL injury. Rehabilitation to include hamstring strengthening can improve function with an ACL instability. Adductors and rotators provide additional stability.

MECHANISM OF INJURY

Means by which knee ligaments are injured vary with the activity and the stresses the activity places on the knee. A valgus stress on the knee, caused by either a direct blow or fixation of the foot on the field, can produce tension on the medial supporting structures including the medial collateral ligament and the medial capsular structures. The anterior cruciate ligament and posterior cruciate ligament can also be injured with this mechanism. Studies have indicated that the ACL is a primary stabilizer to valgus loads on the knee. Additionally, the anterior cruciate ligament is a secondary stabilizer that can compensate when the MCL is sectioned or previously injured [17, 24, 30, 53]. Kurosaka et al. [27] and Noyes et al. [29–31] have indicated that the maximum tensile strength on the anterior cruciate ligament exceeds 500 newtons when tested in a laboratory. This indicates a significant stress on the knee.

Houseworth et al. [22] suggests that a narrow posterior arch in the intercondylar notch may predispose to anterior cruciate ligament tears in extension because of the impingement on the anterior cruciate ligament in this position. A varus configuration can produce stress on the lateral aspect of the knee and disrupt the lateral collateral ligament, the iliotibial band, as well as the anterior cruciate and posterior cruciate ligaments. Rotational configurations with these stresses can produce additional injuries. Other mechanisms producing injury to the ligaments of the knee include a position of abduction or valgus of the knee with external rotation, particularly with the foot fixed, as can occur with a caught ski tip. Stress is placed on the medial supporting structures as well as the anterior cruciate and the posterior cruciate ligaments. Varus stress with internal rotation can produce disruption of the lateral supporting structures with or without the anterior cruciate ligament or posterior cruciate ligament being injured. Hyperextension of the knee can cause disruption of the anterior cruciate ligament, the posterior cruciate ligament, and the posterior capsule. Hyperextension, particularly in situations such as landing from a jump, can result in injury ranging from a mild sprain to dislocation of the knee.

A direct posterior blow to the tibia can cause disruption of the anterior cruciate ligament. A posterior lateral blow producing abduction and external rotation can cause the medial collateral ligament and anterior cruciate ligament to be torn. A common mechanism of injury to the PCL is a direct anterior blow to the tibial tubercle, such as a fall on the knee or a direct blow by another participant in a contact sport.

Two-thirds of anterior cruciate ligament injuries occur without any contact, but instead are related to foot fixation, hyperextension, and torsional stresses. Many of these situations include a deceleration mechanism. One study shows that 96% of anterior cruciate ligament injuries are sports related and 75% occur in varsity athletes [20].

INJURY PREVENTION

Factors to consider in preventing injuries include: (*a*) conditioning, (*b*) technique, (*c*) surface, (*d*) rules, and (*e*) protective equipment.

Conditioning

Training alone is not the only answer to prevention of ligament injuries, although it can be helpful in terms of producing strength, flexibility, and endurance. Specific activities must be pursued that strengthen the ligaments. Ligaments can be strengthened, within limits, over a period of time with improved conditioning activities including specific activities to strengthen muscles.

Cahill and Griffith [6, 7] indicated that a conditioning program prior to contact activity in football strengthened the extremities dynamically but also had the effect of producing increased strength of the ligaments. This cannot be statistically supported; however, it appears plausible. Tipton and colleagues [48, 49, 52] in animals demonstrated that the strength of the medial collateral ligament could be influenced by an exercise program. They found that the MCL strength, as measured in the laboratory, was increased in animals after a period of exercise compared to that in animals not exercised.

Technique

Improper technique can result in a significant increase in the injury rate with a predictable pattern. Both deceleration and hyperextension when landing from a jump may increase the rate of anterior cruciate ligament injury. In an effort to prevent ACL injuries, Henning [20] has developed a program of modification of the deceleration activities in competitive athletics, modifications that can be applied to basketball, football, gymnastics, soccer, and other sports. The principles of his program include acceleration around turns, a two-step stop, and bent knee landings, which are modifications of the plant and cut, one-step stops, and straight knee landing, respectively.

The plant and cut may produce a sudden decelerating maneuver with a twisting movement. This can load the anterior cruciate ligament, causing a tear. The one-step stop is a sudden decelerating movement that places the ligament in a dangerously tight position and may end in a tear of the anterior cruciate ligament. Deceleration with one step and with the leg near extension is particularly dangerous. The approved training technique is to practice accelerating around turns such as in pass pattern situations. The competitor accelerates off the inside foot while making the turn. It is important to enter the turn under control and accelerate through the turn. Straight knee landings occur during a jump. The player lands stiff legged and does not continue to bend the knees as he or she lands, thus being likely to damage the anterior cruciate ligament.

Bent knee landings involve a two-step landing technique. When making the bent knee landing on one leg, the individual takes another step with the other leg before initiating a turn off the inside leg. When landing on the right leg, he/she takes another step on the left to initiate a turn toward the left. The first step after landing must be a light touch. The individual must land on the toes and let the knees bend. Ideally, individuals must have a 2-yard landing zone and a second foot on the ground before beginning the turn. Then they must lean into the turn and accelerate through the turn.

A three-step stop is used when a player needs to come to a stop or change direction. This may be used when, for example, a running back in football is in a situation where he needs to make a sudden deceleration in order to avoid the defensive players. The approved technique allows the player to reduce his forward speed, lower his center of gravity by bending his knees and decelerate with at least three steps. The player is now in a position of balance, which prepares him for any directional change or an explosive move into a defender.

Henning has implemented the new technique with a program involving young gymnasts and basketball and soccer players. He finds that the injury rate to the anterior cruciate ligament is 2.5 times less after establishing prevention skills [20]. Although not statistically proven, the program has merit and further study is appropriate.

Sports-specific Injuries

Athletic competition can be divided into collision, contact, and noncontact activities. Sports such as football and lacrosse are collision sports because of the high impact loads associated with these activities. Other sports involving contact without frequent collisions include soccer and basketball. Noncontact sports are best represented by activities such as tennis, volleyball, and gymnastics. The injury mechanism seen varies in degree based on the sport classification. Activities such as tennis are safer for all competitors and are better tolerated by people who have had a previous anterior cruciate ligament injury than are sports such as basketball. Tennis tends to be a shuffling sport with one foot on the ground most of the time. Sports such as soccer, basketball, and volleyball are best represented as leaping sports and result in landings that can be uncontrolled, resulting in hyperextension and rotation, which may be dangerous to the ligaments of the knee. Football incorporates some of the other mechanisms with the added stress of periodic impact loads to the knee.

Some of the epidemiologic studies of the injuries associated with specific sports include the following. Keller et al. [25] indicated that knee and ankle ligament injuries accounted for one-third of all soccer injuries in their study. Halpern and Colleagues [18, 47] studied football injuries in high school and found that 25% of all injuries involved the ligaments of the ankle and knee. Rovere et al. [40] found an incidence of ACL injury of 4.0/100 football players during the nonbrace period and 4.8/100 players during the brace period. The incidence for all knee injuries was 6.1/100 football players during the nonbrace period and 7.5/100 players during the brace period. Derscheid and Garrick [10] in a study of college football injuries found that 73% of all the injuries were either grade I or grade II MCL sprains. Whiteside et al. [55] at Pennsylvania State University found that the incidence of MCL ligament injuries was 7.5/100 football players. Epidemiologic studies done on gymnasts indicated that ligament injuries to the knee were a common source of disability. Weiker and Canim [54] found that in gymnasts ligament injuries to the knee were the most common type of disabling injury. Garrick and Requa [14] and Pettrone and Ricciardella [36] indicated that ligament injuries of the knee were the second most common injury diagnosed in gymnastics.

Running Surface

The surface of the field during activity makes a significant difference in terms of foot fixation. Grass, by far, is the most commonly used surface for outdoor activities. In the past, long cleats, so called "mud cleats," were used, which produced foot fixation and rotational stresses associated with cutting activities. A study by Torg and Quedenfeld [51] was one of the first to report that the conventional football shoe could create a situation that was dangerous to the athlete. These researchers found that the incidence and severity of knee and ankle injuries were greatly reduced when a soccer shoe with a 3/8 inch long and 1/2 inch diameter cleat was used. They concluded that the conventional football shoe was a major factor responsible for the incidence of knee injuries. Mueller and Blyth [28] suggested that a possible related factor would be the condition of the playing field. A randomized study of schools with modified playing fields and footwear showed a reduction of knee and ankle injuries of 30.5% when compared to injuries reported from schools with no changes in playing surface or the modification of footwear. Rules in football currently provide for cleats similar to those used in soccer with a molded 5/8-inch cleat. Artificial turf for outdoor activities can also produce a foot fixation problem because of the stickiness of some of the turf shoe/surface interfaces. This can produce torsion with hyperextension or abduction and external rotation stresses on the knee, which may result in disruption of the MCL and ACL as outlined previously.

Indoor surfaces include wood, which tends to produce less of a foot fixation problem, and rubberized surfaces. The rubberized surfaces in combination with certain types of footwear can produce a foot fixation problem and torsional stress. There have been recent mini epidemics, among women basketball players in particular, with disruption of the anterior cruciate ligament associated with foot fixation on rubberized surfaces.

Snow can produce an injury by catching the ski tip. A ski with the tip caught can produce an abduction and external rotation injury or the "caught ski tip" mechanism as described previously.

Rules

Rules that prevent contact activities that are statistically likely to produce injury can be significantly helpful in reducing the rate of injury to the knee ligaments. A number of these rules have been instituted in football.

The clipping injury is one maneuver where there is blocking at the posterior lateral aspect of the knee. The rule against clipping should be consistently enforced in an effort to prevent injury to the knee. Another maneuver is downfield blocking below the waist [35]. The rule forbidding this maneuver is currently enforced by the National Collegiate Athletic Association and the National Football League and does empirically appear to reduce the rate of ligament injury. Another rule includes the elimination of the crack back block. This is a type of maneuver in which a wide receiver in football goes down field and then comes back and blindly hits the defensive player at the knee level producing an exorbitantly high rate of injury to the knee [35]. A rule that is not always enforced is high/low double teaming of a defensive player. A lineman will block another individual at the shoulder level and then the second offensive player will block the player at the knee level. This is a dangerous maneuver. Whip kicking or rotating with your legs against the knees of another individual is dangerous and technically outlawed, but not always enforced.

Protective Equipment: Bracing Issues

Braces have been proposed as a stabilization effect for use before injury occurs in the competitive athlete as well as for use after injury has occurred. There is speculation about the usefulness of braces in preventing injury and limited information from clinical and laboratory studies. The definition of brace types includes (*a*) prophylactic, (*b*) rehabilitation, and (*c*) functional. A *prophylactic* brace is defined as one that is used to prevent injury in previously uninjured players. Prophylactic braces are commonly single upright lateral braces with one or more hinges and strapping over the thigh and lower leg area [11]. A *rehabilitation* brace is one that is used post surgical or post injury prior to return to competition in an effort to limit range of motion. It produces static stability and is not used for competitive athletics. A *functional* brace is one that has been specifically molded for the individual involved. Most common functional braces are double upright custom-fitted braces with rigid crossing struts with significant plastic or rubberized soft tissue containment [11]. These are most commonly used by individuals who have sustained a previous injury with or without a surgical procedure. These braces include models manufactured with brand names such as Lenox-Hill, CTI from Innovation Sports, Donjoy, Generation II, and others. A number of in vivo, in vitro, and epidemiologic studies have been conducted in an effort to shed light on the potential for a protective effect by these braces. Currently, there is no study available that truly represents the on-field situation.

The epidemiologic studies done in the recent past include studies by Taft et al. [45] of the University of North Carolina, Rovere et al. of Wake Forest University, Hewson et al. [21] of the University of Arizona, and Teitz et al. [46] of the University of Washington. Other studies were done by the Big Ten Conference and at the U.S. Military Academy at West Point by Sitler et al. [43].

Taft et al. [45] studied the use of prophylactic bracing and suggested that there was a reduction in the frequency of medial collateral ligament injuries associated with football when the braces were worn. Hewson et al. [21] at Arizona revealed no difference in injury rate between those individuals wearing braces and those without braces. Rovere et al. [40] at Wake Forest suggested that there was an increased rate of injury associated with the use of braces, when compared to no bracing. All of these studies were conducted with prophylactic braces. Teitz et al. [46] from Washington reviewed 71 institutions and their information concerning knee injuries associated with and without bracing. Their conclusions were that, at best, there was no protection of the medial collateral ligament or anterior cruciate ligament associated with the use of bracing. There was some suggestion that a prophylactic brace may produce additional injuries.

The randomized study conducted by Sitler et al. [43] at the U.S. Military Academy at West Point involved full contact eight-person college intramural football. This study was conducted over 2 years, with half of the players wearing a prophylactic brace 1 year with the remaining half not wearing braces. The subsequent year, the players reversed their status. The most common injury was to the medial collateral ligament, with the next most common injury being to the anterior cruciate ligament. The injury was defined as acute trauma to ligaments or menisci that resulted in the athlete's inability to participate in football 1 day after the injury. The severity of ligament injury was not affected by the use of a prophylactic brace. Those individuals not wearing braces had a greater number of MCL and ACL injuries than those who did wear a brace. Analysis revealed that there was no statistical difference in injury rate comparing offense to defense. On defense, braced players had statistically fewer knee injuries than control unbraced players; whereas on offense, there was no statistical difference between the braced and unbraced participants. Additionally, a Big Ten Conference unpublished study suggests that there may be some improvement in terms of reduction of injuries associated with isolated positions such as offensive and defensive linemen.

A cadaver biomechanical evaluation was completed by Baker et al. [2, 3]. A two-stage project was proposed. The first stage involved a static abduction external rotation force on the cadaver knee simulating a fixed foot with upper body contact with and without prophylactic or functional braces [2]. Force transducers were placed on the anterior cruciate and medial collateral ligaments, and an electrogoniometer on the extremity with an abduction force applied. It was found that functional braces have some capacity to control the abduction angle whereas prophylactic braces did not. Prophylactic braces had no effect on reducing medial collateral ligament transducer loads, and there was an increased anterior cruciate ligament load above the no brace measurement with one prophylactic brace, suggesting a prestressing effect.

The second stage model involved the use of the cadaver lower extremity with a fixed foot, suspended femur with a free knee, and a lateral impact load simulating a clipping injury [3]. Functional braces and prophylactic braces were tested. The cadaver knee was cast and the mold sent to the manufacturer. The extremity was frozen and subsequently thawed when the braces were available. All braces were applied by a certified orthotist according to the manufacturer's specification. The cadaver extremity, which was disarticulated at the hip, had a fixed foot with a Steinmann pin in the calcaneus and a suspended femur at the hip joint with a free knee. This was supported in a wooden frame. The femoral head was seated in a plastic socket, and force springs were attached to the socket at the proximal femur. The femoral head and socket were free to move vertically. A constant downward vertical load was applied to the head of the femur, and various forces were applied to the quadriceps mechanism via pulley systems that balanced the knee at the desired angles of flexion.

At each test position, internal femoral rotation was limited by a bar clamped to the plastic socket and contacting a foam pad attached to the wooden frame. Force transducers were applied to the anterior cruciate and medial collateral ligaments. An electrogoniometer, with 6 degrees of freedom, was attached to the femur and tibia with Steinmann pins and bone screws. The force and motion data were sampled by a minicomputer. A lateral impact was applied to the knee with a fixed weight mounted inside of a modified football helmet. The helmet and weight were held at a fixed angle away and then released to swing as a pendulum to contact the knee at the level of the joint line. The impact load was first applied directly lateral to the knee. The foot plate was internally or externally rotated 20° to allow anterior oblique or posterior oblique blows. This study was performed with and without braces.

Results without bracing indicated the largest ACL and MCL forces occurred at full extension when the impact was a direct lateral or anterior oblique blow. The maximum MCL forces for a direct lateral blow were 200% larger when the knee was extended as compared to when the knee was at 20° of flexion. In general, at full extension, the MCL forces were short in duration as compared to those measured in flexion. The ACL forces were larger with the knee extended than with it flexed, regardless of the direction of impact. This effect was largest with an anterior oblique impact. The maximum abduction angles were consistently greater with the knee flexed than with it extended, regardless of the direction of impact. The maximum tibial rotation angles were greater with the knee flexed, than with it extended, regardless of the direction of impact. In general, the ACL force reached a maximum value before the MCL force, the abduction angle, or the tibial rotation angle reached their respective peak values, regardless of the type of impact or flexion angle. The abduction and tibial rotation angles frequently peaked last.

With the braces applied, the abduction angle caused on impact by a blow to the cadaver knee was decreased after application of a functional brace and, to a limited extent, with a prophylactic brace. The effect of the braces was decreased with the MCL cut. There was a significant decrease in the effect of the prophylactic brace on the abduction angle when the blow was applied anterolateral or posterolateral with the prophylactic brace. The protective effect rapidly decreased to zero and a similar result was seen when the flexion angle was changed to 20°. The magnitude of the MCL transducer force was again affected by the angle of flexion of the knee as well as the direction of the applied force. There was a limited capacity to reduce the stress on the MCL by the prophylactic brace. This was reduced to zero with flexion of the knee or an oblique angle of application of the load. Transducers on the anterior cruciate ligament revealed that at full extension, regardless of the angle of impact or whether the MCL was attached or cut, the force readings were reduced more with a functional brace than with a prophylactic brace.

The effect of braces on tibial rotation varied. In general, the functional braces had some capacity to control rotation while the prophylactic braces did not.

Paulos and associates [34] conducted laboratory studies on the effect of bracing on cadaver extremities. Ligament tensions and joint displacements were measured at static nondestructive valgus forces as well as at low rate destructive forces. The effects of lateral bracing were analyzed according to valgus force, joint line opening, and ligament tensions Valgus forces with or without braces consistently produced medial collateral ligament disruption at ligament tensions higher than the anterior cruciate ligament and higher than or equal to the posterior cruciate ligament. Bundle disruption in the MCL, ACL, and PCL was noted at much smaller joint openings than those required for complete disruption of the structures. No significant protection could be documented with the two preventive braces used in this study.

A subsequent study by France and associates [13] involved the use of a surrogate model instrumented to measure ligament/tendon tension and medial joint openings. Six models of prophylactic braces were tested with this device. The tests were conducted for three impactor masses, two flexion angles, and free or constrained limb positions. Impact safety factors were calculated for each test condition and brace type. The results were: (*a*) brace-induced MCL preload in vivo was negated by joint compressive forces; (*b*) the ideal brace should increase the lateral force at MCL injury by 80%; (*c*) at a 1000% strain/s strain rate, MCL failure force was increased by 28%; and (*d*) one brace exceeded the minimum impact safety factor. Of the variables analyzed, impactor mass, leg constraint, and knee flexion angle most greatly influenced overall lateral brace effectiveness. In general, braces were most effective for larger mass, lower velocity impacts with both the hip and foot fixed and the knee extended. On the other hand, braces were least effective for smaller mass, higher velocity impacts with free hip and ankle motion, and the knee at 30° of flexion. These trends were consistent for all braces tested.

As an extension of Baker's studies [57], static in vivo studies have been done on the use of functional braces on individuals with ligament instability. When tested on a Genucom, there was no difference in terms of anterior-posterior (AP) laxity or rotational control associated with the functional braces [57]. These braces do not appear to reduce AP translation. One positive effect from a functional brace may be the use of a hyperextension stop at 10 or 15°. This may help to reduce the potential for producing the position of hyperextension, which is known to be dangerous to the ACL.

Several organizations have taken a position in regard to bracing. These include the American Academy of Orthopaedic Surgeons, The Medical Society of the State of New York, and the *Journal of Bone and Joint Surgery* [9]. The position of these institutions is that, because the current clinical and laboratory studies available do not support the contention that prophylactic braces have the capacity to reduce injury to the knee, they cannot support the use of this type of bracing.

CONCLUSIONS

There is no ideal way to evaluate bracing in the laboratory. In addition, there is no accurate way to simulate the on-field situation. Large numbers are needed, as many as 50,000 players during one season epidemiologically, requiring 500 teams over 1 year or 50 teams over a 10-year period, to provide meaningful numbers. The studies that produce static loading do not have the capacity to simulate the dynamic effect on the field. Dynamic loading is destructive and results in difficulty in comparison cadaver studies.

Current thinking is that most functional braces have some capacity to protect the medial collateral ligament and may have some effect on external rotation but a very limited effect on AP translation. They may resist hyperextension with a 10° extension stop. Prophylactic braces are probably not useful and, until further studies support the contention that these braces protect the knee from injury, they should not be promoted for general use.

Rules modifications in sports such as football need to be enforced. They definitely help reduce the rate of knee ligament injury, but in many situations are not enforced.

Modification of footwear in certain situations is appropriate. Players themselves may prefer a less "sticky," shoe such as a sneaker, in an effort to decrease this potential for foot fixation and subsequent injury.

Training, with conditioning, including strength, endurance, and flexibility are important, as is modification of technique as suggested by Henning [20]. If these techniques were taught from an early age, the theory would suggest that a reduction of knee injuries could be achieved with this approach.

Substantial additional evaluations both epidemiologically and in the laboratory are required to provide data for the production of a more functional brace. This is particularly true when considering the ability of braces to control anterior translation of the tibia on the femur with chronic anterior cruciate ligament insufficiency. There is probably no way to totally statically stabilize the knee with significant previous ligament disruption, short of immobilizing the extremity in a cast (bracing is a modification of total immobilization). However, concentrated mechanical studies could provide information leading to substantial improvement in protective equipment. Additionally, combined studies of large conferences of intercollegiate football teams could be used to gain the epidemiologic data necessary to test newly designed equipment following initial evaluation in the laboratory by unbiased sources. Until these types of studies are done, controversy will continue concerning the efficacy of bracing.

SUMMARY

Disruption of the ligamentous structures of the knee are commonly seen in competitive sports. Factors affecting the rate of injury include the sport, the participant, conditioning and technique, the level of competition, rules enforcement, the type of playing surface, and footwear. The role of prophylactic and functional bracing is controversial. Currently, prophylactic bracing has not been shown, conclusively, to be protective. Functional braces appear to have a capacity to provide some protective effect.

ACKNOWLEDGMENTS

The author acknowledges the technical assistance of Reatha Baker, Sherri Dundon, and Carrie Mosher.

REFERENCES

1. Anderson G, Zeman SC, Rosenfeld RT: The Anderson Knee Stabler. *Physician Sportsmed* 7:125–127, 1979.
2. Baker BE, VanHanswyk E, Bogosian S, Werner M, Murphy D: A biomechanical study of the static stabilizing effect of knee braces on medial stability. *Am J Sports Med* 15:566–570, 1987.
3. Baker BE, VanHanswyk E, Bogosian S, Werner M, Murphy D: The effect of knee braces on lateral impact loading of the knee. *Sports Med* 17:182–185, 1980.
4. Bassett GS, Fleming BW: The Lenox Hill brace and anterolateral rotatory instability. *Am J Sports Med* 11:345–348, 1983.
5. Beck C, Drez D, Young J: Instrumented testing of functional knee braces. *Am J Sports Med* 14:253–256, 1986.
6. Cahill BR, Griffith EH: Effect of preseason conditioning on the incidence and severity of high school football knee injuries. *Am J Sports Med,* 6:180–184, 1978.
7. Cahill BR, Griffith EH: Exposure to injury in major college football. A preliminary report of data collection to determine injury exposure rates and activity risk factors. *Am J Sports Med* 7:183–185, 1979.
8. Coughlin L, Oliver J, Berretta G: Knee bracing and anterolateral rotatory instability. *Am J Sports Med* 15:161, 1987.
9. Cowell HR: College football: To brace or not to brace? (Editorial). *J Bone Joint Surg* 69A:1, 1987.
10. Derscheid GL, Garrick JG: Medial collateral ligament injuries in football. Nonoperative management of Grade I and Grade II sprains. *Am J Sports Med* 9:365–368, 1981.
11. Drez D: *Knee braces.* Seminar report of Orthopaedic Surgeons. American Academy of Orthopaedic Surgeons, Chicago, 1984.
12. Ellsasser JC, Reynolds FC, Omohundro JR: The nonoperative treatment of collateral ligament injuries of the knee in professional football players. An analysis of seventy-four injuries treated nonoperatively and twenty-four injuries treated surgically. *J Bone Joint Surg* 56A:1185–1190, 1974.
13. France SP, Paulos LE, Jayaraman G, Rosenberg TD: The biomechanics of lateral knee bracing. Part II: Impact response of the braced knee. *Am J Sports Med* 15:430–438, 1987
14. Garrick JG, Requa RM: Injuries in high school sports. *Pediatrics* 61:465–469, 1978.
15. Garrick JG, Requa RK: Prophylactic knee bracing. *Am J Sports Med* 15:471, 1987.
16. Grant J, Boileau C: *An Atlas of Anatomy.* Baltimore, Williams & Wilkins, 1956.
17. Grood ES, Noyes FR, Butler DL, Suntay WJ: Ligamentous and capsular restraints preventing straight medial and lateral laxity in intact human cadaver knees. *J Bone Joint Surg* 63:1257–1269, 1981.

18. Halpern B, Curl WW, Andrews JR, Hunter SC, Boring JR: High school football injuries: identifying the risk factors. *Am J Sports Med* 15:316, 1987.

19. Hansen BL, Ward JC, Diehl RC: The preventive use of the Anderson knee stabler in football. *Physician Sportsmed* 13:75–81, 1985.

20. Henning C: Injury prevention of the anterior cruciate ligament. Proceedings of the American Orthopaedics Society for Sports Medicine: 15th Annual Meeting, Traverse City, MI, June 20, 1989.

21. Hewson GF Jr, Mendini RA, Wang JB: Prophylactic knee bracing in college football. *Am J Sports Med* 14:262–266, 1986.

22. Houseworth SW, Mauro VJ, Mellon BA, Kieffer DA: The intercondylar computer graphics study. *Am J Sports Med* 15:221, 1987.

23. Indelicato PA: Nonoperative treatment of complete tears of the medial collateral ligament of the knee. *J Bone Joint Surg* 65A:323–329, 1983.

24. Inoue M, McGurk-Burleson E, Hollis JM, Wood SL-Y: Treatment of the media collateral ligament injury. *Am J Sports Med* 15:15, 1987.

25. Keller CS, Noyes FR, Buncher CR: The medical aspects of soccer injury epidemiology. *Am J Sports Med* 15:230, 1987.

26. Knee braces to prevent injuries in football. A round table. *Physician Sportsmed* 14:108–118, 1986.

27. Kurosaka M, Yoshiya S, Andrish JT: A biomechanical comparison of different surgical techniques of graft fixation in anterior cruciate ligament reconstruction. *Am J Sport Med* 15:225, 1987.

28. Mueller FO, Blyth CS: North Carolina high school football injury study: equipment and prevention. *J Sports Med* 2:1–10, 1974.

29. Noyes FR, Butler DL, Grood ES: Biomechanical analysis of human ligament grafts used in knee-ligament repairs and reconstructions. *J Bone Joint Surg* 66A:344–352, 1984.

30. Moyes FR, Dorvik PJ, Hyde HB: Biomechanics of ligament failure. An analysis of immobilization, exercise, and reconditioning effects in primates. *J Bone Joint Surg* 56A:1406–1418, 1974.

31. Noyes FR, Butler GL, Grood ES: Biomechanical analysis of human ligament grafts used in knee-ligament repairs and reconstructions. *J Bone Joint Surg* 66A:344–352, 1984.

32. Pansky B, House EL: *Review of Gross Anatomy.* ed. 3. New York, Macmillan, 1975.

33. Paulos LE, Drawbert FP, France P: Lateral knee braces in football: Do they prevent injury? *Physician Sportsmed* 14:119–126, 1986.

34. Paulos LS, France EP, Rosenberg TD, Jayaraman G, Abboty PJ, Jaen J: The biomechanics of lateral knee bracing. Part I: Response of the valgus restraints to loading. *Am J Sports Med* 15:419–429, 1987.

35. Peterson TR: The cross-body block, the major cause of knee injuries. *JAMA* 211:449–452, 1970.

36. Pettrone FA, Ricciardelli E: Gymnastic injuries: the Virginia experience 1982–1983. *Am J Sports Med* 15:59, 1987.

37. Pritchitt JW: A statistical study of knee injuries due to football in high school athletes. *J Bone Joint Surg* 64A:240–242, 1982.

38. Pritchitt JW: High cost of high school football injuries. *Am J Sports Med* 8:197–199, 1980.

39. Prophylactic knee braces fail to curtail football injuries. *Orthop Today* 5:1, 22–35, 1985.

40. Rovere DD, Haupt HA, Yates CS: Prophylactic knee bracing in college football. *Am J Sports Med* 15:111–116, 1987.

41. Schriner JL, Schriner DK: The effectiveness of knee bracing in preventing knee injuries in high school athletes. Presented at the American College of Sports Medicine Annual Meeting, Nashville, TN, May 26–29, 1985.

42. Singer KM, Henry J: Knee problems in children and adolescents. *Clin Sports Med* 4:385–397, 1985.
43. Sitler DI, Ryan JB, Wheeler JG: The efficiency of prophylactic knee brace to reduce knee injuries in football: a prospective randomized study. Proceedings of the American Orthopaedic Society for Sports Medicine: 15th Annual Meeting, Traverse City, MI, June 21, 1989.
44. Solomonow M, Barratta R, Zhou BM, Shoji H, Bose H, Beck C, D'Ambrosia R: The synergistic action of the anterior cruciate ligament and thigh muscles in maintaining joint stability. *Am J Sports Med* 15:207, 1987.
45. Taft TN, Hunter S, Fundurbeck CH, Jr: Presentation at the American Orthopaedic Society for Sports Medicine, Nashville, TN, July 2, 1985.
46. Teitz CC, Hermanson BR, Kronmal RA; Evaluation of the use of braces to prevent injury to the knee in collegiate football players. *J Bone Joint Surg* 69A:2–9, 1987.
47. Thompson N, Halpern B, Curl W, Andrews J, Hunter S, McLeod, W: High school football injuries evaluation. *Am J Sports Med* 15:117, 1987.
48. Tipton CM, James SL, Mergner W: Influence of exercise on strength of the medial collateral ligament of dogs. *Am J Physiol* 218:294–302, 1970.
49. Tipton CM, Matthes RD, Maynard JA: The influence of physical activity on ligaments and tendons. *Med Sci Sports Exerc* 7:165–175, 1975.
50. Torg JS, Conrad W, Kalen V: Clinical diagnosis of anterior cruciate ligament instability in the athlete. *Am J Sports Med* 4:84–93, 1976.
51. Torg JS, Quedenfeld T: Effect of shoe type and cleat length on incidence and severity of knee injuries among high school football players. *Res Q* 42:203–211, 1976.
52. Vailas AC, Tipton CM, Matthes RD: Physical activity and its influence on the repair process of medial collateral ligaments. *Connect Tissue Res* 9:25–31, 1981.
53. Warren RF, Marshall JL, Girgis F: The prime static stabilizer of the medial side of the knee. *J Bone Joint Surg* 56A:665–674, 1974.
54. Weiker GG, Canim RJ: A prospective statistical analysis of gymnastic injuries on the club gymnastic level. *USGF Technical Journal:* 13, December 1982.
55. Whiteside JA, Fleagle SB, Kalenak A: Manpower loss in football: a 12-year study at the Pennsylvania State University. *Physician Sportsmed* 13:103–114, 1985.
56. Zarins B, Nemeth VA: Acute knee injuries in athletes. *Clin Sports Med* 2:149–166, 1983.
57. Zogby RG, Baker BE, Seymour RJ, VanHanswyk E, Werner FW: A biomechanical evaluation of the effect of functional braces on the anterior cruciate ligament, using the Genucom analysis system. Proceedings of the Orthopaedic Research Society, Las Vegas, February 1989.

11
Determinants of Exercise Behavior

JAMES F. SALLIS, Ph.D.
MELBOURNE F. HOVELL, Ph.D., M.P.H.

In this chapter we will familiarize readers with the challenges of conducting exercise determinants research and set a research agenda for this area of investigation. Most research on the determinants of exercise has been conducted within the "exercise adherence" framework, and it has therefore focused on only a portion of the natural history of exercise. We attempt to broaden the scope of exercise determinants research by proposing a descriptive model of the natural history of exercise behavior.

While there have been recent applications of theory to the study of exercise determinants, most of the theories have been narrow in scope, postulating just a few variables that influence exercise. We view exercise behavior as the result of a complex causal web, but that causal web has been inadequately described. To guide research in this area, we have borrowed from two very general theories of behavior change, and we propose a multivariate model of exercise determinants that we hope will be useful to investigators in this area.

Throughout this chapter we have adopted a public health perspective. The public health perspective leads one to emphasize data, theories, and methods that lead to the greatest health benefits for the largest possible proportion of the total population. The public health emphasis leads us to (a) address each major phase in the natural history of exercise behavior, (b) only consider types of exercise that have been shown to have health benefits, and (c) focus on determinants that may be subject to change for intervention purposes. While studying determinants of exercise behavior may be justified solely on the basis of improving theories and generating basic research data, we are particularly interested in exercise determinants research because advances in this area should allow one to design more effective exercise promotion programs that would benefit public health.

One additional note on terminology is in order. In a strict sense, "determinants" is used inappropriately throughout this chapter. Very few variables have been isolated as determinants or "causes" of physical activity. Instead, most studies have identified only correlates or "potential determinants" of exercise, and determinants should be understood in that context.

307

DEFINING THE AREA OF STUDY

There would be no need to study the determinants or influences on exercise behavior if there were no particular benefits of exercise and physical activity. However, there are many well-documented beneficial physiological and psychological benefits of exercise that are well known. Briefly, exercise has therapeutic effects and is commonly used in the treatment of coronary artery disease [49, 62], hypertension [10], diabetes mellitus [73], obesity [11, 27], and psychological disorders such as depression [70]. Numerous studies have indicated that regular exercise can significantly reduce risk for coronary artery disease [48] and hypertension [46] and can extend the life span [45]. Data are emerging that suggest that exercise may reduce the incidence of selected types of cancer [66]. Thus, exercise is now widely accepted by professionals and the public alike as a behavior with many important health benefits. The current problem is that relatively few individuals in the United States and other industrialized nations are taking advantage of the health-protecting effects of regular exercise.

While it is difficult to estimate the prevalence of regular vigorous physical activity in the population, available data indicate that the prevalence is well below the 60% participation rate that was targeted in the 1990 fitness objectives for the nation [72]. For example, a large representative sample of U.S. adults were interviewed in the 1985 National Health Interview Survey. Caspersen et al. [13] reported that only 8.1% of men and 7% of women in that study reported being regular participants in vigorous physical activities. About 25% of men and 30% of women reported no participation in any activity. These data agree with the results of other national surveys of the United States and Canada [68] showing the low degree of participation in regular vigorous exercise.

Public health and exercise science professionals view this situation with alarm, because a very large percentage of the population are increasing their risks for several major chronic diseases by their failure to regularly engage in physical activity. These concerns have stimulated interest in studying the determinants of exercise behavior. In general, the goal of this area of research is to identify the various factors that appear to influence the degree of participation in exercise, with a common rationale being that identification of such factors could be used to improve the effectiveness of exercise intervention programs.

The initial problem faced by those who study exercise determinants is that it is difficult to both define and measure exercise and physical activity. The distinctions between exercise and physical activity and their definitions have been discussed previously [14], but agreement on these issues has not yet been reached. Measurement of physical activity is complicated by variations in type, intensity, frequency, duration, and intermittency. Over 30 different methods for assessing physical activity have been reported, including self-report, direct observation, and mechanical and electronic monitoring [34], and new measures are proposed with regularity. Few of these measures combine affordability, practicality of use, and high validity, so physical activity is usually measured with considerable error. These definitional and methodological problems have the effect of making the study of exercise determinants an imprecise science.

The Natural History of Exercise

Few investigators have carefully considered the probable natural history of exercise behavior. However, Figure 11.1 displays a simplified diagram of the four major phases of the natural history of exercise. Research on exercise determinants seeks to predict and explain the three transitions between phases. One simplification used in constructing the model is that exercise is treated as a dichotomous variable, even though it is continuously variable. A second simplification is that the model begins at the sedentary state. In reality, people will be distributed across all stages of the model at any given time, but because the vast majority of adults in industrialized countries are currently sedentary, it is reasonable to assume that sedentary behavior is the baseline state.

SEDENTARY → ADOPTION. The first transition is from being a nonexerciser to being an exerciser, however defined. Using continuous variables, one could specify an increase in exercise behavior. Given that less than 10% of the U.S. adult population engages in sufficient vigorous exercise to produce increases in cardiovascular fitness and maximum protection from chronic diseases [13] this transition point may be the

FIGURE 11.1
Four major phases of the natural history of exercise.

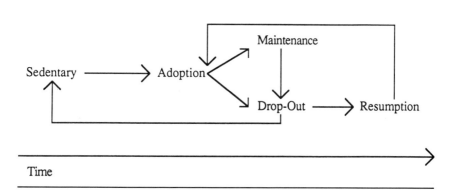

most important. However, as discussed later, the determinants of adoption of exercise have seldom been studied.

ADOPTION → DROP-OUT OR MAINTENANCE. There is widespread agreement that exercise must be practiced consistently for the health and fitness benefits to be achieved. However, there is substantial evidence to indicate that of those people who adopt regular exercise, approximately 50% drop out within 1 year. This percentage appears to apply to clinical cardiac rehabilitation patients [41] and to the general population [54]. The high rate of drop-out is clearly an important issue, especially because few people seem to be adopting exercise. The bulk of the exercise determinants research has focused on this transition.

DROP-OUT → RESUMPTION. Not everyone who drops out of exercise remains sedentary. Some unknown proportion of drop-outs resume exercise. This transition has been almost totally ignored, but it may be very important to know how dynamic the exercise cycle is. If many people start and stop exercise programs several times over their lifetimes, then exercise interventions need to focus on shortening the interval between drop-out and resumption. If very few drop-outs resume exercise, that suggests that more intervention resources should be directed to preventing drop-out.

Obviously, people vary widely in the amount of time that they spend at the various phases and in how many times they drop-out and resume exercise. Behavioral epidemiologists are encouraged to collect data on the dynamic nature of exercise, because simple prevalence estimates will not provide information on past exercise experience.

Those who study determinants of exercise behavior must carefully define which transition they are studying, because the determinants are likely to be different at each transition point. It is certainly not justifiable to assume that the determinants of adopting exercise are the same as resuming exercise after dropout. There may even be different determinants for resuming exercise after, for example, 2 months versus 2 years of drop-out. To maximize the relevance of determinants research to intervention design, determinants researchers must eventually provide information on all transition points.

Differentiating Types of Exercise

Another challenge facing exercise determinants researchers is the variety in types of exercise. Most determinants research has focused on the general category of regular vigorous exercise, on the justifiable assumption that the physiological effects of exercise are more dependent on overall degree of participation than on the specific type of exercise. This approach has been productive in increasing our understanding of the determinants of regular vigorous exercise, but there are at least two limitations to this approach.

First, while equivalent amounts of different types of exercises may produce similar physiological effects, the determinants of different types of exercises may be quite distinct. For example, factors that influence an indoor exercise like stationary cycling may be different from those that influence cross-country cycling. Likewise, jogging and aerobic dance may differ in their pattern of determinants, because the behaviors themselves have different characteristics and occur in very different settings. While it should not be assumed that all vigorous exercises have the same determinants, the assumption should be tested.

Second, there is the issue of the intensity of the exercise. Most studies of the health effects of exercise and most studies of exercise determinants have focused on aerobic activities requiring 60% or greater of cardiorespiratory capacity. There is ample justification for this focus, but there are also limitations [28]. There are two major lines of evidence that suggest that it is important to study the determinants of "moderate-intensity" activities. Moderate-intensity activities are those that require less than 60% of maximal capacity, and the most common example is walking. Accumulating evidence indicates that moderate-intensity physical activity has many of the health protective effects as vigorous exercise [31, 55]. For example, Paffenbarger and colleagues have reported that large amounts of walking and stairclimbing protect one from cardiovascular disease mortality [47] and extend longevity [45] significantly, but not to the same extent as more vigorous activities. It also appears that moderate-intensity activities increase cardiovascular fitness, but not as rapidly as vigorous activities [28]. Thus, there is a health rationale for studying determinants of moderate-intensity physical activity.

A second reason for studying determinants of moderate-intensity physical activity is that moderate and vigorous activities have many important differences. In virtually all studies of adults, walking is the most common type of physical activity [68]. Participation in walking and other moderate-intensity activities is relatively stable across the adult age range, while participation in vigorous activities declines dramatically with age [56]. Several authors have hypothesized that because moderate-intensity activities like walking and stairclimbing can be easily incorporated into one's daily routine, there are fewer barriers to participation, and maintenance should be enhanced [11, 22]. These behavioral differences between moderate and vigorous physical activities strongly suggest that determinants of moderate-intensity physical activities should be studied separately.

Focusing on Population Subgroups

The available data indicate that the patterns of physical activity differ substantially by age, sex, education, income, and possibly by race [13, 68]. Thus, it is reasonable to hypothesize that the determinants of exercise differ somewhat by population subgroup. In order to understand the determinants of exercise for the entire population, it may be necessary to study the determinants in each major population segment. In fact, much of the exercise determinants literature is based on studies of specific population segments. However, some segments have been studied extensively, such as middle-aged Caucasian men, cardiac rehabilitation patients, and college students. Other important population groups have been severely understudied. Included in this group are many of the subgroups with the lowest exercise participation rates and highest risks for exercise-related diseases, such as blacks, Latinos, the elderly, obese individuals, the poor, and children.

SUMMARY OF STUDIES OF EXERCISE DETERMINANTS

There have probably been close to 200 studies conducted in the past 20 years on some aspect of the determinants of exercise behavior [17]. Since there have been numerous excellent reviews of those studies in recent years [15–17, 19, 21, 35, 37, 38, 40, 63] it is not necessary to repeat the detailed consideration of the individual studies. Instead, interested readers are referred to the reviews cited above. In this section, we summarize the major findings of the previously published reviews and discuss selected studies that address important issues that have not been covered elsewhere. The review is organized by summarizing current knowledge regarding the determinants of each of the three major transition points in the natural history of exercise behavior.

Determinants of the Adoption of Exercise Behavior

Very few studies have been conducted on this topic, although from a public health perspective it is vital to know what influences a person to move from a sedentary life-style to regular exercise. Because approximately 90% of the U.S. adult population is not vigorously active, the problem of adoption of exercise is a critical one. Several studies claimed to study predictors of adoption of exercise. Unfortunately most had serious flaws such as only self-selected participants were studied [36, 64] or actual exercise was not used as the dependent variable [71]. One large multicenter study invited middle-aged men at risk for heart disease to participate in a program of moderate exercise [29]. Volunteers were less likely to be smokers and more likely to be married and already active [50]. Most studies had subjects report their reasons for joining the various programs, but these reports cannot be considered determinants. Thus, these studies of selected populations produced limited data on determinants of adoption of exercise.

One study employed a true prospective design with a representative community sample [54]. Over 1400 adults were assessed with a battery of measures of potential determinants, and their exercise behaviors were remeasured 1 year later. In univariate analyses, several predictors of adoption of vigorous exercise were found for women and/or men: exercise self-efficacy (i.e., confidence in one's ability to exercise regularly), health knowledge, attitudes toward exercise, and participation in moderate-intensity activity at baseline. This study also examined predictors of increases in moderate-intensity physical activity. Significant predictors were: moderate exercise self-efficacy, health knowledge, exercise knowledge, perceived self-control, attitudes toward exercise, and body mass index (i.e., lighter subjects were more likely to adopt exercise). While this study indicated that determinants of adoption of exercise could be identified, the incomplete list of potential determinants and lack of a theoretical focus limited the utility of the findings.

Overall, it must be concluded that we understand almost nothing about why some people begin exercising. This is a topic of great importance in need of serious investigation.

Determinants of the Maintenance of Exercise

The large exercise adherence literature addresses the question of determinants of exercise maintenance. Many studies examined predictors of adherence to specialized worksite, cardiac rehabilitation, and adult fitness programs, and relatively few studies investigated predictors of exercise maintenance in more representative population samples. A wide variety of determinants have been studied, and the general pattern of results is presented in Table 11.1, which is reprinted from Dishman et al. [19]. Results are separated according to the population studied. For participants in supervised programs there is strong evidence that blue collar workers, overweight persons, those who have discomfort during exercise, smokers, and those with mood disturbances are especially likely to drop out. Strong determinants of continued participation are self-motivation, behavioral skills, spouse support, available time, access to facilities, perception of good health, and (paradoxically) high risk for heart disease. Both personal and environmental variables appear to influence maintenance of exercise. However, relatively few of these determinants can be manipulated in intervention programs. Determinants that could be altered in exercise promotion programs include behavioral skills, social support, and perceptions of available time.

The many blank spaces in the spontaneous activity program column reflect that fewer studies have been conducted on community samples. Only mood disturbance was found to be reliably correlated with dropout. Maintenance was associated with high educational attainment and various supports and influences by peers and family members. Most of the population-based surveys were cross-sectional, and only one prospective study examined predictors of maintenance of exercise over

TABLE 11.1
Summary of Variables That May Determine the Probability of Exercise

Determinant	Changes in Probability	
	Supervised Program	Spontaneous Program
Personal characteristics		
Past program participation	++	
Past extra-program activity	+	
School athletics, 1 sport	+	0
School athletics, >1 sport		+
Blue-collar occupation	--	-
Smoking	--	
Overweight	--	
High risk for coronary heart disease	++	
Type A behavior	-	
Health, exercise knowledge	-	0
Attitudes	0	+
Enjoyment of activity	+	
Perceived health	++	
Mood disturbance	--	--
Education	+	++
Age	00	-
Expect personal health benefit	+	
Self-efficacy for exercise		+
Intention to adhere	0	0
Perceived physical competence	00	
Self-motivation	++	0
Evaluating costs and benefits	+	
Behavioral skills	++	
Environmental characteristics		
Spouse support	++	+
Perceived available time	++	+
Access to facilities	++	0
Disruptions in routine	--	
Social reinforcement (staff, exercise partner)	+	
Family influences		++
Peer influence		++
Physical influences		+
Cost		0
Medical screening	-	
Climate	-	
Incentives	+	
Activity characteristics		
Activity intensity	00	-
Perceived discomfort	--	-

KEY: ++ = repeatedly documented *increased* probability; + = weak or mixed documentation of *increased* probability; 00 = repeatedly documented that there is *no change* in probability; 0 = weak or mixed documentation of *no change* in probability; - = weak or mixed documentation of *decreased* probability; -- = repeatedly documented *decreased* probability. Blank spaces indicate no data.
From Dishman RK, Sallis JF, Orenstein DR: The determinants of physical activity and exercise. *Public Health Rep* 100:158–172, 1985. Copyright 1985 by the U.S. Public Health Service. Reprinted by permission.

1 year [54]. Predictors of vigorous exercise in women and/or men were self-control, attitudes toward exercise, self-efficacy for exercise, and education. Predictors of moderate-intensity physical activity were health knowledge, exercise knowledge, self-control, activity attitudes, self-efficacy for moderate exercise, and education. Some differences in predictors of maintenance of vigorous versus moderate exercise are interesting. Knowledge about health and exercise predicted maintenance of moderate activity only, while self-control, attitudes and education predicted maintenance of both types of exercise. The value of self-efficacy perceptions was emphasized by the finding that, in general, perceptions of self-efficacy for moderate activity strongly predicted moderate activity, and ratings of vigorous activity self-efficacy strongly predicted vigorous activity.

The results of the spontaneous activity studies suggest that interventions should target family and peer support, activity attitudes and self-efficacy. However, because so many potentially important determinants have not been adequately studied, there are insufficient data upon which to base populationwide exercise interventions.

Determinants of Resumption of Exercise after Drop-out

This phase of the natural history of exercise has been completely neglected by both theoreticians and empirical investigators. The extent to which drop-outs resume exercise later has never been studied, to our knowledge. Thus, there are no studies on the determinants of resumption of exercise. Research on these issues is desperately needed with both participants in specialized programs and with the general population.

Determinants of Exercise in Children and Adolescents

The need to study determinants of exercise in children has been recognized [18] but very few studies in this area could be located. Although they appear to the casual observer to be quite active, most data indicate that children ranging in age from preschool [61] to school age, [24, 30] to adolescence [69] are surprisingly inactive. Two categories of determinants of exercise in children have been studied. First, obese children have been found to be less active than thin children in most [7, 33] but not all [75] studies.

Second, a number of family influences appear to be important determinants of children's activity. Parent's obesity status and physical activity [61], parent's exercise beliefs [25], father's education [69], and direct parental encouragements [33] have been associated with activity levels in children. Two studies found that parental exercise is an important correlate of the physical activity of teenagers [26, 60].

Based on an excellent series of treatment studies of obese children, Epstein et al. [21] found that sex, age, height, obesity indices, and fitness did not predict adherence to exercise during the treatment. However, adherence was higher among children assigned to low-intensity exercise regimens.

One adherence issue in need of study is the apparent decrease in physical activity in late adolescence. National surveys indicate that one of the sharpest age-related decreases in exercise participation may be after high school and after college [68], as young adults are making the transition to independent living. At this time, relatively active adolescents appear to become increasingly inactive working adults. This phenomenon needs to be verified with improved measures, and specific determinants of these decreases need to be identified.

The Role of Intervention Studies

Experimental demonstrations that manipulating a specified parameter increases adoption, maintenance, or resumption of exercise provide the most compelling evidence regarding determinants of exercise. Virtually all behavioral intervention studies have been conducted with small select groups, but some of the principles derived from these studies may be applicable to larger samples or entire communities. The earlier exercise intervention studies were reviewed by Martin and Dubbert [38], worksite studies were reviewed by Sallis et al. [57], and Epstein et al. [21] have reviewed their series of studies with obese children. Wankel [74] has reviewed his series of studies of discrete strategies. These and other studies [5, 9, 32, 39] have demonstrated that several behavioral strategies appear to increase adherence to exercise programs over brief intervals. The specific behavioral techniques that have been shown to increase exercise adherence in experimental programs are listed in Table 11.2. These few studies generally indicate that the same methods of behavior change that are effective for most human behaviors [76] can also be applied to exercise.

Experimental intervention studies will continue to play a special role in the development of knowledge of exercise determinants because attribution of causality can be made unambiguously. A fruitful application of intervention studies would be to experimentally test hypotheses about exercise determinants that are generated in the observational studies.

Gaps in the Exercise Determinants Literature

Many of the gaps in the exercise determinants literature have been summarized previously [15–19, 35, 37] so only the needs most related to the public health perspective are discussed here.

1. Two of the three major transition points in the natural history of exercise have not been studied in any meaningful sense. The deter-

TABLE 11.2
Behavioral Strategies That Have Increased Adherence to Exercise in Experimental Studies

Study	Population	Behavioral Intervention
Wysocki et al., 1979 (77)	College students in an exercise group	Contracts detailed the amount of exercise that was expected. Deposited items were returned based on attendance at classes.
Epstein et al., 1980 (23)	College women in exercise classes	Signed contracts detailed the amount of exercise that was expected. Deposit money was returned for each week of attendance. In the lottery condition, participants deposited money and earned chances to win the entire pool based on attendance at classes.
Oldridge and Jones, 1983 (42)	Cardiac rehabilitation patients	Written agreements (contracts) were signed by patients in which they agreed to participate in the program for 6 months. Self-monitoring diaries regarding exercise heart rates, diet, physical activity, weight, and smoking were kept, and the diaries were discussed regularly with the program coordinator.
King and Frederiksen, 1984 (32)	College women in a jogging class	Relapse prevention training included behavioral skills such as rescheduling missed jogging sessions and cognitive skills such as challenging negative thoughts.
Martin et al., 1984 (39)	Healthy sedentary adult enrollees in an aerobic exercise course	*Study 1.* Personalized feedback and praise during exercise sessions were delivered by leaders. Shaping (gradual increases) of running time was based on time rather than distance goals. *Study 2.* Flexible goals allowed subjects to modify instructor-recommended goals based on how subjects felt on a particular day. *Study 5.* Dissociative cognitive strategies were encouraged in which subjects attended to the environment and other pleasant distractions rather than exercise-related sensations.
Wankel, 1984 (74)	Healthy participants in various fitness programs	The decision balance sheet approach leads the participant to consider the positive and negative outcomes of exercising. The interviewer reinforces the positive outcomes and buffers anticipated negative outcomes. Social support was facilitated by class leaders who encouraged a buddy system for class members and elicited support from family members.
Belisle et al., 1987 (5)	Healthy enrollees in "beginners" exercise groups	Charts for monitoring attendance and support were displayed in class. A multicomponent program focused on relapse prevention skills but also included self-monitoring of exercise and anticipating situations that might lead to relapse.

minants of adoption of exercise and resumption of exercise after drop-out need to be investigated.

2. Although there are important health-related benefits of moderate-intensity physical activity, very few studies of the determinants of this type of exercise have been reported. Studies of the determinants of moderate-intensity physical activity should be a high priority.

3. The most conclusive data on determinants of exercise behavior come from controlled intervention studies. More intervention studies targeting adoption, maintenance, and resumption of exercise are needed both to test hypotheses arising from observational determinants studies and to demonstrate the utility of interventions that could be applied to increase physical activity in the population.

4. More studies are needed on determinants of exercise in specific population subgroups, such as minorities, children, and the elderly.

5. Determinants studies should include measures of personal and environmental determinants that have relevance to intervention design. That is, determinants should be subject to change through educational, behavioral, or policy interventions. Studies of demographic variables, psychological traits, and health status as exercise determinants are interesting, and they may identify subgroups in need of special interventions, but studies of such variables do not guide the design of the intervention programs.

6. While some exercise determinants research has been based on behavioral theories, the theories that have typically been used are not comprehensive enough to encompass the measurement of the entire range of variables that probably influence exercise behavior. Thus, there is a need for a comprehensive model of exercise behavior.

A THEORETICAL APPROACH TO EXERCISE DETERMINANTS RESEARCH THEORIES OF HEALTH BEHAVIOR

A number of social/psychological theories concerning health behavior are in wide use. Most notable among these are the Health Belief Model [51] and the Fishbein and Ajzen Reasoned Action Model [1, 44]. These assume that individuals make rational decisions regarding the "cost/benefits" of performing a given behavior, including physical activity. Their attitudes and perceptions are prerequisite to performance. Thus, the person who believes that they will benefit more than they will "suffer" (cost) will perform exercise reliably. These theories lead to persuasion efforts to change individuals' perception of cost/benefits and their general attitudes toward the behavior of concern. These theories have face validity, but they focus almost exclusively on cognitive variables. These theories also ignore influences from the physical environment, learning processes, and genetic variables [67].

Learning theories have provided a more complete basis for explaining and controlling behavior, in that they include environmental factors and focus on the learning processes that both exert powerful influence over behavior and are modifiable. Most notable among the learning theories are operant conditioning [65] and social learning theory, recently revised and named social cognitive theory [3, 4].

Operant conditioning asserts that consequences are the primary determinants of behavior. Reinforcing (i.e., rewarding) consequences increase behavior; punishing consequences (e.g., discomfort) decrease behavior. There is truly a massive literature on animals and humans indicating that reinforcement is the most effective means of altering behavior [6]. Social learning theory assumes the same principles of behavior held by operant conditioning but emphasizes bidirectional influences in which the person can alter the environment in addition to the environment controlling the person's behavior. Social learning theory also elevates the importance of social modeling as important antecedents and social consequences as especially powerful reinforcers or punishers. The concept of self-efficacy is a central element of social cognitive theory [4]. This concept assumes that persons who are confident in their ability to perform a specific behavior (e.g., jogging) are more likely to actually perform it. Similarly, those who are confident that they will obtain commonly expected benefits are more likely to perform the behavior. These beliefs are specific to the behavior in question, as opposed to general traits such as self-esteem. Self-efficacy perceptions have been shown to be powerful predictors of many types of behaviors [2, 4].

Physical Activity, Learning Theory, and Genetics

For over 90% of the time on this planet, Homo sapiens have lived in a fashion where relatively intense physical activity was required in order to attain important reinforcers [8]. Gathering food, hunting, and escaping the occasional tiger required constant walking and frequent running [12]. It may be presumed that these physical activities produced some pain and discomfort. However, it must also be assumed that these would-be punishing consequences were offset by the competing reinforcers of food or avoidance of more extreme pain (e.g., being eaten by a tiger).

Modern society has eliminated the need for much of the physical activity previously necessary for survival. Machines provide the physical labor for food acquisition and machines and housing provide protection from the physical environment. Under these modern conditions, the more intense physical activity may be expected to result in immediate noxious consequences, with essentially no competing rewards or avoidance of more serious noxious consequences. Depending on the intensity and duration, these consequences may range from minor nuisances such as perspiration, to fatigue and discomfort, to serious pain and injury. These consequences are likely to be punishing and would tend to suppress the frequency, duration, and intensity of physical activity. The low prevalence rates of vigorous activity in the U.S. population noted earlier are exactly what might be expected given this interaction between learning and our evolutionary background. Under modern circumstances the punishing aspects of exertion are not offset by perceptible reinforcers.

Genetic differences also interact with learning theory to account for some of the variation among individuals in their likelihood of exercising. The genetically endowed tall and lean individual may find running "easy," while the short and relatively rotund somatotype may find running considerably more difficult. Genetically determined somatotypes and possibly other physiological differences, may make a given intensity or duration of physical activity more or less "painful," or more or less punishing. In this way, genetics may interact with learning processes, making it more likely for some individuals to learn to engage in more intense or longer duration exercises than others.

Learning processes might interact with acquired physiological conditions in a manner that could influence the likelihood of exercise. Individuals who perform aerobic exercise routinely, regardless of their genetic background, will acquire a greater degree of cardiovascular fitness that makes a given intensity of activity less difficult (i.e., less punishing) than would be true for the less physically fit. Fit individuals presumably experience less discomfort from a given degree of intensity or duration of physical activity compared to untrained individuals. Thus, the degree of punishing consequences "naturally" occurring as a consequence of exercise will decrease as one acquires physiological fitness.

This somewhat speculative background serves to emphasize the inherent difficulties in initiating and maintaining regular exercise habits. The historical utilitarian reinforcers of physical activity no longer exist for urban populations. The punishment of vigorous exertion remains immediate and salient, while the reinforcers of improved health or weight loss are greatly delayed and silent.

Learning theory, taken in the context of both genetic interactions and the development of modern society, may provide the most comprehensive explanation of physical activity and the most useful prescriptive model for increasing physical activity in sedentary subpopulations. Indeed, social learning theory has served as the basis for all the major community heart disease prevention studies in both the United States and other western nations [20].

A Model of Exercise Determinants Based on Learning Theory

Because exercise is a complex behavior with multiple determinants, it is necessary to use theories and models to guide research on exercise determinants. Several models have been used by investigators in the field [67], but most of them dealt almost exclusively with cognitive variables. Because learning theories indicate that environmental, social, and other factors are also important, there is a need for a more comprehensive model.

The authors, with substantial input from our colleagues, Dr. John P. Elder and Dr. C. Richard Hofstetter, have developed a model based on operant and social learning theories that is presented in Table 11.3. Variables that were selected for inclusion represent only a partial list of those that might be selected for study. The variables are by no means definitive, but they do illustrate the types of influences that learning theory would lead one to consider.

The most useful feature of the model may be its structure. Potential determinants of exercise are classified as either antecedents or consequences, and operant learning theory would predict that consequences would be more powerful influences in general [65]. Within those categories, variables are further grouped as distal or proximal in time, space, or concept to exercise. Other things being equal, proximal influences are expected to be more important determinants of exercise. For example, the climate may affect the overall probability of exercise, but the weather would be expected to have a stronger effect on exercise for a given day. While a distal reinforcer such as compliments for losing weight may be very important to an individual, such events that are separated in time from the exercise behavior are likely to have much less influence on exercise than encouragement from an exercise partner during or just after the exercise session.

Five types of variables are categorized according to the framework described above, but many variables could reasonably fit into more than one category. *Environmental* factors are characteristics of the physical environment that might influence exercise behavior. While climate, terrain, and air quality may have some effects, convenient access to facilities and equipment may serve as cues or may reduce barriers to exercise. Some of these same environmental variables may interact with exercise itself to alter the consequences. Hot temperatures and steep terrain may create a punishing exercise experience while beautiful scenery may be reinforcing.

Social variables are the dominant influences on many types of behavior [52], and modeling is a central process in Bandura's theories [3, 4]. The model implies that the past history of modeling is less influential than modeling by current friends and relatives. Modeling influences can be transmitted via the media as well as face to face. Social support for

TABLE 11.3
A Model of Determinants of Physical Activity Based on Learning Theory

	Antecedents		Consequences	
	Distal	*Proximal*	*Proximal*	*Distal*
	I. Environmental Factors		I. Environmental Factors	
	Climate	Convenience of facilities and equipment	Rough terrain (increased work)	
	Terrain	Safety of neighborhood	Equipment failure	
	Air quality	Weather	Hot/cold temperature	
			Pleasantness of exercise setting	
	II. Social Factors		II. Social Factors	
	Past modeling and support	Family models	Praise	Physical attractiveness "shape"
		Friend models	General attention	
		Media influences	Criticism	
		Competing responsibilities	Competing opportunities	
			Solitary or social exercise	
	III. Cognitive Factors		III. Cognitive Factors	
	Normative beliefs	Exercise knowledge	Proprioceptive feedback	Anticipated health benefits
		Self-efficacy	Pain	Fear of injury
		Behavioral intentions	Pleasure	
			Exhaustion	
			Positive/negative mood or affect	
	IV. Physiological Factors		IV. Physiological Factors	
	Age		Effort/work	Weight change
	Gender		Perspiration	Fitness
	Somatotype		Acute injury	Chronic injury
	Handicapping illness/injury		Heart rate	
	Health status		Breathing rate	
	Coordination			
	V. Other Personal Factors		V. Other Personal Factors	
	Exercise history	Diet	Smoking	
	Weight control history	Other health-related behavior	Alcohol consumption	
	Injury history		General risk-taking	
	Education		Other health behavior	
	Income			

exercise appears to be an important determinant [53]. Whereas praise for exercise is one social consequence for exercise, the exerciser can also be criticized for spending time away from the family, for wasting money at a health spa, for inviting injury, etc. Distal social consequences may be related to an improved social life accompanying exercise-induced changes in appearance.

Cognitive factors have been studied extensively, and only a few variables have been listed here. Normative beliefs concern perceptions about whether exercise is the norm in the population, so this variable was classified as a distal antecedent. More proximal antecedents are exercise self-efficacy and intentions to exercise. Positive and negative sensations, thoughts, and moods during and just after exercise are probably very important determinants of exercise maintenance, but they have not been adequately studied. Anticipated health benefits or fear of injury may be thought of as distal cognitive consequences.

Physiological influences are likely to play a major role in determining exercise habits, but it is difficult to classify them as proximal or distal, because they are basically constant. Somatotype and health status are pervasive physiological influences. The acute physiologic response to exercise and the perception of that response are likely to be important determinants. The literature suggesting that low intensity exercise promotes better adherence [15, 19, 21, 22, 54] is consistent with a physiologic influence. Weight and fitness changes are delayed consequences of exercise.

There are a variety of other personal factors such as exercise history and weight control history. Other health behaviors such as diet, smoking, and alcohol use may affect one's probability of exercise. However, behaviors such as smoking and alcohol use may also influence the consequences of exercise.

RESEARCH BASED ON THE LEARNING THEORY MODEL OF EXERCISE DETERMINANTS

The learning theory model clearly reflects that exercise behavior is the result of a complex causal web. The model implies that exercise determinants research should assess several types of variables, rather than study only one type. Contrasting the relative strengths of environmental, social, cognitive, and physiological variables on the adoption, maintenance, and resumption of exercise may provide information that will help in the design of appropriate interventions.

A program of research in exercise determinants is being conducted by researchers in San Diego, California, in collaboration with Dr. Kenneth E. Powell and Dr. Carl J. Caspersen at the Centers for Disease Control in Atlanta, Georgia. The purpose of the San Diego Health and Exercise

Project is to study exercise determinants using a multidimensional learning theory-based model such as the one described above.

Survey research methodology with a mailed questionnaire was used to collect cross-sectional data on the frequency of vigorous exercise, the amount of walking for exercise, and 24 potential determinants of exercise that were selected to represent different categories of variables in the model. A random sample of households in San Diego were sent three waves of surveys, and various prompts and incentives were used to increase the response rate. A final response rate of 43.4% yielded 2053 adult subjects. The sample over-represented affluent, educated, Caucasians, so generalizations should be limited to that segment of the population. Three analyses have been conducted that are particularly relevant to this chapter, and they are summarized briefly.

Study 1 assessed the relationships between the 24 potential determinants and the frequency of vigorous exercise with a duration of at least 20 min per session [59]. The 24 determinants and their classification in the model are listed in Table 11.4. Bivariate correlations indicated that self-efficacy had the highest correlation with frequency of vigorous exercise. For the subsequent stepwise multiple regressions, self-efficacy was excluded because in a cross-sectional study it is confounded with the dependent variable.

TABLE 11.4
Determinants Included in the San Diego Health and Exercise Project

Antecedents		Consequences	
Distal	*Proximal*	*Proximal*	*Distal*
I. Environmental Factors		I. Environmental Factors	
	Home equipment		
	Neighborhood environment		
	Convenience of facilities		
II. Social Factors		II. Social Factors	
Modeling history	Modeling	Friend support	
	Media influences	Family support	
III. Cognitive Factors		III. Cognitive Factors	
Normative beliefs	Self-efficacy	Barriers	Benefits
	Exercise knowledge		
IV. Physiological Factors		IV. Physiological Factors	
Age			
Gender			
Body mass index			
Coordination			
V. Other Personal Factors		V. Other Personal Factors	
Education	Smoking	Smoking	
Exercise history	Alcohol	Alcohol	
Injury as a child	Diet	Diet	
Injury as an adult			

In the regression analyses, the only significant environmental variable was home exercise equipment (positive association; $p < 0.001$). Modeling and friend support were the two significant social factors (positive; $p < 0.0001$), and benefits (positive; $p < 0.002$) and barriers (negative; $p < 0.0001$) were significant cognitive factors. Significant physiological variables were age (negative; $p < 0.0001$) and coordination (positive; $p < 0.003$). Other significant variables were smoking (negative; $p < 0.001$) and heart-healthy diet (positive; $p < 0.0001$). The overall regression accounted for 27% of the variance in frequency of vigorous exercise.

Significant variables were identified in all categories of determinants, confirming the need for multidimensional studies of exercise determinants. Results suggested that proximal variables may be more important than distal variables and this finding confirms a prediction of learning theory.

Study 2 assessed the relationships between determinants and walking for exercise in the same population [31]. Walking for exercise was defined as the product of reported frequency times average duration over the past 2 weeks. Those subjects who reported regular vigorous exercise were excluded from this analysis so that the study could focus on those who were obtaining only low-intensity exercise ($N = 1080$).

Only three significant correlates were identified in the multiple regression analysis: self-efficacy for exercise (positive; $p < 0.0001$), heart-healthy diet (positive; $p < 0.0002$), and age (negative; $p < 0.05$). The regression accounted for 12% of the variance in walking for exercise.

The 24 potential determinants explained much less variance in low-intensity exercise than in high-intensity exercise. This indicates again that different determinants appear to be important for different types of exercise. Much more work is needed to understand the influences on walking for exercise. Of the few significant correlates, each was classified as a different type of variable. This implies that walking is a multiply determined behavior as well.

Study 3 assessed correlates of relapse from vigorous exercise [58]. Subjects reported the number of times in their life they had exercised for at least 6 months and then stopped exercising for at least 3 months. This criterion was chosen to define a full relapse from a well-established exercise program. A major finding from this study was that relapse patterns were identical in both current exercisers and current nonexercisers. This result highlights the dynamic nature of vigorous exercise and indicates that many people who are identified in cross-sectional studies as sedentary have been regular exercisers in the past. The most common reason for the last relapse was "injury." Multiple regression analyses for the nonexerciser subgroup revealed that age (negative; $p < 0.001$), injury as an adult (positive; $p < 0.002$), education (positive; $p < 0.001$); history of exercise models (positive; $p < 0.002$), and home exercise equipment (positive; $p < 0.02$) were significant correlates of number of relapses. This regression only accounted for 11% of the variance. Among exercisers, self-efficacy (negative; $p < 0.001$), injury as a child (positive; $p < 0.001$), and education (positive; $p < 0.01$) were the significant correlates. This regression accounted for 8% of the variance in relapse from exercise.

This study emphasized the role of injury in relapse from exercise, but again, the significant correlates were distributed across categories rather than concentrated within categories.

The San Diego Health and Exercise Project surveys illustrate the value of using a learning theory-based model to study determinants of physical activity. The study also illustrates many of the challenges of conducting exercise determinants research.

Multidimensional models require the assessment of many variables, placing large burdens on the subjects. Because the determinants of low- and high-intensity activities appear to be very different, even more potential determinants may have to be identified and measured in future studies. Growing understanding of the determinants of exercise is leading to the need for more complex research methodology.

The current studies were based on survey methodology. In addition to the problems of the reliability and validity of self-reports, it is simply not possible to obtain self-reports of some variables. Unfortunately, reinforcing and punishing social and environmental consequences are likely to be the most important determinants of physical activity, yet it is not feasible to study these processes by self-report methods. Untrained observers are not able to observe and report the consequences of their behaviors. For a learning theory-based study, this limitation has been an important one. Fortunately, there are well-developed methods for studying the effects of reinforcement on behavior in experimental intervention studies. Several intervention studies have been reported, confirming that reinforcement is effective [38, 39] but additional studies are needed to refine the methods so they can be applied on the community level.

CONCLUSIONS

Learning theory appears to be a fruitful model upon which to base exercise determinants research. However, the use of survey research methods to identify learning-based determinants is limited, because subjects are unable to evaluate and report adequately the role of behavioral consequences, which are the most powerful determinants of behavior. Only intervention trials that manipulate the contingencies of reinforcement (i.e., the conditions under which exercise behavior is rewarded) and the nature of rewards will be able to fully describe these important determinants.

We believe the principal role of exercise determinants research should be to provide data that can be used to guide the design of educational and policy-related exercise promotion interventions. Although over 200 studies on exercise determinants research have been published, our knowledge of determinants is rudimentary and imprecise. Social, cognitive, physiological, and environmental factors all appear to be related to the maintenance of exercise, and the specific determinants of adoption, maintenance, and resumption may be different. Thus, there is unlikely to be a simple final answer to the question, "Why do people exercise?" Nevertheless, this remains an important field of inquiry, given the health benefits of exercise and the low rate of participation in exercise in industrialized nations.

ACKNOWLEDGMENTS

Our colleagues in the San Diego Health and Exercise project have influenced both the conceptualization of the model of exercise determinants and the conduct of the studies. The contributions of Dr. John P. Elder and Dr. C. Richard Hofstetter from San Diego State University and Dr. Kenneth E. Powell and Dr. Carl J. Caspersen from the Centers for Disease Control are especially appreciated. Project coordinators Patricia Faucher, Vivien Spry, and Elizabeth Barrington have also contributed. Sheila Dowe assisted in manuscript preparation.

This work was partially supported by a Cooperative Agreement from the Associated Schools of Public Health/Centers for Disease Control and National Institutes of Health Grant HL 40575.

REFERENCES

1. Ajzen I, Fishbein M: Understanding attitudes and predicting social behavior. Englewood Cliffs, NJ, Prentice-Hall, 1980.
2. Bandura A: Self-efficacy: toward a unifying theory of behavior change. *Psychol Rev* 84:192–215, 1977.
3. Bandura A: Social learning theory. Englewood Cliffs, NJ, Prentice-Hall, 1977.
4. Bandura A: Social foundations of thought and action. Englewood Cliffs, NJ, Prentice-Hall, 1986.
5. Belisle M, Roskies E, Levesque MM: Improving adherence to physical activity. *Health Psychol* 6:159–172, 1987.
6. Bellack AS, Hersen M, Kazdin AE: International handbook of behavior modification and therapy. New York, Plenum, 1982.
7. Berkowitz RI, Agras WS, Korner AF: Physical activity and adiposity: a longitudinal study from birth to childhood. *J Pediatr* 106:434–438, 1985.
8. Blair SN: Exercise within a healthy lifestyle. In Dishman RK (ed): *Exercise Adherence: Its Impact on Public Health*. Champaign, IL, Human Kinetics, 1988.
9. Blair SN, Piserchia PV, Wilbur CS, Crowder JH: A public health intervention model for work-site health promotion: impact on exercise and physical fitness in a health promotion plan after 24 months. *JAMA* 255:921–926, 1986.

10. Boyer JL, Kasch FW: Exercise therapy in hypertensive men. *JAMA* 211:1668–1671, 1970.

11. Brownell KD, Stunkard AJ: Physical activity in the development and control of obesity. In Stunkard AJ (ed): *Obesity*. Philadelphia, WB Saunders, 1980, pp 300–324.

12. Burke EJ: Thoughts on heredity and the environment, preliminary to a study of exercise. In Burke EJ (ed): *Exercise, Science and Fitness*. Ithaca, NY, Mouvement Publications, 1980.

13. Caspersen CJ, Christenson GM, Pollard RA: Status of the 1990 physical fitness and exercise objectives—Evidence from NHIS 1985. *Public Health Rep* 101:587–592, 1986.

14. Caspersen CJ, Powell KE, Christenson GM: Physical activity, exercise, and physical fitness: definitions and distinctions for health-related research. *Public Health Rep* 100:126–131, 1985.

15. Dishman RK: Compliance/adherence in health-related exercise. *Health Psychol* 1:237–267, 1982.

16. Dishman RK: Exercise compliance: a new view for public health. *Physician Sports Med* 14:127–145, 1986.

17. Dishman RK: Overview. In Dishman RK (ed): *Exercise Adherence: Its Impact on Public Health*. Champaign, IL, Human Kinetics, 1988, pp 1–9.

18. Dishman RK, Dunn AL: Exercise adherence in children and youth: implications for adulthood. In RK Dishman (ed): *Exercise Adherence: Its Impact on Public Health*. Champaign, IL, Human Kinetics, 1988, pp 155–200.

19. Dishman RK, Sallis JF, Orenstein DR: The determinants of physical activity and exercise. *Public Health Rep* 100:158–172, 1985.

20. Elder J, Hovell MF, Lasater J, Wells B, Carleton R: Applications of behavior modification to community health education: the case of heart disease prevention. *Health Educ Q* 12:151–168, 1985.

21. Epstein LH, Koeske R, Wing RR: Adherence to exercise in obese children. *J Cardiac Q Rehabil* 4:185–195, 1984.

22. Epstein LH, Wing RR, Koeske R, Valoski A: A comparison of lifestyle exercise, aerobic exercise, and calisthenics on weight loss in obese children. *Behav Ther* 16:345–356, 1985.

23. Epstein LH, Wing RR, Thompson JK, Griffin W: Attendance and fitness in aerobic exercise: the effects of contract and lottery procedures. *Behav Modif* 4:465–479, 1980.

24. Gilliam TB, Freedson PS, Geenen DL: Physical activity patterns determined by heart rate monitoring in 6- to 7-year-old children. *Med Sci Sports Exerc* 13:65–67, 1981.

25. Godin G, Shephard RJ: Normative beliefs of school children concerning regular exercise. *J Sch Health* 54:443–445, 1984.

26. Gottlieb NH, Chen MS: Sociocultural correlates of childhood sporting activities: their implications for heart health. *Soc Sci Med* 21:533–539, 1985.

27. Hagan RD, Upton SJ, Wong L, Shittam J: The effects of aerobic conditioning and/or caloric restriction in overweight men and women. *Med Sci Sports Exer* 18:87–94, 1986.

28. Haskell WL, Montoye HJ, Orenstein D: Physical activity and exercise to achieve health-related physical fitness components. *Public Health Rep* 100:202–212, 1985.

29. Heinzelman F, Bagley RW: Response to physical activity programs and their effects on health behavior. *Public Health Rep* 85:905–911, 1970.

30. Hovell MF, Bursick JH, Sharkey R: An evaluation of elementary students' voluntary physical activity during recess. *Res Q* 49:460–474, 1978.

31. Hovell MF, Sallis JF, Hofstetter CR, Spry VM, Elder JP, Faucher P, Caspersen CJ: Identifying correlates of walking for exercise: an epidemiologic prerequisite for physical activity promotion. *Prev Med* (in press).

32. King AC, Frederiksen LW: Low-cost strategies for increasing exercise behavior: relapse preparation training and social support. *Behav Modif* 8:3–21, 1984.

33. Klesges RC, Coates TJ, Moldenhauer-Klesges LM, Holzer B, Gustavson J, Barnes J: The FATS: an observational system for assessing physical activity in children and associated parent behavior. *Behav Assess* 6:333–345, 1984.
34. LaPorte RE, Montoye HJ, Caspersen CJ: Assessment of physical activity in epidemiologic research: problems and prospects. *Public Health Rep* 100:131–146, 1985.
35. Lee C, Owen N: Uses of psychological theories in understanding adoption and maintenance of exercising. *Aust J Sci Med Sport* 18:22–25, 1986.
36. Long BC, Haney CJ: Enhancing physical activity in sedentary women: information, locus of control, and attitudes. *J Sport Psychol* 8:9–24, 1986.
37. Martin JE, Dubbert PM: Adherence to exercise. In Terjung RL (ed): *Exercise and Sport Sciences Reviews*. Syracuse, NY, MacMillan, 1985, pp 137–167.
38. Martin JE, Dubbert PM: Exercise applications and promotion in behavioral medicine: current status and future directions. *J Consult Clin Psychol* 50:1004–1017, 1982.
39. Martin JE, Dubbert PM, Kattell AD, Thompson JK, Raczynski JR, Lake M, Smith PO, Webster JS, Sikora T, Cohen RE: Behavioral control of exercise in sedentary adults. Studies 1 through 6. *J Consult Clin Psychol* 52:795–811, 1984.
40. Oldridge NB: Compliance and exercise in primary and secondary prevention of coronary heart disease: a review. *Prev Med* 11:56–70, 1982.
41. Oldridge NB: Compliance of post-myocardial infarction patients to exercise programs. *Med Sci Sports* 11:373–375, 1979.
42. Oldridge NB, Jones NL: Improving patient compliance in cardiac exercise rehabilitation: effects of written agreement and self-monitoring. *J Cardiac Rehab* 3:257–262, 1983.
43. Owen N, Lee C: Why people do and do not exercise. Adelaide, Australia, Sport and Recreation Ministers' Council, 1984.
44. Olson JM, Zanna MP: Understanding and promoting exercise: a social psychological perspective. *Can J Public Health* 78:S1–S8, 1987.
45. Paffenbarger RS, Hyde RT, Wing AL, Hsieh C: Physical activity, all-cause mortality, and longevity of college alumni. *New Engl J Med* 314:605–613, 1986.
46. Paffenbarger RS, Wing AL, Hyde RT: Chronic disease in former college students. XX. Physical activity and incidence of hypertension in college alumni. *Am J Epidemiol* 117:245–257, 1983.
47. Paffenbarger RS, Wing AL, Hyde RT: Physical activity as an index of heart attack risk in college alumni. *Am J Epidemiol* 108:161–175, 1978.
48. Powell KE, Thompson PD, Caspersen CJ, Kendrick JS: Physical activity and the incidence of coronary heart disease. *Annu Rev Public Health* 8:253–287, 1987.
49. Rechnitzer PA, Sangal DA, Cunningham GR: A controlled perspective of the effect of endurance training on the recurrence rate of myocardial infarction. *Am J Epidemiol* 102:358–365, 1975.
50. Remington RD, Taylor HL, Buskirk ER: A method for assessing volunteer bias and its application to a cardiovascular prevention program involving physical activity. *J Epidemiol Commun Health* 32:250–255, 1978.
51. Rosenstock IM. Historical origins of the health belief model. *Health Educ Monogr* 2:328–335, 1974.
52. Rosenthal T, Bandura A: Psychological modeling: theory and practice. In Garfield SL, Bergin AE (eds): *Handbook of Psychotherapy and Behavior Change*. ed, 2 New York, John Wiley & Sons, 1978, pp 621–658.
53. Sallis JF, Grossman RM, Pinski RB, Patterson TL, Nader PR: The development of scales to measure social support for diet and exercise behaviors. *Prev Med* 16:825–836, 1987.
54. Sallis JF, Haskell WL, Fortmann SP, Vranizan KM, Taylor CB, Solomon DS: Predictors of adoption and maintenance of physical activity in a community sample. *Prev Med* 15:331–341, 1986.

55. Sallis JF, Haskell WL, Fortmann SP, Wood PD, Vranizan KM: Moderate-intensity physical activity and cardiovascular risk factors. The Stanford Five-City Project. *Prev Med* 15:561–568, 1986.

56. Sallis JF, Haskell WL, Wood PD, Fortmann SP, Rogers T, Blair SN, Paffenbarger RS: Physical activity assessment methodology in the Five-City Project. *Am J Epidemiol* 121:91–106, 1985.

57. Sallis JF, Hill RD, Fortmann SP, Flora JA: Health behavior change at the worksite: cardiovascular risk reduction. In Hersen M, Eisler RM, Miller PM (eds): *Progress in Behavior Modification*. Vol. 20. New York, Academic Press, 1986, pp 161–197.

58. Sallis JF, Hovell MF, Hofstetter CR, Elder JP, Faucher P, Spry VM, Barrington E, Hackley M: Lifetime history of relapse from exercise. *Addict Behav* (in press).

59. Sallis JF, Hovell MF, Hofstetter CR, Faucher P, Elder JP, Blanchard J, Caspersen CJ, Powell KE, Christenson GM: A multivariate study of exercise determinants in a community sample. *Prev Med* 18:20–34, 1989.

60. Sallis JF, Patterson TL, Buono MJ, Atkins CJ, Nader PR: Aggregation of physical activity habits in Mexican-American and Anglo families. *J Behav Med* 11:31–41, 1988.

61. Sallis JF, Patterson TL, McKenzie TL, Nader PR: Family variables and physical activity in preschool children. *J Dev Behav Pediatr* 9:57–61, 1988.

62. Shaw LW: Effects of a prescribed supervised exercise program on mortality and cardiovascular morbidity in patients after a myocardial infarction. The National Exercise and Heart Disease Project. *Am J Cardiol* 48:39–46, 1981.

63. Shephard RJ: Factors influencing the exercise behavior of patients. *Sports Med* 2:348–366, 1985.

64. Shephard RJ, Morgan P, Finucane R, Schimmelfing L: Factors influencing recruitment to an occupational fitness program. *J Occup Med* 22:389–398, 1980.

65. Skinner BF: *Science and Human Behavior*. New York, The Free Press, 1953.

66. Slattery ML, Schumacher MC, Smith KR, West DW, Abd-Elghany N: Physical activity, diet, and risk of colon cancer in Utah. *Am J Epidemiol* 128:989–999, 1988.

67. Sonstroem R: Psychological models. In Dishman RK (ed): Exercise adherence: its impact on public health. Champaign, IL, Human Kinetics, 1988, pp 125–153.

68. Stephens T, Jacobs DR, White CC: A descriptive epidemiology of leisure-time physical activity. *Public Health Rep* 100:147–158, 1985.

69. Sunnegardh J, Bratteby LE, Sjolin S: Physical activity and sports involvement in 8- and 13-year-old children in Sweden. *Acta Pediatr Scand* 74:904–912, 1985.

70. Taylor CB, Sallis JF, Needle R: The relation of physical activity and exercise to mental health. *Public Health Rep* 100:195–202, 1985.

71. Teraslinna P, Partanen T, Koskela A, Oja P: Characteristics affecting willingness of executives to participate in an activity program aimed at coronary heart disease prevention. *J Sports Med* 9:224–229, 1969.

72. U.S. Department of Health and Human Services: Surgeon General's Report: Promoting Health-Preventing Disease, 1990 Objectives for the Nation. Washington D.C.: National Institutes of Health, 1980.

73. Vranick M, Berger M: Exercise and diabetes mellitus. *Diabetes* 28:147–167, 1979.

74. Wankel LM: Decision-making and social support strategies for increasing exercise adherence. *J Cardiac Rehab* 4:124–135, 1984.

75. Waxman M, Stunkard AJ: Caloric intake and expenditure of obese boys. *J Pediatr* 96:187–193, 1980.

76. Wilson T, O'Leary D: *Principles of Behavior Therapy* Englewood Cliffs, NJ, Prentice-Hall, 1980.

77. Wysocki T, Hall G, Iwata B, Riordan M: Behavioral management of exercise: contracting for aerobic points. *J Appl Behav Anal* 12:55–64, 1979.

12
Moral Development in Sport

MAUREEN R. WEISS, Ph.D.
BRENDA JO LIGHT BREDEMEIER, Ph.D.

Traditional quotes associated with sport participation include: "It's not whether you win or lose but how you play the game," "Sport builds character," and "A sound mind in a sound body." Indeed, the world of sport, from youth through professional levels and for both males and females, is an extremely visible and salient institution. It is for this reason that phrases such as those above seem to conflict with daily portrayals of sport by the mass media. For example, most people will never forget the Rosie Ruiz caper at the 1982 Boston Marathon. Rosie, a virtual unknown runner, crossed the finish line far ahead of the next woman runner. It turned out that Rosie hopped on a bus and covered most of the 26-mile distance on wheels. In a story involving youth sports, Gibson (cited in Ref. 77) details in an article titled "Watergate on Wheels" how a young boy, with the help of his engineer father, rigged his makeshift vehicle to gain an unfair advantage in the Soapbox Derby. Finally, in a recent *Sports Illustrated* article [110] titled "The Death of an Athlete", a former high school player is portrayed in his coffin as a result of sudden death following collapse at a football practice. Although the pathologist's report technically attributed his death to cardiac arrhythmia, anabolic steroids were found to be the major cause. It's not whether you win or lose? Sport builds character? Sound mind in a sound body? Such adages are difficult to accept in light of such frequent and tragic stories.

The purpose of this chapter is to critically review the literature focusing on moral development and education in sport and physical activity contexts. Despite the prevalence of popular stories that suggest sport promotes unethical thoughts and behaviors, we strongly believe that the sporting world is a significant arena for studying moral development. Our perspective as researchers in this area views the possibilities for moral growth through sport as optimistic. This stance is based on the premise that moral development theory, research, and education are viable and necessary areas of study and application for sport scientists and practitioners alike. When structured purposefully and guided by sound educational principles, sport *can* build character and develop a sound mind in a sound body.

There are several reasons, we feel, for the current dearth of moral development literature in the sport domain, especially in comparison to

331

other research areas within sport psychology. First, the development of theoretical models of morality has been relatively recent, especially structural-developmental or contructivist approaches. Closely linked with this reason is the commonly held belief that morality is a personal or philosophic concern and not one appropriate for scientific investigation [103].

A second reason for the lack of sport morality literature is that some individuals question whether, in fact, research on morality can be useful. Can findings from empirical studies actually be applied in the real world of physical education classes or organized competitive sport? For example, such practical concerns as special teacher training, realistic time periods for implementation of intervention strategies, and effective approaches with large numbers of students readily surface. Perhaps the most important question is: "Can moral development curricula within sport actually make a difference?"

A third reason for little research on moral development is the question of whether it is appropriate for teachers and coaches to employ strategies to enhance participants' moral growth. Many feel that the job of nurturing moral growth should be left to parents, academic classrooms, and religious institutions. However, in response to this argument, one might question whether the "parameters of morality" are even recognized by practitioners in sport. For example, the first author was asked to address several hundred physical educators at a state convention on strategies for enhancing social development through physical education. The state curriculum guide was consulted for background, terminology, and objectives. These were the stated social development objectives: respect for self and others, sense of fair play, appreciation of individual differences, cooperation, controlling aggression, and resolving conflicts. What the curriculum specialists were labeling social development we would label moral development! Thus, the topic of moral development may be "hidden" as social development objectives within physical education curriculum guides across America. Intimately related to the problem of morality parameters is that the empirical literature primarily has focused on theoretical issues and descriptive data, and less on practical applications. Thus, sport practitioners are less likely to recognize the value or potential for applying moral development content into their curricula.

Finally, because there is relatively little research on moral development in sport and it has been received with some ambivalence, students have not been exposed to this research to the extent that they have to other social science topics. For example, topics such as exercise adherence, competitive anxiety, and mental imagery are currently "hot" topics in the sport psychology literature. Thus, journal articles, text chapters, and review papers abound with these content areas. In contrast, moral development in sport is infrequently included as a chapter in sport psychology and sport sociology textbooks. Thus, the neglect of sport morality is perpetuated as many students are not aware of the issues that exist and the research that needs to be completed.

In conclusion, we have suggested that research and application issues in the area of moral development in sport are recognized by few. From an empirical perspective, the potential for learning more about moral development in the microworld of sport resides in relatively few journal articles and physical education-related texts. From an applied perspective, few practitioners have taken the opportunity to translate to practice current understandings in an attempt to promote moral growth in their athletic classrooms. Thus, it is our intent to bridge the research and application gap in moral development by framing the historical underpinnings of moral development with the most current research in moral growth through sport and to provide recommendations for translating these findings to practice.

To accomplish these goals, the remainder of the chapter is divided into five sections. First, a historical overview of the important place that moral development has held in sport will be described. Additionally, a historical account of the scientific literature in moral development will be characterized. Second, the theoretical models that have been used to understand moral development will be reviewed. Third, concepts linked to the moral thought-moral action relationship are grounded within a four-component interactive model of moral functioning proposed by Rest [94]. Using this model as a conceptual framework, two subtopics will be discussed: research related to moral reasoning and athletic aggression, and factors influencing the thought-action relationship. The factors to be included in this subsection are gender, cognitive-developmental differences, and significant others. The final two sections will explore the potential for moral education within physical education and sport-related contexts, and directions for future research.

MORAL DEVELOPMENT: ITS PLACE IN THE HISTORY OF SPORT

The notion that sport participation and moral development are intimately related has been around for a very long time. References date as far back as the mid-19th century. For example, in an article in *The American Annals of Education and Instruction* in 1833, a teacher stated that the character of one's students could best be studied on the playground, and that in this context a teacher may be able to "mold" their characters most effectively (cited in Ref. 95, p. 1).

Arnold [1] suggests that the assumed positive relationship between participation in sport and the development of moral values emanated from the English public schools in the 19th century. One hypothesis for the sport-moral values connection rests in sport's educational usefulness in developing such desirable moral virtues as honesty, generosity, and courage. A second hypothesis is based on the premise that moral training on the playing fields generalizes to life skills. This is especially exemplified in the well-known adage: "The battle of Waterloo was won on the playing fields of Eton."

In a comprehensive review of the history of children's sport in America, Wiggins [116] also acknowledges the 19th century as a time period when references to the character-building function of sport emerged. Specifically, Wiggins attributes this connection to the muscular Christianity movement by the YMCA and the influential leadership of Luther Gulick in promoting the contribution of sport to the harmonious development of mind, body, and spirit. Indeed, these ideals still exist in the philosophy of YMCA and YWCA organizations worldwide. Wiggins also acknowledges Clark Hetherington and his Demonstration Play School at Berkeley as contributing to opportunities for children to develop physically, socially, *and* morally. His school consisted of a wide variety of activities ranging from vocal and social to dance and team activities, and established itself as a model school for others emerging across the country.

Despite these early held beliefs about the connection between sport participation and moral development, the rise of highly competitive sport for children around the turn of the century called into question the character-building function of sport [116]. Organized competitive school programs for children and adolescents continued to escalate until the 1930s when professional educators voiced opposition to the practice of interschool competition for elementary-age children. In 1938, the Association for Health, Physical Education, and Recreation passed a resolution to condemn interscholastic sport for elementary school children. In spite of these efforts to curtail the competitive opportunities for young children, numerous nonschool competitive sport organizations were established between 1939 and the late 1960s. McCloy [80], in the inaugural issue of *Research Quarterly*, stated: ". . . it is no wonder that character results have failed to come through physical education when methods used were not specifically planned to secure changes in character, or were not in harmony with sound educational techniques. We have in far too many cases trusted rather blindly to an all-wise Providence" (p. 41). This sentiment seems to accurately reflect that of many individuals today.

It has only been over the last decade that empirical research studies of moral development in sport have emerged. This research is also associated with an increase in curiosity about the role that sport participation can play in social and moral development. Along with the ever-present negative media through popular journals and newspapers, contributors to this increased interest include the refinement and reformulation of moral development theories such as those of Piaget, Kohlberg, Gilligan, and Haan; and, the emergence of social psychology as a subdiscipline within the sport and exercise sciences [95]. The consequences of this increased interest in moral development have been the establishment of various "sportspersonship codes" and ethics programs such as The Bill of Rights for Young Athletes [79], The Code of Ethics for Youth Sport Coaches [99], and the "On Target" program of the National Federation of State High School Associations designed to facilitate drug education for adolescents.

Perhaps one of the most significant events to occur among physical education researchers and educators was the position statement drafted in 1983 by the American Academy of Physical Education. The statement was an intent to target moral education in sport as an explicit goal of the profession, especially amid the controversies about the character-building role of sport. Specifically, it was stated: "Because of the opportunities to teach ethical values and to influence moral behavior of students through sports and games, it is thought that physical educators might well place an increased emphasis on the problems of ethical judgements and morally responsible behavior in sports" (see Ref. 89, p. 53). In addition to charging physical education teachers and athletic coaches with emphasizing moral and ethical values among their stated curricula, the Academy also recommended that criteria be established for the selection of appropriate ethical and moral values, developing formal plans of instruction, and developing methods for the assessment of results.

Given the charge to place moral education closer to center stage in physical education curricula, it is necessary to integrate a variety of resources for the purpose of designing programs to promote moral growth. These resources must include theoretical principles, research findings, and intuitive and experiential knowledges of practitioners. During the 20th century and especially over the last decade, a number of theories and research studies have emerged in order to understand the relationship between participation in sport and moral development.

Today, researchers are exploring how different approaches to fostering moral growth yield effects on moral thought and action. Moral development research is gaining momentum, partly because of more refined theoretical insights and careful empirical work based on operationalized terms. In the next section, we will briefly overview several theoretical perspectives that can be seen as exemplifying one of the two major approaches introduced in this section: internalization and constructivist.

THEORETICAL MODELS OF MORAL DEVELOPMENT

The internalization and constructivist theoretical approaches depict the two major research traditions in moral development and education.

These complementary frameworks have contributed valuable insights into the psychological nature of morality. Each of these approaches offers a unique and comprehensive picture of the processes by which individuals develop into mature moral beings.

Internalization Approaches

Proponents of the internalization approach view moral development as the learning of socially accepted values and behaviors. Learning is posited to occur through transmitted social norms that govern how a moral course of action is to be defined. Thus, an individual's moral growth is seen as a process of enculturation or socialization by significant others and institutions. Both psychoanalytic and social learning theories of moral development may be categorized as internalization approaches.

The earliest theoretical perspective offering a comprehensive understanding of moral development was Freud's [38] psychoanalytic theory. Freud posited that internal dynamic processes tied to the id, ego, and superego functioned as moral prohibitions of an individual's aggressive and sexual instincts. He believed that the superego, informed through internalized parental and societal values, served to control primitive, hedonistic impulses by censoring pleasure-seeking instincts (the id) and personal thoughts and decisions (the ego). The regulation of internalized standards, Freud argued, occurred through the process of guilt, defined as self-targeted aggressive instinctual energies.

Freud hypothesized that the critical event in children's moral development is the resolution of the oedipal complex. This process is associated with the child's identification with the same-sex parent, leading to the internalization of the parent's superego prohibitions and ideals as the child's own. Through the process of identification, conformity is promoted to familial and societal role expectations.

More recently, social learning theorists have offered an alternative interpretation of the internalization approach to moral development. Similar to psychoanalytic theorists, morality is viewed as equivalent to social norms and expectations. Specifically, moral values are seen as deriving through identification with a socializing agent, and moral development is seen as the process by which an individual comes to adopt social regulations. The theorists diverge, however, in their view of the processes by which the internalization of social norms occurs. While psychoanalytic theorists highlight the internal processes tied to the id, ego, and superego, proponents of social learning theory point to the role of significant others in transmitting social norms through operant conditioning [2], modeling [3–5, 74], and reinforcement [73, 82]. The reader is directed to Burton [28] and Marantz [76] for comprehensive reviews of learning-behavioral approaches to moral development.

Individuals who advocate either of the internalization approaches are strong proponents of "character development" programs to facilitate moral growth. The term "character," which originally referred to personality structure [39], has come to represent culturally valued attributes deemed morally appropriate by society [91]. For example, teachers using a character development approach explain in no uncertain terms the difference between right and wrong, preaching such virtues as social responsibility, reciprocity, honesty, the letter of the law, and competitiveness. The objective is for teachers to explicitly define values for children, and to consistently model and reinforce desired behaviors associated with those values.

Individuals who identify character development as an explicit outcome of physical education and sport experiences assume that it occurs "naturally" or automatically among participants. Others are convinced of the premise stated by Tutko and Ogilvie [112] in their well-known article: "Sport: If you want to build character, try something else." Social learning researchers, intrigued by the possibility that sport-related contexts are mediums through which character development can be influenced, have focused on prosocial behavior or value orientation studies. Prosocial behaviors are defined as those enacted solely to positively influence others, with no anticipated benefits for oneself [76]. For example, altruism, sharing, and cooperation are examples of prosocial behaviors employed in sport-related morality studies [41, 65, 88]. Value orientations, conversely, generally refer to understanding character development through the professionalization of values [113] and power value orientations [13].

Constructivist Approaches

The constructivist approach to moral development focuses on how people think about values and behavior; in short, how they construct their own moral understandings. In contrast to internalization theorists, constructivists do not equate morality with societal norms. Rather than viewing moral development as a process of internalizing values transmitted by significant others, they believe that individuals create personal moral conceptions about their social world through interactions with others.

The major proponents of a constructivist approach to moral development are structural developmental theorists. Their perspective can be better understood by analyzing the two components of the term "structural development." First, these theorists believe that underlying the specific content of a person's moral judgments and actions exists a moral reasoning structure. Second, this moral reasoning structure undergoes a regular sequence of transformations as a result of a combination of maturation and environmental experiences. Thus, moral growth consists not only of a quantitative increase in moral content or knowledge, but more importantly a qualitative transformation in how the moral content is organized or structured. There have been several structural developmental "pioneers" of moral development: those most influential include Piaget, Kohlberg, Gilligan, and Haan.

JEAN PIAGET. The structural developmental understanding of morality originated with Piaget's observation of Swiss children's play in the microcosm of the common Geneva street game of marbles. His pioneering efforts to delineate stages of moral reasoning in children yielded a two-stage model of moral development [92]. This model moved from an attitude of unilateral respect for adult authority (called the heteronomous stage) to relationships of mutual respect among peers (called the autonomous stage). At the heteronomous stage, children not only were constrained by nonmutual respect for adult authority but expressed rigid beliefs that game rules are unalterable and must be followed. At the autonomous stage, an orientation toward mutual respect and cooperation with peers superseded conformity to adult authority. In addition, rules were viewed as flexible products of mutual agreement, serving to facilitate cooperative interaction in play.

LAWRENCE KOHLBERG. Of all the morality theorists, Kohlberg has had the greatest influence on the study of moral development. He expanded the scope of Piaget's inquiry and thoroughly revised his model [67–70]. He hypothesized a six-stage sequence of moral development, seen as invariant and culturally universal. The first two stages characterize an egocentric approach to moral problems. Kohlberg termed this the "preconventional" level because the individual does not yet comprehend the way social norms and rules impact on moral responsibility. The next two stages comprised the "conventional" level, during which time an individual approaches problems through the eyes of one's social group or society as a whole. Finally, at the "postconventional" level, an individual recognizes universal values that are not tied to particular societal norms. Table 12.1 depicts sport examples for each of Kohlberg's six stages.

In addition to his six-stage sequence, two principles characterize Kohlberg's approach to understanding moral development. First, moral growth was believed to occur as a result of "cognitive disequilibrium." The increase in an individual's ability to take the role of others results in one's own reasoning becoming inadequate. Consequently, new principles are slowly formulated to guide moral reasoning at the next stage. Second, "justice" is identified by Kohlberg as the single moral norm from which all others are derived. Each subsequent stage represents a more adequate understanding of the way in which justice can resolve moral conflicts. Thus, Kohlberg's theory of moral judgment represents an abstract, deductive, and logically consistent way of structuring moral values.

When Kohlberg died in 1987, the fields of moral psychology and education lost the person who has contributed more to these areas than anyone else in this century. Beyond the legacy of his own significant

TABLE 12.1
Kohlberg's Moral Stages with Sports Illustrations

Stage 1:	*The punishment-and-obedience orientation.* The physical consequences of action determine its goodness or badness, regardless of the human meaning or value of these consequences.
Illustration:	When asked about whether or not a pitcher should use an illegal pitch, one player reasons, "No, it's wrong; it can get the pitcher expelled from the game."
Stage 2:	*The instrumental-relativist orientation.* Right action consists of that which instrumentally satisfies one's own needs and occasionally the needs of others.
Illustration:	Two runners make a deal to each false-start twice in an attempt to tire out a third competitor.
Stage 3:	*The interpersonal concordance or "good boy-nice girl" orientation.* Good behavior is that which pleases or helps others and is approved by them.
Illustration:	In the third quarter, when his team is far ahead, a football coach removes his best players because that is appropriate sportsperson-like behavior.
Stage 4:	*The "law-and-order" orientation.* Right behavior consists of doing one's duty, showing respect for fixed rules and authority, and maintaining the given social order for its own sake.
Illustration:	Even though he is sure he could get away with it, a boxer refuses to throw any "kidney punches," because one ought to fight by the rules.
Stage 5:	*The social-contact, legalistic orientation.* Right action, aside from what is constitutionally and democratically agreed upon, is a matter of personal "values" and "opinions."
Illustration:	When it becomes apparent that certain "legal" drugs are being used to improve athletic performance even though the long-range effects of the drugs are unknown, a group of athletes join to seek a change in the rules so that their use will be forbidden. The athletes reason that drug use violates the spirit of the game and is not in keeping with their rights as individuals.
Stage 6:	*The universal-ethical-principle orientation.* Right is defined by the decision of conscience in accord with self-chosen ethical principles appealing to logical comprehensiveness, universality, and consistency.
Illustration:	In a very close gymnastics meet, the leading gymnast on the losing team decides he is going to attempt a routine he has been working on but has not yet done without safety apparatus. When the judge learns of the gymnast's intention, he refuses to allow the performance, reasoning that all persons have an unforfeitable right to life and safety and that forfeiting basic human rights cannot be justified by an appeal to lesser goods associated with athletic victory.

Moral level and stage typing is a difficult and involved process. Whereas these illustrations are typical of the level indicated, no claim is made that the information provided is adequate for definitive moral scoring.

work, one testament to Kohlberg's intellectual interests and capabilities is reflected in the wide range of ongoing contributions by those he mentored and/or those who have engaged in related research to his conception of the processes of morality. (See the *Journal of Moral Education*, Vol. 17, No. 3, October 1988 and *Counseling and Values*, Vol. 32, 1988 for journal issues that honor Kohlberg and feature (*a*) references to much of the work he had a central hand in authoring but which has appeared after his death, and (*b*) contributions illustrating some of the current directions in morality research that have resulted from contact with Kohlberg and his ideas.)

CAROL GILLIGAN. One researcher who has added a significant dimension to the constructivist contributions of Kohlberg is Carol Gilligan [42–22, 84]. She developed an alternative to Kohlberg's model that highlighted a feminine expression to the construction and resolution of moral problems. Her framework evolved from her study of women contemplating the real life moral decision of whether to have an abortion. An analysis of the women's interview responses delineated a developmental sequence that paralleled Kohlberg's three levels of morality, from an egocentric to societal to principled orientation.

In contrast to Kohlberg's principle of justice, however, Gilligan discovered that these women employed principles of responsibility and care to guide their postconventional reasoning. She contends that these principles are as flexible and differentiated as Kohlberg's justice principle. Optimal growth-producing experiences, according to Gilligan's model, demand coordination of autonomy and interdependence, and the need to care for both self and other. Table 12.2 depicts sport examples for Gilligan's moral development model.

Support for Gilligan's model has recently been attained in a study with men [44]. She found that men who value intimacy and relationships also give primacy to these moral principles, supporting her claim that "two moralities" exist. Kohlberg and his colleagues [54, 71, 87], however, argue that Gilligan's findings are not reflective of two different kinds of morality, but rather of two distinguishable but related kinds of moral judgments. These two kinds of moral judgments are revealed when one reasons about personally experienced moral dilemmas. One is called "deontic judgments," which are abstract judgments of "rightness" derived from rules or principles, and the other is called "judgments of responsibility," which affirm the will to act in terms of that judgment. Blasi [12] contends that moral reasoning about personally experienced situations goes through two phases reflected in these two types of moral judgments and addresses the question, "To what extent is that which I have judged to be morally right also good for myself?" Thus, according to these scholars, the relationship between judgment and action is supported by the tendency toward self-consistency, a proposition elaborated on more fully in a later section.

NORMA HAAN. Whereas Kohlberg's theory has dominated the study of moral development for the last two decades, and Gilligan's work has revealed new insights into moral experience, Norma Haan's interactional model has been the dominant one for exploring moral development in sport. According to Haan, morality is interpersonally constructed during the processes of social living [46, 48, 49]. Her model evolved from an investigation of people's interactive behavior in everyday life situations and simulation game contexts.

TABLE 12.2
Gilligan's Moral Levels with Sports Illustrations

Level 1:	*Self-orientation.* At the first level, the individual's moral concern is focused primarily on the needs and desires of the self. Survival and self-protection are dominant themes.
Illustration:	A basketball coach tells a recruiter from a competing institution that she is not interested in a particular athlete when in reality she has been recruiting her heavily. The coach feels justified in the deception because her job security depends upon coaching success.
Transition:	*From selfishness to responsibility.* During the transition from the first to second level, selfishness versus responsibility becomes a focal problem. The issue is one of attachment or connection to others. The person's understanding of self-interest broadens in a way that allows for an integration of responsibility and care.
Illustration:	In a one-sided basketball contest, the high-scoring center begins to pass frequently to her less-experienced forward to give her an opportunity to gain experience and recognition. She does this because she feels she's been selfish in shooting so frequently.
Level 2:	*Goodness as self-sacrifice.* Whereas at the first level morality is seen as a matter of sanction imposed by a society in which one is more subject than citizen, at the second level moral judgment comes to rely on shared norms and expectations. Here the conventional feminine voice emerges with great clarity, defining the self and proclaiming one's worth on the basis of the ability to care for and protect others. The strength of this position lies in its capability for caring; its limitation is the restriction it imposes on direct expression.
Illustration:	In a close softball game an injured player risks more serious injury by returning to the game when the coach asks her to go to bat. The player does not want to let down the other players or the coach.
Transition:	*From goodness to truth.* The second transition begins with the reconsideration of the relationship between self and other, as the woman starts to scrutinize the logic of self-sacrifice in the service of a morality of care. The issue of selfishness reappears; the person wonders whether responsibility should include care of the self. To make the transition to the postconventional level, the individual must carefully distinguish between personal needs and views from those of others. The criterion for judgment thus shifts from "goodness" to "truth" as the morality of action comes to be assessed not on the basis of its appearance in the eyes of others, but in terms of the realities of its intention and consequence.
Illustration:	A scholarship athlete decides to stop participating in extra practices for gymnastic competition even though it has been paying off in improved performance. She has decided that her participation in gymnastics has largely been to win approval from others and she would prefer to use the time to improve her grades.
Level 3:	*The morality of nonviolence.* By elevating nonviolence—the injunction against hurting—to a principle governing all moral judgment and action, one is able to assert a moral equality between self and others. Care then becomes a universal obligation and the basis for a positive assertion of responsibility.
Illustration:	A swimmer in a water polo match refuses orders to deliberately aim her goal shot at the goalie's head. She reasons that all people are entitled to a life free from deliberate harm and that she is entitled to play free from the fear of possible retaliation.

Moral level and stage typing is a difficult and involved process. While these illustrations are typical of the level indicated, no claim is made that the information provided is adequate for definitive moral scoring.

Three major concepts provide the scaffolding for Haan's model of moral development: moral balance, moral dialogue, and moral levels. Moral balance refers to a situation in which all individuals are in basic agreement about respective rights and obligations. For example, a player and coach are in moral balance if they have a shared understanding about such issues as the amount of practice required, the type and quality of the coach's input, and the seasonal goals. When moral balance exists, the interpersonal exchanges function smoothly and require little or no reflection on the part of the participants. When two or more people disagree about mutual rights and obligations, they are said to be in a moral imbalance. Because interpersonal exchanges are characterized by changing expectations, selective perceptions, and affective and behavioral changes, moral imbalances occur frequently. A player and coach may enter moral imbalance, for example, when the coach demands extra effort from the player, but the player's own expectations do not show a parallel shift. Moral life can be described as a continuous process or fluctuation of moral balances and imbalances.

Moral dialogue, according to Haan, refers to the collective strategies for reestablishing moral balance when imbalances occur. The most obvious way to reestablish moral balance is through an open, verbal negotiation. An example of moral dialogue would be the effort by a professional athlete's representative to negotiate a contract with an athletic team. Moral dialogue, however, can take many other forms in addition to explicit verbal negotiation. For example, if a soccer player is fouled in violation of both game rules and informal player norms, then the two players involved are in moral imbalance. Under such circumstances, moral dialogue may take the form of the offended player retaliating during a later play to communicate, "I didn't like what you did to me and don't do it again." The result may be a restored moral balance. If the communication is unsuccessful at restoring balance, however, further "dialogue" may continue until balance is achieved or until the relationship (or game) ends. In sum, moral dialogue is any communication—direct or indirect, verbal or nonverbal—intended to convey information about one's needs or desires in an effort to maintain or restore moral balance.

Five moral levels define the development of moral maturity in Haan's theoretical model. Each level reflects a different understanding of the appropriate structuring of the moral balance. The first two levels comprise what is called the "assimilation phase," during which time the person seeks to establish moral balances that give preference to one's own needs and concerns. This is not because the person is "selfish," but because the person is unable to comprehend with equal clarity the needs and desires of others. This situation is reversed during the "accommodation phase." People reflecting levels 3 and 4 generally seek to give to the moral exchange more than they receive. Finally, at the "equilibration

TABLE 12.3
Haan's Moral Levels with Sports Illustrations

Level 1:	At this level there is no real view of moral interchange between people. The moral balance is seen as an exchange of power: the person of greater power thwarts the person of lesser power. All are entitled to what they can get.
Illustration:	An athlete is ordered to the showers by an angry umpire.
Level 2:	Balances at this level are established by the self-making trade-offs to get what is desired. It is assumed that the self and others want similar things and that others, like the self, are after their own benefit.
Illustration:	A football lineman intentionally injures another player because "that's just the way the game is played."
Level 3:	The person now thinks of herself or himself as part of a human collectivity. This appreciation for social existence leads to the assumption that everyone recognizes the need for good faith and moral responsibility. The person naively assumes others will behave morally and so tries to create moral balances that consist of harmonious exchanges of good.
Illustration:	A shot-putter fails to call the official's attention to a shot that has not been weighed-in because she assumes that no one would try to cheat.
Level 4:	The naive assumptions of Level 3 inevitably result in disappointment and harm to the self. The person reasoning at Level 4 structures the moral balance through attempts to regulate it with external impartial formulations that assign everyone the same rights or duties. It is thought that the "common interest" of all is best secured by submitting to external regulation, or systematized structured exchange.
Illustration:	A new curfew rule is strictly enforced—no exceptions—because it is in the best interest of the whole team that everyone get a good night's sleep.
Level 5:	At the final level, the individuality of persons and the complexity of social life are given full consideration. The external regulation of the "common interest" is abandoned in favor of situationally specific balances that optimize the potential of all parties in a manner consistent with the particular context. All interests are taken into account and coordinated in a way that is mindful of the participants' future lives together.
Illustration:	A coach plans a heavy and strenuous workout for her team in preparation for an important game, but after a team discussion, excuses one of her star players from part of the practice because the player needs to study for a final exam.

More level and stage typing is a difficult and involved process. While these illustrations are typical of the level indicated, no claim is made that the information provided is adequate for definitive moral scoring.

phase," the level 5 person gives equal recognition to all parties' interests. Table 12.3 depicts sport examples for Haan's model of moral development.

Haan places her moral theory within a broader model of psychological functioning in order to explain the discrepancy that often occurs between thought and action [46, 47, 49]. This model features both moral structures and ego processes. In Haan's view, ego processes perform two critical psychological tasks: they coordinate the contributions of various psychological structures (e.g., cognitive and moral structures), and they coordinate internal functioning with environmental experience. Ego processes influence a person's interpretation of the morally relevant elements of a situation and they coordinate the weighing, organizing, deciding, and acting on moral information.

Haan's ego processing model synthesizes Freud's discovery of the pervasiveness of self-deception through ego defense mechanisms with Piaget's observation that normal functioning people accurately perceive environmental and intrapsychic events. Freud postulated that people use defensive mechanisms, such as repression and projection, to reduce anxiety. Haan reasoned that if defense mechanisms are processes that lead to reality distortion, then there must be corresponding "coping" mechanisms that lead to accurately perceiving reality. She has identified 10 pairs of coping and defending ego processes. Coping processes reflect accurate and faithful interchange among intrapsychic structures, and between intrapsychic structures and the environment. Conversely, defending processes reflect a breakdown in accuracy. A person must remain coping in her or his ego processing in order for action to reflect the most mature reasoning capabilities. Sometimes, however, accuracy is abandoned for the sake of maintaining a coherent and positive sense of self. For example, coping may give way to defending, particularly under stress, and the quality of moral action may deteriorate.

MORAL DEVELOPMENT RESEARCH IN PHYSICAL EDUCATION AND SPORT

Research pertaining to moral development in sport can be categorized into two major approaches. *Internalization* or "bag of virtues" approaches view moral development as the learning of socially acceptable behavior through transmitted values. They claim that morality can be defined by a list of character traits or virtues that reflect prominent cultural values. For example, virtues such as honesty, sharing, cooperation, and peer encouragement are all potential candidates in a study taking an internalization approach. Studies grounded in social learning theory [3, 4], for exampie, which emphasize the *content* of moral knowledge and behavior characterize an internalization approach to moral development. In contrast, *constructivist* approaches advocate that moral growth occurs as a result of the interaction between developmental capabilities and characteristics of the observer and the environmental experiences that provide information about social reality. These approaches employ research designs that consider the *structure* of moral knowledge and reasoning. These studies have tested hypotheses based on theories by Piaget [92], Kohlberg [67–70], Gilligan [42–45], and Haan [46–49].

Internalization Research

Internalization studies fall into three classifications: personality characteristics, value orientations, and prosocial behaviors. An early study by

Blanchard [10] is illustrative of personality trait research. She examined the effects of physical education programs on the cooperation, self-control, and sociability characteristics of children over a 2-year period. Results revealed significant increases in these character traits from pre- to posttesting, with positive changes especially indicative of girls. Although Blanchard concludes that physical education activities contributed to positive character development, the lack of a control group and lack of a theoretical basis for choosing the outcome variables severely limit the generalizations of this study. For example, the pronounced effects found for girls could easily be a function of the selection of expressive character traits.

The second classification of internalization studies is identified by a focus on value orientations of sport participants. According to Webb [113], attitudes toward sport tend to evolve from a play orientation to a professional orientation. The play orientation consists of a value hierarchy of fairness, skill, and success in that order; these priorities are reversed in a professional orientation. As children get older and acquire more experience within organized competitive sport, they tend to move from a play to a professional orientation [9, 113]. In addition, males have been found to score higher on a professionalization orientation than females [97].

A recent study by Dubois [36] investigated sport-related value orientations in children 8- to 10-years-old, playing in either an instructional or competitive soccer league. Subjects responded to a 13-item fixed alternative response interview schedule prior to and following an 8-week season for 2 successive years. Findings revealed that competitive athletes placed a greater emphasis on winning, competing against others, and social status than did recreational athletes. Emphasis on competing against others, fair play, improving fitness, and improving social status increased from pre- to post-season in competitive athletes, whereas competing against others and being part of a social group increased for recreational athletes.

Duda et al. [37] investigated the relationship between motivational goal orientation (task and ego incentives) and sportspersonship attitudes. Morality was operationalized as responses to a self-report attitude measure depicting cheating (e.g., faking an injury to stop the clock) and sportspersonship (e.g., helping a player up off the floor) behaviors. Results revealed a significant negative relationship between task orientation and cheating, and a positive relationship between task orientation and fair play. Ego orientation showed a positive relationship with self-reported cheating behaviors. The authors conclude that there appears to be a motivational interpretation to the observed differences in disapproval of rule violating behavior and the endorsement of sportspersonlike play.

The value orientation approach provides limited insight to the moral growth-sport participation relationship. Although one's orientation may change from one of fairness to success, or competing against others to sportspersonship (i.e., Dubois), it is not known whether this is a value change per se, changes based on cognitive maturity, or changes based on experiences apart from the sporting environment. The possibility also exists that adoption of a more professional attitude reflects an individual's conformity to the social norms and regulations of competitive sport itself as a result of experience (i.e., Duda et al.). Another important point is that value orientation studies suffer from a superficial conceptualization of morality, and by relying on self-report measures of sportspersonship without contextual or measurement validation [66].

The third classification of internalization studies entails a focus on prosocial behaviors as a result of sport-related experiences. Using this perspective, morality is defined in terms of observable behaviors such as altruism, turn-taking, and cooperation with peers. Studies of prosocial play behavior have been conducted for the purpose of establishing relationships between participation in sport and a particular measure of moral behavior, such as altruism.

Kleiber and Roberts [65] investigated the effect of sport competition on social character, operationally defined in their design as the prosocial behaviors of cooperation and altruism. Children in the 4th and 5th grades were randomly assigned to either an experimental group who competed in a kickball tournament during recess period for 8 days, or to a control group. Analyses of pre- and posttournament prosocial behaviors using a self-report measure revealed that boys in the experimental group reported significantly less altruistic behavior than boys in the control group. The conclusion that competition can cause decrements in prosocial behavior should be viewed with extreme caution. Limitations of this study include failure to validate the self-report measure with observations of actual behavior, a single measure of morality in altruism, the very short intervention period, and the use of a recess kickball tournament as analogous to organized competitive sport.

Orlick [88] also employed a prosocial behavior design to investigate the relationship between physical activity and moral development. Children ($N = 71$), all 5 years of age, were assigned to either an experimental group, which consisted of an 18-week program of cooperative games, or a control group, which consisted of an 18-week program of traditional games. The effects of participating in these physical activity programs on sharing behavior was assessed by asking children to indicate how many pieces of candy they would share with children in another class by placing the number of pieces in a brown paper sack. Conflicting results were found: a cooperative games program in one of the two schools showed a significant increase in willingness to share while the other school showed no change. The traditional games program in one school showed a significant decrease in willingness to share, while no difference from pre- to posttest was found for the other school. These inconsistent results may be attributed to the single measure of morality in willingness to share, or possibly to different instructional styles or curricula for these two types of programs.

Another example of an internalization study that took a prosocial behavior perspective is an investigation by Giebink and McKenzie [41]. These researchers employed a case study design to modify negative social interaction behaviors in four boys during physical education and recreation activities. Intervention strategies included instructions, praise, modeling, and a contingent reward system. Results revealed that the effect of the interventions varied across the four boys, but all strategies increased sportspersonlike and decreased unsportspersonlike behaviors. However, attempts to generalize from the physical education to the recreation setting were unsuccessful. Limitations in research design are also apparent in this study, including the single measure of morality, the small sample size, and the inability to determine which of the intervention techniques contributed to the observed behavior changes.

Constructivist Research

Constructivist studies can be classified according to whether the investigation focused on description and explanation of the relationships among morality and other variables, or on intervention strategies focused on the practical applications of morality research [104]. One of the first descriptive studies testing hypotheses from moral development theory to sport was conducted by Jantz [63]. Specifically, he modified Piaget's marble experiment to test children's knowledge of the rules of basketball. Results revealed that children in grades 1 and 2 interpreted rules using a morality of constraint, while children in grades 3–6 primarily viewed rules using a morality of cooperation. The results of this study supported Piaget's developmental stages.

The overwhelming majority of constructivist morality research has been conducted by Bredemeier and her colleagues. This line of research can be divided into four categories: (*a*) life-sport reasoning differences, (*b*) sport participation and moral reasoning maturity, (*c*) moral reasoning and behavioral tendencies, and (*d*) moral education [24]. Most of these studies will be appropriately discussed in the section on the moral thought-moral action relationship in sport. Thus, only short synopses of some of these studies will be presented here to illustrate the types of research conducted to date from a constructivist approach to morality in sport.

Several investigations have examined the relationship between sport participation or nonparticipation and moral reasoning maturity [18, 21, 50]. Bredemeier and Shields [21], for example, found that college nonathletes recorded significantly higher moral reasoning scores for both life and sport situations than did basketball players. No significant differences in moral reasoning, however, were found for high school age athletes and nonathletes on either life or sport scores.

Bredemeier et al. [25] investigated the relationship between sport involvement and moral reasoning maturity. Sport involvement was operationalized by sport participation (e.g., the number of years of experience in high, medium, and low contact sports) and sport interest (e.g., favorite athlete and most enjoyable sport, both classified as high, medium, or low contact sport). Results revealed that boys' participation and interest in high contact sports and girls' participation in medium contact sports (the highest level that they reported) were related to less mature moral reasoning and greater reported tendencies to aggress.

Bredemeier and colleagues [26] also investigated the relationship between children's judgments regarding the legitimacy of potentially injurious sport acts, their moral reasoning, and aggression tendencies. Results revealed that boys' legitimacy judgments were significantly related to their moral reasoning maturity for sport and tendencies to aggress, but for girls only nonsport reasoning scores were related to their legitimacy judgments. Additionally, children's aggression tendencies were found to be the best predictors of their legitimacy judgments.

Three studies to date have employed intervention strategies in order to observe changes in moral reasoning and/or behaviors [27, 33, 96]. Bredemeier et al. [27] conducted a field experiment to examine the effect of three instructional strategies on children's moral reasoning and distributive justice levels. Children ($N = 81$), ages 5–7 years, in a summer sport program were randomly assigned to either a structural developmental group based on Haan's framework, a social learning group, or a control group. During the 6-week program, groups were provided identical physical education curricula and exposure to the same weekly themes of fair play, sharing, verbal aggression, physical aggression, and righting wrongs. Results revealed that significant pre- to postprogram changes in moral reasoning levels occurred for the structural developmental and social learning groups but not for the control group. Between-group differences, however, only approached significance.

In a follow-up study, Romance et al. [96] employed older children (10–11-year-olds) for a slightly longer intervention period (8 weeks) in a school physical education setting. Only structural developmental and control groups were used in this study. Using a more sophisticated measure of moral reasoning than Bredemeier et al., strong group differences were found. Children in the structural developmental group recorded significantly higher moral reasoning scores for both nonsport and sport hypothetical dilemma stories. The Romance et al. study is particularly noteworthy for two reasons. First, the study was conducted in actual physical education classes as part of the normal school curriculum. Second, the theoretically based design and concomitant teaching strategies, combined with the trained professional who taught the classes, demonstrated that physical education can be an appropriate setting for promoting moral development.

Finally, a recent study by DeBusk and Hellison [33] employed a self-responsibility model based on constructivist principles to effect changes in 10 boys identified as behavior problems. At the end of the 6-week program, results revealed that the teaching strategies based on the model produced affective, behavioral, and knowledge changes in the boys. Additionally, the special program resulted in changes of the teacher's attitudes and values regarding both delinquency-prone youth and the applicability of the self-responsibility model for nondelinquency-prone youth.

In summary, researchers employing a constructivist approach have provided new paradigms for studying morality in sport and physical education settings. First, morality is defined as the underlying moral reasoning, cognitions, and affect associated with behavioral tendencies, and not as an arbitrary virtue or trait. Second, testable hypotheses based on any of the several constructivist theories have been conducted at the description, explanation, and intervention levels. Finally, and most importantly, the line of research on the relationship between moral development and sport participation allows us to move closer to realizing the goals identified by the Academy of Physical Education: selection of appropriate ethical and moral values, formal plans of instruction, and methods for the assessment of results.

Several questions regarding the structure of moral development programs in sport and physical education remain unanswered. Damon [32] poses the questions: "Which values should we teach our children?" and "How should we do it?" In short, he is alluding to whether a "bag of virtues" or a constructivist approach should be embraced, or perhaps a combination of both. The internalization approach puts an emphasis on identifying and reinforcing selected values. Conversely, constructivist approaches put an emphasis on engaging children in activities and discussion that challenge them to think autonomously about resolutions to moral issues. To date, neither approach has proven to be singularly successful.

THE MORAL THOUGHT-MORAL ACTION RELATIONSHIP

The relations between moral thought and moral action represent a key issue for social scientists seeking to understand moral development and to promote growth through moral education. In an impressive review of studies relating moral thought to moral action, Blasi [11] presented evidence of both consistency and inconsistency between relatively high levels of moral reasoning and behaviors typically defined as moral (i.e., altruism and honesty). Blasi's comprehensive review suggests a significant judgment-action link, yet it is evident that many factors in addition to moral reasoning must be considered in an analysis of the processes involved in moral action.

It is ironic that this crucial issue has received relatively little theoretical attention until recently. This is an exciting time to be engaged in theoretical and empirical work on moral development because the field is undergoing a dramatic transformation, an evolution that reflects a growing recognition of the role of social interaction as it influences moral cognition and behavior. Traditional theoretical approaches are undergoing significant changes and new perspectives are emerging. In addition to the evolutionary aspects of change in the content area of morality, growth is also evident in the size and scope of the literature focusing on moral issues. A number of books have been published recently in an effort to detail the innovative contributions of prominent scholars and researchers and to highlight the emerging issues that define current literature. Two volumes that offer substantive contributions in this regard are edited by Kurtinez and Gerwitz (*Morality, Moral Behavior, and Moral Development* was published in 1984 and *Moral Development Through Social Interaction* was published in 1987).

These books and other recently published volumes emphasize the richness and diversity of newly emerging perspectives. Yet they also underscore how independently formulated models of moral development are strikingly compatible. Collectively these models offer significant insights into the thought-action relationship and illuminate promising research themes for investigating interdependent factors that mediate that relationship. We have selected one of these models to provide a framework for our discussion of the moral cognition-moral behavior relationship in the context of sport. The model is an inclusive conceptualization of moral functioning derived by James Rest [94], a professor at the University of Minnesota, who has been a prolific researcher in the area of moral assessment.

Rest [94] has proposed a four-component interactive model of moral functioning by which existing moral research can be organized. While not a linear decision-making model, the four components are presented according to a logical sequentiality. The first component, interpreting the situation and identifying a moral problem, involves imagining possible courses of action in a situation and considering how the consequences of those actions will impact on all parties who are in the situation. This component may involve such issues as one's interpretation of sport actions as moral or nonmoral, one's sensitivity to and ability to make inferences about the interests and needs of self, teammates, or opponents, and the role of one's primary affective responses (e.g., anger) in mediating empathic responses to others.

The second component involves formulating a plan of action that applies the most relevant moral standard or ideal—making a judgment about what *ought* to be done in a particular situation. Internalization theorists focusing on morality in the sport context would postulate that social norms, such as following "the rules of the game" or playing at "the level of the ref," govern how a moral course of action is to be defined. Constructivists would focus on athletes' progressive understanding of the "purpose, function and nature of social arrangements" (see Ref. 94, p. 31) encountered in sport.

The third component, deciding what one *actually intends* to do by selecting among competing values, involves value integration and moral motivation. In sport, it is not unusual for an athlete to choose a course of action that preempts or compromises the moral ideal. As an example, a runner who takes steroids may acknowledge that, in an ideal world, performance-enhancing drugs should not be taken, but the runner may choose to use and/or abuse drugs in order to "even the competitive field" or to win a gold medal for his or her country.

The last component, executing and implementing the moral plan of action, involves ego strength and self-regulation skills. Athletes are challenged to demonstrate ego strength and self-regulation skills—and in Haan's [46] terms, to cope rather than defend—when they attempt to overcome fatigue or frustration, when they strive to resist distractions and delay gratification, and when they struggle to be "good sports." Rest contends that the production of moral behavior requires these four interacting component processes and that deficiencies in any component can result in a failure to act morally. See Table 12.4 for Rest's elaboration of the component processes that influence moral behavior.

Rest's model of factors influencing the moral thought-moral action relationship offers a promising approach to organizing the research on moral development in sport. The number of situational permutations that influence moral behavior in sport makes a general analysis of the thought-action relationship confusing, and the paucity of empirical literature makes such a goal impossible. Thus, we will confine our review to the only example of thought-action research in the context of sport: the line of research conducted by Bredemeier and her colleagues which explores the moral reasoning-athletic aggression relation. This research will be discussed in light of Rest's four components. Following this analysis, we will discuss how selected factors may mediate moral functioning, by reviewing pertinent literature on the possible influence of such factors on one or more of Rest's component processes. The mediating factors to be reviewed include gender, cognitive developmental differences, and significant others.

Moral Reasoning and Athletic Aggression

Research by Bredemeier and her colleagues has focused primarily on athletic aggression. One cluster of studies focused on the major function of Rest's Component 2, moral reasoning, and its relations with aggressive behavior tendencies. Preliminary evidence that moral reasoning ma-

TABLE 12.4
Component Processes of the Moral Thought-Moral Action Relationship [94]

Component 1: Interpretation of the situation

Major function of the process:	To interpret the situation in terms of how one's actions affect the welfare of others.
Factors that influence the process:	Ambiguity of people's needs, intentions and actions; familiarity with the situation and the people in it; time allowed for interpretation; sheer number of elements in the situation and the embeddedness of crucial cues; degree of personal danger and susceptibility to pressure; complexity in tracing out cause-effect chains.

Component 2: Formulating a plan of action

Major function of the process:	To formulate a moral course of action; to identify the moral ideal in a specific situation.
Factors that influence the process:	Factors affecting the application of social norms or moral ideals; delegation of responsibility to others; prior conditions or expectancies that affect role responsibilities and reciprocity; the combination of moral issues involved; prior commitments to some ideology.

Component 3: Deciding what to actually do

Major function of the process:	To select among competing value outcomes of ideals the one to act on; deciding whether or not to try to fulfill one's moral ideal.
Factors that influence the process:	Motivations other than moral ones; mood states that affect decision-making; estimating costs and benefits; estimates of the probability of certain outcomes; factors that affect one's self-esteem.

Component 4: Implementing a moral plan of action

Major function of the process:	To execute and implement what one intends to do.
Factors that influence the process:	Physical barriers to executing the moral plan of action; distractions or fatigue; cognitive transformations of the goal; timing difficulties in managing more than one plan at a time.

turity is related to athletic aggression came from a pilot study [18] employing Rest's Defining Issues Test [93], a measure based on Kohlberg's stage theory. In addition to obtaining athletes' moral reasoning maturity scores, coaches provided ratings and rankings of their players' athletic aggression. The operational definition of aggression used in the study—the initiation of an attack with the intent to injure—was carefully explained to the coaches so they would not confuse assertive or competitive play with aggression. As hypothesized, moral reasoning was found to negatively correlate with coaches' evaluations of aggressiveness. Thus, this study provided some support for the contention that athletic aggression is a moral issue: Athletes with less mature moral reasoning were described by their coaches as more likely to try to hurt people in a sport context, and athletes with more mature moral reasoning were described as exhibiting significantly lower levels of athletic aggression.

The relationship between moral thought and sport action was also investigated with children. Bredemeier [15] administered four hypothetical moral dilemmas, together with pencil-and-paper measures designed to assess children's self-described action tendencies (assertion, aggression, submission) in response to conflict situations encountered both in everyday life [34, 35] and sport. Since assertion is a conflict resolution strategy that reflects a balancing of one's own needs with those of others, and aggression places personal interests above the needs or rights of others, it was hypothesized that assertive behaviors would be associated with more mature moral reasoning and aggressive behaviors with less mature reasoning. This, in fact, turned out to be the case. Children (ages 9–13 years) who were relatively mature in their moral reasoning described themselves as significantly more assertive and less aggressive in response to conflict situations than children who exhibited lower levels of reasoning. These findings may reflect the conceptual congruence between Haan's formulations of moral structures and the definitions of assertion and aggression. Assertion is congruent with the construction of nonegocentric moral balances; aggression, in contrast, is difficult to reconcile with equity.

In another facet of this research project, the relationship of children's sport participation with their reasoning maturity and aggression tendencies was examined [25]. Children responded to a sport involvement questionnaire, as well as the moral dilemmas and behavior tendency measures. Analyses revealed that boys' participation in high contact sports and girls' participation in medium contact sports (the highest level of contact sport experience girls reported) were associated with less mature moral reasoning and greater self-reported tendencies to aggress. A constructivist interpretation of these relationships incorporates the interaction between the environment of contact sports and the meanings constructed by sport participants. Sport structures that allow higher levels of contact encourage rough physical play that can sometimes be interpreted as aggressive. It is not surprising that participation in these sports was associated with children's reports of higher levels of aggressiveness in sport. The fact that participation also was related to self-reported aggression in daily life suggests that these sport experiences may be related to behavioral tendencies that generalize beyond the boundaries of the playing field. Also, these findings point to the importance of identifying those factors within sport structures that are key to the relationships among sport involvement and morality variables. Differentiating sports according to the degree of physical contact allowed by their normative structures, for example, appears to be one helpful means of categorizing types of sport experience.

As Rest's model suggests, the relationship between moral reasoning structures and aggressive behavior is complex and mediated by numerous factors. In Bredemeier's research program, the role of "legitimacy judgments" in mediating this thought-action relationship has been a factor of central focus. Legitimacy judgments, identified as a stated belief about whether an action is justifiable or not, is a factor that may influence moral reasoning and behavior. In one study of moral reasoning maturity and legitimacy judgments, children (ages 9–13 years) were administered moral interviews and shown slides of potentially injurious sport behaviors [26]. The slide series featured athletes performing four legal and five illegal sport acts. All the acts, whether within or outside the rules, were judged by the children to carry a high risk of injury. Results revealed that boys (but not girls) with less mature moral reasoning accepted a greater number of potentially injurious sport acts to be legitimate ($r = -0.43$) than their more mature peers. This moderate correlation suggests that judgments about the legitimacy of potentially injurious sport acts can be considered moral judgments. These results underscore Rest's contention that the component processes in his model are interactive in that moral reasoning maturity (Component 2) can influence one's interpretation of actions within a situation (Component 1).

In a related study, 40 female and male high school and college basketball players were given moral interviews and were twice asked to make judgments about the legitimacy of six increasingly aggressive behaviors [14]. The acts ranged from nonphysical intimidation through attempting to permanently disable an opponent. The two sets of legitimacy judgments were made at different times and under differing conditions. In the midweek interview, athletes offered judgments about what acts they thought would be okay for a fictitious football player. In another interview, immediately following a postseason game, athletes made judgments about what would be appropriate for their own basketball play. The first interview was labeled the "hypothetical" condition, and the second the "engaged" condition. Similar to the studies with children, results indicated an inverse relationship between players' levels of moral reasoning and the number of intentionally injurious sport acts they judged to be legitimate. Those athletes with more mature moral reasoning accepted fewer aggressive acts as legitimate.

A second issue examined in this study was differences in legitimacy judgments as a function of sex, school level, and judgment context. Male athletes were found to accept a greater number of aggressive acts as legitimate than did female athletes, and college athletes a greater number than did high school competitors. Results also indicated that athletes judged significantly more aggressive acts as legitimate in the engaged condition than in the hypothetical condition. One likely interpretation of these results, reflecting both the third and the fourth component of Rest's model, is that the immediate stresses of competitive sport may temporarily erode an athlete's capacity to make clear judgments consistent with that person's most mature reasoning.

The contextual nature of legitimacy judgments about aggressive behavior was elaborated more fully in a qualitative analysis of the moral distinctions employed by athletes to interpret the meaning of their aggression experiences [22, 23]. Most athletes accepted some limited degree of athletic aggression as a legitimate aspect of the egocentricity of sport. However, they interpreted acts involving the intentional infliction of serious injury and injurious acts causing less serious harm but occurring outside the rules as illegitimate.

Moral exchange is an intimate aspect of sport experience, but it may arise from different moral norms than characterize nonsport morality. Empirical study of moral reasoning and athletic aggression suggests that movement into the sport world involves a transformation of moral meaning. In cross-sectional studies involving 4th–7th grade youth sport participants [16] and high school and college athletes [19], it was found that at approximately the 6th or 7th grade, participants' moral reasoning about sport issues begins to diverge significantly from their general reasoning patterns in daily life contexts. For those whose "life" and "sport" reasoning diverged, moral reasoning employed to resolve sport dilemmas was significantly less mature than the reasoning they used in response to daily life dilemmas. Bredemeier and Shields [20, 22, 23, 102, 103] have proposed a theory of "game reasoning" to make sense of the contextualized legitimacy judgments about aggression, and the finding that adolescents' and adults' sport reasoning is significantly lower than their corresponding life reasoning. Still in its early stages of development, the theory holds that the unique context of sport may allow for the temporary suspension of the typical moral obligation to equally consider the interests of all. Within the clear boundaries of sport, egocentric moral engagement may be accepted or even celebrated as an enjoyable and nonserious moral deviation.

Game reasoning may have significant implications for the thought-action relationship, potentially impacting on each of Rest's model components. This moral transformation may influence four issues: (a) one's definition of aggression as a moral or nonmoral issue; (b) the adequacy of one's moral reasoning about athletic aggression; (c) one's interpretation of athletic aggression as a valued or even required social norm within the spatial and temporal boundaries of sport; and (d) one's self-regulation in response to the ambiguous meaning of an opponent's physical contact. The interactive nature of these components increases the complexity of the moral functioning relationships. For example, an athlete may reappraise her or his interpretation of a moral situation in light of the personal cost experienced by a teammate who has been a victim of an opponent's aggressive act (Component 3 influencing Component 1). Moral development, according to Rest, entails gaining proficiency in all of these component processes.

Factors Influencing the Thought-Action Relationship

GENDER. Gilligan [42–45], Noddings [86], and others have suggested that gender influences how we meet each other morally. They have proposed that the feminine approach to relatedness has an intrinsically moral quality, meaning that to be in relationship with another individual or collective creates moral responsibilities, obligations, and aspirations. Building on this contention, Gilligan [42] contrasts two orientations to moral judgment, one an ethic of care and responsibility typically integral to the female gender role, and one an ethic of rights and justice, more closely associated with the male gender role. Lyons [75] has developed a reliable method for classifying care and rights orientations to personally experienced moral dilemmas. She found that females' framing of dilemmas tends to reflect an orientation of care and males' an orientation of rights, but that a majority of females and males employ both orientations.

In the context of sport, moral judgments may be made solely on the basis of a care orientation. An act of moral sacrifice, for example, such as advantaging one's team in a way one perceives to be unfair, may be done out of obligation to a coach or team members. Similarly, an act of social responsibility–like agreeing to be tested for drugs—may be undertaken with the intent to enhance the team's public image in spite of one's belief that the test violates personal rights. Moral judgments also may be made solely on the basis of a rights orientation, as in the case of an athlete who contends that disabling an opponent is acceptable as long as the action is within the "letter of the law." Or an athlete may appeal to the rules of the game or basic human rights to disobey a coach's orders to "take an opponent out of the game." Finally, moral judgments may be influenced by both care and rights orientations. As an example, in a close softball game, an injured player may struggle to decide whether to risk further injury by returning to the game when her coach asks her to go to bat, or to let her coach and teammates down by not going to bat.

Judgment orientations appear to be gender related, although they are certainly not confined to one sex or the other. Because one's judgment orientation may potentially influence the first three components of Rest's model, we would expect that gender may influence one's interpretation of the moral situation, formulation of an ideal course of action, and decision about which action will actually be taken. The empirical literature examining moral development among female and male athletes and nonathletes, although scant, suggests that this expectation may be accurate [14, 18–20, 25, 26]. Unfortunately, none of these studies were designed to ascertain cause-effect relationships so interpretations must be qualified and tentative.

Familiarity with the sport context and with norms for acceptable sport behavior could potentially influence one's interpretation of moral situations within that realm (Rest's Component 1). Investigators report a greater degree of sport involvement and interest for males than females [25, 78]; organized sport is still dominated by male involvement and is often characterized as an activity that socializes boys into men in our culture. Males who are more at home in the sport world than females may be more able to imagine possible courses of action in a particular sport situation and more able to trace out the consequences of that action for all the parties involved. On the other hand, male familiarity with sport norms may have a down side: aggression and other moral defaults may lose their moral valence and come to be seen as part of conventional sport behavior. It may be easier, for example, for females to empathize with coparticipants than to objectify them.

Males also have been found to have greater experience and interest in high contact sports than females [25]. There are several likely reasons for this. For example, higher contact sports are more congruent with the traditional male gender role, and girls are given little opportunity or encouragement to participate in them. Similarly, there are few professional or visible female models in these sports; such sports remain organized and coached almost exclusively by males.

More experience and interest in sport in general, and in high contact sport in particular, are related to findings that males report more expressed aggression in sport and at home and school, and accept more athletic aggression as legitimate [14, 15, 18, 21–23, 25, 26]. These findings suggest that gender may influence Rest's second component, determining what course of action ought to be undertaken. An internalization approach to moral action postulates that social norms govern how a moral course of action is to be defined (i.e., see Ref. 8), while a constructivist approach focuses on the progressive understanding of the purpose, function, and nature of social relationships [49]. The expression and acceptance of aggression is more consistent with the male gender role [62], a fact that may influence male and female interpretations of aggression as a moral issue as well as their consideration of aggression as a legitimate or desirable action within the sport context.

In a related vein, a study referred to earlier suggests that gender may influence the meanings children attach to physical contact experiences within similar sport structures [25]. Analyses revealed that boys' participation in high contact sports and girls' participation in medium contact sports were positively related to less mature moral reasoning and greater reported tendencies to aggress. If the sport structure itself were the only significant factor, we would have expected participation in medium contact sports to be similarly related to aggression tendencies for boys and girls. The finding that participation in medium contact sports was significantly related to girls' but not boys' aggression tendencies leads us to posit that the girls and boys in this sample attached different meanings to actions within similar sport structures. Because medium contact sports were the roughest that girls had experienced, girls may have been more likely than boys to interpret acts within these sports as aggressive.

Familiarity with sport and the acceptance of athletic aggression may also influence Rest's third component, deciding what one actually will do by selecting among competing values. Veteran sport participants are aware of a variety of possible outcomes of different courses of action, each representing different values and activating different motives. The rewards for success in competitive sport create an environment where nonmoral values are so strong and attractive that athletes are frequently tempted to choose a course of action that preempts or compromises their moral ideal. This is particularly true for male athletes who enjoy many more extrinsic rewards than do females. Thus, factors both external to the game context and factors intrinsic to the sport experience may differentially influence female and male estimates of the costs and benefits of ideal moral action and may differentially activate motives other than moral motives.

COGNITIVE-DEVELOPMENTAL DIFFERENCES. Age-related changes in cognitions and social experiences are another factor that may influence the relationship between moral thought and moral action. It would appear that consideration of cognitive-developmental factors falls into Component 1 (interpretation of the situation) and Component 2 (defining a moral course of action) of Rest's interactive model. Changes in general cognitive development and social cognition have a considerable bearing on the patterns of moral reasoning expressed by individuals across the life span.

Researchers who adopt a structural-developmental perspective have investigated the development of judgments in order to chart the course of age-related transformations in the organization of moral thought [30, 67, 68, 92]. According to these researchers, developmental changes in moral reasoning and behaviors occur as a function of maturity in cognitive abilities, the ability to take the perspective of others, and social interaction experiences. Kagan [64] has also recently stated that sensitivity to what is morally right or wrong cannot appear until children are capable of a certain level of maturity in being able to infer the possible causes and affective consequences in others and to anticipate the reactions of adults to their actions.

Piaget's [92] studies were the first to extensively examine the ontogeny of children's moral judgments. His explanation of moral development was tied closely to explanations of nonsocial cognitive development, which was an ongoing goal in his attempts to formulate a theory of mental development. Piaget's conception of morality centered on two qualitatively different forms, one based on constraint (a heteronomous orientation) and one based on cooperation (an autonomous orientation). These two types of morality, Piaget maintained, formed a developmental sequence. The basis for the morality of constraint was a nonmutual, unilateral respect for adults, and emerged during the ages of 3–8 years. The basis for the morality of cooperation, in contrast, was characterized by reason, justice, and cooperation with equals and was thought to occur after 8 years of age.

Kohlberg [67–70] extensively revised Piaget's developmental formulations of moral growth. He studied the ways in which children, adolescents, and young adults made moral decisions by responding to hypothetical stories dealing with moral conflicts. On the basis of the analyses of these responses, Kohlberg formulated his sequence of six stages of moral judgment. Whereas Piaget maintained that there are two kinds of morality, Kohlberg contends that three kinds of morality form a developmental sequence. These are a morality of restraint, a morality of rules, authority, and convention, and a morality of justice and principle. The first kind of morality, the preconventional level, is representative of children 6–11 years of age. This level is associated with the link between morality and sanctions, emanating from the fact that children of these ages do not differentiate morality from punishment or prudence. The second type of morality is the conventional level, representative of individuals 12–17 years of age, and it is characterized by the emergence of a concept of morally good persons and an orientation toward social approval. At this level, according to Kohlberg, there is a failure of adolescents to clearly distinguish between fairness or justice and the demands of the social system. The third kind of morality, the postconventional level, does not emerge until late adolescence or early adulthood. This level is characterized by distinguishing moral judgments from prudence and punishment (level 1) or social order and convention (level 2). Moral rights are defined in terms of rules and laws that are based on consensus and that serve to maximize social welfare.

The ability to take the perspective of others and social interaction skills are highlighted by structural-developmental theorists in attaining mature moral growth [111]. The give-and-take types of social interaction among peers fosters a recognition of the reciprocity of cooperation and facilitates opportunities for role-taking that are critical for moral growth [30, 68, 101]. According to Selman, social perspective-taking abilities can be described through five developmental stages. The first stage is labeled the egocentric stage, in which children have very little understanding of other people's motives, and is reflective of children ages 4–6 years. The next stage is called social-informational (ages 6–8 years) where children have begun to think about the intent of the actions of others. Self-reflective role-taking typifies the third stage (ages 8–10 years) in which children are aware that their own perspective is not necessarily the only valid one. The fourth stage, mutual role-taking (ages 10–12 years), sees the realization that other people are also aware of the self-reflective process. Finally, in the generalized other stage (ages 12 and older) children go beyond individual perspectives and take the perspective of society. Selman [100, 101] has also shown that children's moral judgments are influenced by their ability to take the perspective of others.

Evidence of age-related changes in morality is provided by Damon [30, 31]. Children ages 4–10 years were interviewed with regard to distributive justice. Hypothetical stories dealt with conflicts over how to distribute resources among a group of people. For example, one story provided information about children who made drawings to be sold at a school fair. The way in which the money earned is to be distributed among the children is the focus of investigating developmental differences. Damon identified six stages of distributive justice development based on analyses from his studies. Children ages 4–5 years distribute rewards based on either who wants the money the most or on certain external characteristics, such as who is older or bigger (levels 1 and 2). At about ages 6–7 years, Damon found that children have formed concepts of equality, in which rewards are distributed so that everyone gets the same amount regardless of other characteristics. At the next level, reciprocity enters into the child's decision. The child takes into account compensation for good work and believes that those who work harder should get more money. At the fifth level, a central issue is rewarding *need*, in order to maintain the equality of persons. Thus, the child believes that those who are poorer than others should get the most money. Finally, the most mature level is characterized by a concern for both individuals' actions and needs. In this case, a child distributes money equally between those who drew the most paintings and those who need the money the most. These findings represent evidence for developmental changes in one element of moral judgment. However, more research is needed to examine the potential for developmental change in other aspects of children's moral judgments, as well as in other domains or settings.

Given this general overview of what is known about cognitive-developmental differences that influence moral development, what does the sport-related literature tell us about the topic? Unfortunately, only a few studies have been conducted that allow an analysis of possible age differences in moral thought and action. These studies, however, do lend some insight and support for the important role that cognitive development, perspective taking, and social interaction skills play in the development of morality across the life span.

Jantz [63] was the first to conduct a moral development study in the sport setting based on Piaget's cognitive-developmental theory. Boys spanning the ages of 5–12 years were interviewed about the rules of basketball, similar to the way Piaget interviewed children about the rules in the game of marbles. Responses were classified according to characteristics defining a morality of constraint or a morality of cooperation, and compared among age groups. Results revealed that responses by the

5–7-year-old boys were significantly less mature than those 8–12 years of age, lending support to Piaget's developmental stages.

The field experiment by Bredemeier et al. [27] described earlier investigated the relative effects of social learning, structural developmental, and control group instructional strategies on moral growth over a 6-week summer sport program. Children ranged in age from 5 to 7 years ($M = 6$ years, 7 months); this age group was deliberately selected because it has been identified as a transition period in moral growth from a heteronomous to autonomous orientation in Piaget's scheme of moral development. Specifically, moral issues such as intentionality (objective consequences versus subjective intent) and distributive justice (criteria for the distribution of rewards) were morality variables of interest in this study.

The age-related findings are of special interest in this section. First, over 80% of the children were classified in Piaget's autonomous rather than heteronomous level of morality at the outset of the program based on scores on the intentionality task. This was unexpected, as Piaget suggested that children up to age 8 years are more likely to display a morality of constraint, rather than one of cooperation. Another finding, consistent with Damon's [30, 31] stages of development of distributive justice, was that children as a group scored midway between stage 3 and stage 4 (distribution based on equality and behavioral reciprocity). However, as a result of the intervention program, children in the social learning and structural developmental groups were found to increase an average of approximately one-third of a stage, while the control group stayed the same.

Informal assessments or observations revealed some other interesting age-related findings. Although the motor skills curriculum was designed to incorporate moral dilemmas consonant with the weekly theme, often the children simply failed to recognize situations of inequality. This may have been due to cognitive immaturity with regard to selective attention, role-taking abilities, or attributional style. Moreover, many of the contrived situations were competitive in nature; however, the children rarely responded in a competitive way. For example, in a relay race activity, three groups of children were organized into lines of unequal numbers. They were then instructed to race each other, with the first ones to finish declared the winners. Although the unequal make-up of the group resulted in a predictable order of finish, the children neither verbalized recognition of the unfair conditions nor negative affect in response to losing.

These results are perhaps not surprising given that social comparison processes do not become a primary or preferred source of information for children until about 10 years of age [59–61, 98]. It is possible, therefore, that some of the same situations that were innocuous to the younger children would have presented moral conflict for older children. Finally, instructors in the structural-developmental group reported that children had difficulty engaging in moral dialogue, even in small groups. Many were inexperienced with participating in such activities with peers, and the request to express thoughts and feelings was a difficult one for these children. The overall results that significant change occurred in the experimental groups are nonetheless important in demonstrating that a program specifically designed to target moral growth in a traditional physical education-type curriculum can produce changes in children as young as 5 years old.

Romance and colleagues [96] designed a follow-up study to Bredemeier et al. in a physical education classroom setting. Based on the previous study's findings, older children were used (ages 10–11 years) as well as a longer intervention period (8 weeks). Dialogue activities as a means of developing comfort with speaking in a group were conducted for a longer period of time before the intervention program began. Specific physical activities as well as instructional styles based on Haan's interactional morality were derived and validated by Haan herself. Finally, the measure of morality was more sophisticated than those in the Bredemeier et al. study, consisting of interviews with the children about hypothetical stories that presented moral conflict in both sport and nonsport settings.

Results revealed strong between-group differences on sport, non-sport, and total morality scores for the structural-developmental and control groups. In all cases, the experimental group demonstrated significant pre- to posttest gains in moral reasoning while the control group showed no change. Of noteworthy interest, however, were the behavioral observations that occurred over the 8-week period [95]. For example, children in the structural developmental group became more active in dialoguing and balancing and were more receptive to using this strategy as a means of resolving moral dilemmas in the gymnasium. There were fewer incidents of misconduct and disciplinary problems in the experimental group. Finally, children in the structural-developmental group became more sensitive to the needs of the less skilled and engaged in more cooperative play. For example, one boy low in motor skills was rarely included by the children in team activities at the outset of the program; by the end of the intervention period, however, children were sensitive to his needs and included him as an active participant at all times.

The Bredemeier et al. and Romance et al. studies offer promising directions for moral education within sport-related settings. Children as young as 5 years old were found to mature in their moral reasoning ability. Older children, however, seemed to benefit more substantively from such intervention techniques, and this likely may have been due to their more mature social cognitive abilities, including perspective-taking and peer interaction skills. More research is needed to discover the ways to enhance moral development in the physical domain.

Three other studies by Bredemeier found age differences on measures related to moral growth and behaviors. In two studies investigating the relation among children's moral reasoning, sport involvement, self-reported aggression tendencies, and legitimacy judgments about potentially injurious sport acts, children 12–13 years of age were found to significantly differ on some of these measures in comparison to their younger counterparts [25, 26]. More specifically, 12–13-year-olds accepted more potentially injurious acts as legitimate than did 8–11-year-old children. The older age group was also significantly higher in reported tendencies to express aggressive behaviors than were the 9–10-year-old age group; however, no age differences were found for moral reasoning level. Finally, older children reported more experience in organized sports than did younger children, as indicated by the number of seasons they participated on youth sport teams. In each of these cases, boys also scored higher than girls on legitimacy judgements, aggression tendencies, and sport involvement.

In another study [16], children's moral reasoning about issues in daily life and sport-specific contexts was investigated. It was found that 12–13-year-old children significantly diverged in their moral reasoning scores about sport and nonsport contexts. Specifically, the sport reasoning scores for this age group were significantly lower than their nonsport reasoning scores, and this divergence differed from children 8–11 years of age who did not demonstrate context-specific reasoning patterns.

The results of these three studies taken together demonstrate that at about age 12, children's cognitions about moral conflicts show differences to those of their younger peers. Reasoning about sport and daily life moral dilemmas diverge, greater frequencies of tendencies to aggress are reported, and there is greater acceptance of more potentially injurious acts as legitimate. Also, children's social experiences pertaining to the sport context are more extensive as reflected by a greater number of years of sport participation. From a structural-developmental perspective, then, a significant change in moral cognitions and behaviors appears to frequently occur during the early adolescent period.

These differences are consistent with developmental change in other cognitive abilities, such as memory development, selective attention, and verbal rehearsal strategies [40]. Developmental change during this age period is also evident for perceptions about personal competence and control. For example, children have been found to become more accurate in their perceived competence with age [51, 61, 85]. These increases in accuracy are hypothesized to occur as a result of children becoming more capable of analyzing the causes of behavioral outcomes, distinguishing between effort, ability, task difficulty, and luck as determinants of performance outcomes [85]. Also, children show a developmental pattern in the sources of information that they use to evaluate their competence. Evaluative feedback from adults is primary for children younger than 10 years old, while peer comparison becomes the most salient informational source for 10–14-year-old children. Sometime during or after adolescence, peer comparison decreases somewhat in importance as children utilize multiple sources of information, including internal performance criteria, to judge one's competence. In sum, it appears that, as children enter Piaget's formal operational period of cognitive development [81], numerous cognitive changes occur and these are significantly different from those for their younger counterparts.

In conclusion, it is clear that cognitive-developmental factors affect the moral thought-moral action relationship as reflected by Rest's [94] component model. Component 1, interpreting the situation and identifying a moral problem, entails an individual's ability to take the perspective of others, analyze the causes of behavioral outcomes, utilize a number of informational sources in the social environment, and determine how the consequences affect all parties concerned. Component 2, formulating a plan of action that applies the relevant moral standard, encompasses moral reasoning patterns and the application of social-moral norms. Clearly, the sport-related morality research to date, although sparse, indicates that cognitive development can strongly influence the relation between moral thought and moral action.

SIGNIFICANT OTHERS. "Say it ain't so, Joe!" pleaded the young boy to Shoeless Joe Jackson, a destined Hall of Fame baseball player, as he exited the courthouse and his trial for "throwing" the World Series in the infamous 1919 Black Sox scandal. These words represented the disappointment and broken heart of a child whose most respected hero fell from credibility. For individuals of all ages, social interactions with adults, such as parents, coaches, and professional athletes, as well as peers, in the form of teammates and opponents, are a dominant and influential feature of sporting experiences [29, 117]. The primary means by which moral values are conveyed via significant others are modeling, reinforcement, and interpersonal communication styles.

Within Rest's [94] interactive model of morality, the influence of significant others on the moral thought-moral action relationship appears to fall under Components 1 and 3. Component 1 challenges participants to interpret the situation and identify a moral problem by imagining possible courses of action and considering how the consequences of those actions will impact on all parties residing in the situation. Component 3 involves the individual in decision-making among competing value ideals about what one will actually intend to do. The decision in choosing a moral ideal can depend largely on the salience afforded to particular significant others in the sport social environment.

According to Damon [32], moral growth is influenced through different processes and under divergent situations by adults and peers. During the early childhood years, parents are the most important adults affecting moral and social development. It is also within the family structure that the child is most frequently introduced to sport and encounters his or her first exposure to the social regulations and norms governing athletic endeavors [72].

In a comprehensive review of the developmental psychology literature, Damon [32] contends that parental rearing patterns strongly influence the rate and quality of maturity in children's moral development. In particular, the literature suggests that both authoritative and inductive styles of transmitting values from adults to children appear to be the strongest positive influences of moral growth [6, 7, 56]. Authoritative parenting combines high control, clear communication, warmth and nurturance, and firm but consistent maturity expectations. In contrast, an authoritarian style is characterized by high control, low communication clarity, low warmth and nurturance, and high expectations of socially mature behavior. These points seem especially pertinent for the sport setting. Today, an authoritarian style of coaching is still dominant, especially at high school, college, and professional levels. Additionally, this style is modeled to younger coaches and athletes and reinforced when teams win. If morality is to become an explicit goal of sport programs, communication styles must be carefully considered along with specific instructional activities.

Inductive techniques of communication involve the provision of a rationale for expected behaviors as well as encouraging compliance to rules through the use of minimal adult control [55, 56]. This strategy is contrasted with two others: power assertion and love withdrawal. Power assertion is dependent upon the use of punishment or coercion to promote compliance and is legitimized on the premise that the adult has the power to enforce rules. Love withdrawal draws on verbal and nonverbal signs of disapproval or disappointment for a child's noncompliance to expected social standards. Damon [32] notes that both power assertion and love withdrawal techniques work well in the short run but do not show enduring effects that transmitted values have been internalized. Conversely, induction has been found to foster long-lasting and autonomous beliefs in the child and, thus, is considered a salient communication technique for teaching moral values to children. It would appear then that, along with authoritative coaching styles, induction should be used more frequently in competitive athletic settings so that children are facilitated in their interpretation of conflicting moral situations and their decisions about what they actually should do in such situations.

In the competitive sport setting, a diverse group of adults in the form of coaches, parents, officials, and professional athletes take center stage in the lives of young athletes. Research in developmental psychology (e.g., see Refs. 60 and 109) reveals that children under 10 years of age depend upon adult feedback and reinforcement as their primary source of information about self-perceived abilities. Thus, these adults are a salient and visible means for children to interpret social situations and moral dilemmas, and for deciding upon which moral action to adopt. Of special interest may be the role modeling of high level athletes. In an anecdotal story, Greg Louganis (two-time Olympic gold medalist diver) tells of the time when he walked to his car after a workout. There in the parking lot was a 12-year-old boy smoking a cigarette. Louganis, outraged at this sight, demanded to know the meaning of such inappropriate behavior. The boy calmly exclaimed, "But I wanted to be just like you." This event was enough to motivate Louganis to give up smoking.

Research in sport psychology has shown that coaches can have a strong influence in shaping desirable social behaviors and self-perceptions. Thus, it is reasonable to assume that moral beliefs can be similarly influenced. For example, coaches' use of encouragement, contingent praise, informational feedback, and social support has been found to positively affect self-esteem, perceived physical competence, participation motivation, and group cohesion in children, adolescents, and college-age athletes [58, 108, 114, 115]. Research is needed to explicitly examine how the use of particular coaching communication styles may affect moral reasoning and behaviors in the sport setting. More specifically, the relation between communication styles, children's interpretation of the situation, and their decision-making with regard to intended moral actions needs to be examined.

In contrast to a focus on adult values and rules in early and middle childhood, the peer group takes on increasing salience in later childhood [29, 32, 52]. The primary norm of peer relations in childhood and adolescence is one of reciprocity, in which personal exchanges serve the interests of all parties involved. Reciprocity is the frequent mode of interaction because children perceive that they are equals as peers in status and power. Thus, peer relations represent mutual and intimate standards of interpersonal interaction [32]. Damon suggests that one of the first opportunities to experience an orientation of reciprocity is in the realm of sports and games, where children learn that rules that are fair benefit everyone by enabling the game to be played under orderly social norms and regulations. These negotiations are highly influenced by the child's perspective-taking ability [101] discussed earlier. Thus, it would appear from a constructivist stance that moral dialogue and balance among peers about sport dilemmas should lead to higher or more mature levels of moral growth. The salience of the peer group during later childhood is further supported by the literature, demonstrating that peer comparison and evaluation are preferred sources of competence information for children 10–14 years of age [59–61].

Few studies have investigated the influence of significant others on children's moral growth through sport experiences. Bredemeier et al. [27] employed social learning and structural-developmental instructional strategies in a summer sport program setting. The social learning group consisted of strategies such as teacher and peer modeling, tangible rewards, and symbolic reinforcement, while the structural development group focused on moral dialogue and negotiation among peers with facilitation by teachers only to initiate discussion. Results revealed that both instructional styles enhanced moral growth over a 6-week intervention period.

The visibility of professional athletes with regard to moral cognitions and behaviors has resulted in studies of the relation between modeling and aggression in young athletes. Smith [105] interviewed 83 high school ice hockey players regarding their favorite professional players and also recorded their aggressive behaviors on the ice. He found that players who perceived their favorite National Hockey League player as "rough and tough" exhibited higher levels of athletic aggression than players whose favorite players were perceived as less aggressive. Smith [106] also surveyed 604 young male ice hockey players and found that more than one-third of the boys had learned and used illegal hits by watching professional ice hockey. Mugno and Feltz [83] replicated these results with youth league and high school male football players.

Finally, in a study by Bredemeier et al. [26] previously discussed, children's legitimacy judgments for potentially injurious sport actions were investigated through the use of slides depicting college and professional athletes. Results revealed that children accepted more acts as legitimate for adults than for children, and that boys' involvement in high contact sports was related to legitimizing more actions. These results also point to the influence that significant others, in this case professional and collegiate sport athletes, can have on moral thoughts and behaviors.

In conclusion, it is apparent that significant others can powerfully influence the moral thought-moral action relationship. They do so by affecting how participants interpret the meanings attached to sport situations via modeling, reinforcement, and dialoguing opportunities. Similarly, the decision making processes in selecting appropriate actions are influenced through adult styles of communicating (e.g., authoritative authoritarian, permissive) and inductive reasoning techniques. It is imperative that future research tap the underlying processes influencing participants' interpretation and decisions regarding moral standards and behaviors as they interact with adults and peers in sport-related settings.

FROM THEORY TO PRACTICE: MORAL EDUCATION THROUGH SPORT

At the beginning of this paper, it was stated that one of the reasons for few research studies on moral development in sport is the question of whether it is appropriate for teachers and coaches to target moral growth as a curricular objective in their classrooms. Based on the discussion of the scientific literature, theoretical models, and moral thought-moral action relationship, we believe that we have provided strong evidence for the need and potential for nurturing moral growth in the physical domain. It is the purpose of this section to provide guidelines for strategic planning in moral physical education programs based on theoretical and empirical research knowledges.

Damon [32], in his recent book titled *The Moral Child*, consolidates information from theories and scientific studies of morality to identify general principles of moral development. These principles, according to Damon, provide a framework for establishing content and instructional techniques for moral education curricula. The first principle states that through children's social interaction experiences, they naturally encounter moral dilemmas such as those involving honesty, fairness, and justice. Second, children's moral awareness is shaped and supported by natural emotional reactions to observations and events. Third, relations with parents, teachers, and other adults introduce and reinforce the child with regard to important social standards, rules, and conventions. In contrast, relations with peers introduce children to norms of direct reciprocity and to standards of sharing, cooperation, and fairness. Finally, Damon makes the point that moral growth in school settings is governed by the same developmental processes that apply to moral growth everywhere. That is, children acquire moral values by actively participating in adult and peer relationships that support, enhance, and guide their natural moral inclinations.

We strongly believe that physical education and sport settings provide children, adolescents, and adults with ideal opportunities for realizing optimal moral growth based on Damon's principles. The few studies that have been designed to effect changes in moral reasoning and behaviors through sport-related experiences have been optimistic [27, 33, 41, 96]. In addition, we believe that the theoretical and empirical research knowledge base in moral development offers enough support for translating Damon's principles into practical applications for sport practitioners. The guidelines for moral education through sport emanate directly from constructivist and internalization theoretical approaches and study findings.

Internalization Approaches

Instructional strategies that follow the internalization principles of social learning theory have been popular in sport and physical education. These include positive role modeling by teachers and coaches, positive reinforcement for desirable behaviors, and punishment for undesirable behaviors in the sport setting. While these strategies have been effective in establishing social order in the athletic classroom, Damon [32] warns that a focus on indoctrinization and lecturing by adults will not prepare children for the many diverse situations they will face in life nor will they contribute to the development of making autonomous moral choices. Instead, he maintains, children must learn to find the moral issue in an ambiguous situation, apply basic moral values to unfamiliar problems, and create moral solutions. The only way to do this is to help children develop an autonomous ability to interpet, understand, and manage moral problems by encouraging them to actively engage in peer discussions, which are facilitated by adult guidance.

Heeding such warnings, teachers and coaches should reinforce acceptable and unacceptable behaviors in students by encouraging them to accept responsibility for their actions and to think about the consequences to themselves and others. Inductive approaches should be used whenever possible so that children internalize the reasoning behind their actions. Also, teachers and coaches should be aware of their own actions and ensure that they are positive role models, in thoughts and actions, for their students.

Damon [32] introduced the notion of "moral mentoring" as a strategy for enhancing moral growth opportunities in youth. Moral mentoring requires that individuals who have distinguished themselves through exemplary moral behavior be identified and brought into contact with students. This strategy would enhance moral awareness by modeling the type of moral issues to which these individuals responded. It can also contribute to moral maturity by demonstrating how commitments to moral values can be translated into effective social action.

Constructivist Approaches

According to constructivist proponents, any program of moral development must provide role taking opportunities, experiences with moral conflict, and opportunities for moral dialogue and balance. In the realm of sport, natural moral dilemmas occur frequently, such as ball hogging, verbal and physical aggression, and unfair play. Teachers and coaches must take advantage of these occurrences to encourage discussion about moral dilemmas and negotiation toward resolution of the dilemma. The teacher's role in this case is to initiate and facilitate the discussion in order to draw out students' reasons for their position on the dilemma. The variety of conflicting points of view exposes individuals to alternative ways of thinking about and resolving the conflict. The teacher must encourage children to dialogue among themselves, express their own views, and listen to each other's views and feedback. Although not as powerful as personal moral conflicts, Parsons [90] suggests that coaches prepare scripts of common moral dilemmas in their sport and engage athletes in dialogue and negotiation of possible solutions to each situation.

In addition to taking advantage of naturally occurring moral dilemmas in sport, teachers and coaches can build dilemmas into the motor skills curriculum by creating situations offering unequal opportunity, unfair advantages, or temptations to aggress. Then, moral dialogue and balance in response to these contrived moral conflicts can be encouraged. For example, Romance et al. [96] used a strategy called Built-in Dilemma/Dialogue (BIDD) to engage children in discussion and negotiation about dilemmas occurring in the gymnasium. One of the BIDD strategies was in the form of a "score 10" basketball shooting game. Students, in pairs, were asked to make baskets as a team. The first team to make 10 baskets was declared the winner. After the activity, time for dialogue was provided, in which discussion was focused on how each team decided who was to shoot how many shots and how their decisions were related to individual needs and interests.

Damon [32] calls the productive adult-child interchanges with regard to moral development "respectful engagement." In other words, adults must be aware of individuals' developmental needs and provide the opportunity for full participation in social experiences that will build upon natural moral tendencies. Respectful engagement refers to the cooperation between adult and child in fostering moral growth. The child needs adult guidance but in order for the guidance to make a difference, the child must be productively engaged. In order for such engagement to occur, the child's own initiations and reactions must be respected.

Another instructional strategy based on constructivist approaches is to allow students control in designing their own individual and group experiences in sport. This problem-solving style of teaching affords excellent opportunities for individuals to experience moral dilemmas, take the role of others, and engage in dialogue and balance. As an example, Romance et al. [96] had children, in groups of three, play the game of "pickle in the middle" (basketball passing) according to the following guidelines: "try to pass the basketball back and forth between two players while the third player (in the middle) tries to touch it. Passers must stand on the red lines and if the middle person touches a pass, that person changes places with the passer." Children were encouraged to change the rules in order to improve the game if necessary. Postgame discussions centered on rule changes made and how these changes related to individual needs and interests.

A third general instructional strategy is to link sport moral issues to those found in everyday life. For example, in the activity called "Two Cultures" [96], students are instructed to play a competitive game in which players are eliminated or elevated to more desirable positions according to their performance. After playing according to these rules, students are asked to play the game cooperatively by trying to get as many consecutive passes as possible (a focus on process rather than outcome). Postgame discussions involved comparison of the two games with respect to needs for individual motor skill challenges and playing time.

Another strategy for moral education through sport, employing constructivist principles, is inductive discipline. The process for distributing penalties to students should be explained so that they understand the rationale underlying why their behavior was unacceptable. In addition, when two or more individuals come into moral conflict, teachers can send them off to the "talking bench," where they are encouraged to reach consensus on a solution that meets the needs and interests of all parties involved.

The range of specific instructional strategies based on both constructivist and internalization principles is extremely broad. There are many exciting physical activities and creative teaching styles that offer the potential for moving children toward moral maturity in their reasoning and behaviors. However, the description of such strategies is beyond the scope of this paper. Scholars and practitioners in particular are directed to Bredemeier and Shields [17] and Romance et al. [96] for more detailed accounts of recommendations for class structure, adult-child relationship, and child-child relationship strategies that offer the most optimistic opportunities for effecting moral reasoning and behavior change.

In conclusion, moral growth through physical education and sport is not only possible, but a necessary objective to the success of such programs which claim to be building values and "sportspersonship." Strategies based on constructivist principles especially challenge young learners by encouraging autonomous thinking about one's own values, exposing them to alternative views verbalized by others, and providing opportunities for dialogue, negotiation, and balance of moral conflicts. The sport setting is an especially attractive venue for moral growth, because both naturally occurring and contrived moral dilemmas frequently emerge. Teachers and coaches who want to make a difference in the moral lives of youngsters can no longer stand on the sidelines and wait for growth to automatically unfold. They must become active participants in the game of moral education.

MORAL DEVELOPMENT IN SPORT: FUTURE DIRECTIONS FOR RESEARCH

The knowledge base pertaining to the theoretical and empirical research in moral development has grown considerably over the last decade. We have begun to learn about the relationship between moral reasoning and moral aggression, and how gender, cognitive developmental level, and significant others mediate the moral thought-moral action relationship. Despite these developments in the sport moral development literature, much more research is needed to better understand the nature of morality in sport and to provide informed recommendations for instructional strategies appropriate for sport settings.

The line of research by Bredemeier and her colleagues on the relationships among moral reasoning, self-reported athletic aggression, and legitimacy judgments of injurious acts has been an essential beginning to our understanding of moral development in sport. A necessary extension of these studies is the actual behavioral validation of the self-report aggression and legitimacy measures. How do individuals actually choose to act in situations that offer the opportunity for physical and verbal aggression, or in deciding whether to support the explicit or implicit directives by a coach to potentially injure another player? In addition to determining which behaviors actually align with moral reasoning and cognitions, how do males and females view and act in such situations? Is a morality of care and responsibility, or a morality of rights and justice upheld in these instances? What developmental differences affect the moral thought-moral action relationship?

The majority of sport morality studies to date has been conducted within programs that conform to more of a physical education motor skills curriculum rather than organized, competitive sport. Physical education and competitive sport settings are not identical, and several appropriate questions could be asked. One question might pertain to whether there are differences in moral reasoning and aggression between youth sport participants and nonparticipants. Do differences occur as a function of type of sport, the competitive level of play, or whether it takes place in school or nonschool settings? Can coaches be trained to employ effective strategies for promoting moral growth through competitive sport? And will they accept this important role? These and other questions are in need of systematic inquiry.

A line of research that would be interesting from a developmental perspective is the relation between the development of moral reasoning and the development of other cognitive abilities. Such abilities might include general information processing skills, causal attributions and affective reactions to performance outcomes, perceptions of physical competence and control, sources of physical competence information, and motivational orientation. In addition to examining the parallel developmental processes of these constructs, it is also likely that predictive models of the moral thought-moral action relationship may result in greater explained variance with the inclusion of some of these cognitive variables as well as situational influences.

What may be perhaps the most important direction for future research is implications for moral education through sport. The few studies conducted to date have shown promising results. It is our hope that sport practitioners will take the challenge of the Academy of Physical Education by embracing opportunities to target moral growth in their participants. To this end, research studies are needed to investigate what instructional strategies are effective in physical education and sport settings for potentiating changes in moral reasoning and behaviors. Strategies outlined by Romance et al. [96] and Bredemeier and Shields [17] should be systematically tested and outcomes assessed in order to provide a comprehensive model of moral development curricula in school and nonschool sport settings. Intimately related to this recommendation is the need to conduct longitudinal studies of such instructional programs so that strategy implementation and concomitant developmental growth over extended periods of time can be substantiated.

In conclusion, the area of moral development in sport has progressed a long way since its historical beginnings in the anecdotal literature. A greater understanding of the moral thought-moral action relationship, especially moral reasoning and aggression, is necessary, along with the mediating influence of gender, cognitive developmental differences, and significant others. Most importantly, however, is the need to explicitly accept the Academy of Physical Education challenge: "Physical educators might well place an increased emphasis on the problems of ethical judgements and morally responsible behavior in sports" (see Ref. 89, p. 53). To do this, physical education and sport program curricula must incorporate moral education as an objective, and commit to implementing theoretically grounded instructional strategies for effecting changes in moral judgments and behaviors. When thoughts can be translated into actions on the playing fields and gymnasia floors across America, the potential for moral development through sport will be evident.

REFERENCES

1. Arnold PJ: Moral aspects of an education in movement. In Stull GA, Eckert HM (eds): *Effects of Physical Activity on Children.* Champaign, IL, Human Kinetics, 1986, pp 14–21.
2. Aronfreed J: *Conduct and Conscience.* New York, Academic Press, 1968.
3. Bandura A: *Social Learning Theory.* Englewood Cliffs, NJ, Prentice-Hall, 1977.
4. Bandura A: *Social Foundations of Thought and Action:. A Social Cognitive Theory.* Englewood Cliffs, NJ, Prentice-Hall, 1986.
5. Barrett DE, Yarrow MR: Prosocial behavior, social inferential ability, and assertiveness in children. *Child Dev* 48:475–481, 1977.
6. Baumrind D: The development of instrumental competence through socialization. In Pick AD (ed): *Minnesota Symposium on Child Psychology.* Minneapolis, MN, University of Minnesota Press, 1973.
7. Baumrind D: Rearing competent children. In Damon W (ed): *Child Development Today and Tomorrow.* San Francisco, CA, Jossey-Bass, 1989.
8. Berkowitz L, Daniels LR: Responsibility and dependency. *J Abnorm Social Psychol* 66:429–436, 1963.
9. Blair S: Professionalization of attitude toward play in children and adults. *Res Q Exerc Sport* 56:82–83, 1985.
10. Blanchard B: A comparative analysis of secondary-school boys' and girls' character and personality traits in physical education classes. *Res Q* 17:33–39, 1946.

11. Blasi A: Bridging moral cognition and moral action: a critical review of the literature. *Psychol Bull* 88:1–45, 1980.
12. Blasi A: Bridging moral cognition and action: a theoretical perspective. *Dev Rev* 3:178–210, 1983.
13. Bredemeier BJ: *The assessment of expressive and instrumental power value orientations in sport and in everyday life.* Unpublished doctoral dissertation, Temple University, 1980.
14. Bredemeier BJ: Moral reasoning and the perceived legitimacy of intentionally injurious sport acts. *J Sport Psychol* 7:110–124, 1985.
15. Bredemeier BJ: Children's moral reasoning and their assertive, aggressive and submissive tendencies in sport and daily life. (submitted for publication).
16. Bredemeier BJ: Divergence in children's moral reasoning about issues in daily life and sport specific contexts. (submitted for publication).
17. Bredemeier B, Shields D: *Body and Balance:. The Development of Moral Structures Through Physical Education and Sport.* Eugene, OR, University of Oregon Publications, 1983.
18. Bredemeier B, Shields D: The utility of moral stage analysis in the understanding of athletic aggression. *Sociol Sport J* 1:138–149, 1984.
19. Bredemeier B, Shields D: Divergence in moral reasoning about sport and life. *Sociol Sport J* 1:348–357, 1984.
20. Bredemeier B, Shields D: Values and violence in sport. *Psychol Today* 19:22–32, 1985.
21. Bredemeier B, Shields D: Moral growth among athletes and non-athletes: a comparative analysis. *J Genet Psychol* 147:7–18, 1986.
22. Bredemeier B, Shields D: Athletic aggression: an issue of contextual morality. *Sociol Sport J* 3:15–28, 1986.
23. Bredemeier B, Shields D: Game reasoning and interactional morality. *J Genet Psychol* 147: 257–275, 1986.
24. Bredemeier B, Shields D: Moral growth through physical activity: an interactional approach. In Gould D, Weiss M (eds): *Advances in Pediatric Sport Sciences.* Champaign, IL, Human Kinetics, 1987, pp 145–165.
25. Bredemeier B, Weiss M, Shields D, Cooper B: The relationship of sport involvement with children's moral reasoning and aggression tendencies. *J Sport Psychol* 8:304–318, 1986.
26. Bredemeier B, Weiss M, Shields D, Cooper B: The relationship between children's legitimacy judgments and their moral reasoning, aggression tendencies and sport involvement. *Sociol Sport J* 4:48–60, 1987.
27. Bredemeier B, Weiss M, Shields D, Shewchuk R: Promoting moral growth in a summer sport camp: The implementation of theoretically grounded instructional strategies. *J Moral Educ* 15:212–220, 1986.
28. Burton RV: Honesty and dishonesty. In Lickonco T (ed): *Moral Development and Behavior: Theory Research and Social Issues.* New York, Holt, Rinehart & Winston, 1976, pp 173–198.
29. Coakley JJ: Children and the sport socialization process. In Gould D, Weiss M (eds): *Advances in Pediatric Sport Sciences, Vol. 2: Behavioral Issues.* Champaign, IL, Human Kinetics, 1987, pp 43–60.
30. Damon W: *The Social World of the Child.* San Francisco, CA, Jossey-Bass, 1977.
31. Damon W: Patterns of change in children's social reasoning: a two-year longitudinal study. *Child Dev* 51:1010–1017, 1980.
32. Damon W: *The Moral Child: Nurturing Children's Natural Moral Growth.* New York, The Free Press, 1988.
33. DeBusk M, Hellison D: Implementing a physical education self-responsibility model for delinquency-prone youth. *J Teach Physical Educ* 8:104–112, 1989.
34. Deluty RH: Children's action tendency scale: A self-report measure of aggressiveness, assertiveness and submissiveness in children. *J Consult Clin Psychol* 47:1061–1071, 1979.

35. Deluty RH: Behavioral validation of the children's action tendency scale. *J Behav Assess* 6:115–130, 1984.
36. Dubois PE: The effect of participation in sport on the value orientations of youth athletes. *Sociol Sport J* 3:29–42, 1986.
37. Duda JL, Templin TJ, Tappe MK, Olson LK: *Sportsmanship attitudes and the perceived legitimacy of aggressive acts: a goal perspective analysis.* Paper presented at the annual meeting of the North American Society for the Psychology of Sport and Physical Activity, Kent State University, Kent, OH, 1989.
38. Freud S: *New Introductory Lectures on Psychoanalysis.* New York, Morton, 1933.
39. Freud S: *The Psychopathology of Everyday Life.* London, Hogarth Press, 1960. (First German Edition, 1901).
40. Gallagher JD, Hoffman S: Memory development and children's sport skill acquisition. In Gould D, Weiss M (eds): *Advances in Pediatric Sport Sciences, Vol. 2: Behavioral Issues.* Champaign, IL, Human Kinetics, 1987, pp 187–210.
41. Giebink MP, McKenzie TC: Teaching sportsmanship in physical education and recreation: an analysis of intervention and generalization efforts. *J Teach Physical Educ* 4:167–177, 1985.
42. Gilligan C: In a different voice: women's conceptions of the self and of morality. *Harvard Educ Rev* 47:481–517, 1977.
43. Gilligan C: *In a Different Voice: Psychological Theory and Women's Development.* Cambridge, MA, Harvard University Press, 1982.
44. Gilligan C: On "In a different voice:" an interdisciplinary forum. *Signs: J Women Culture Soc.* 11:324–333, 1986.
45. Gilligan C, Belenky M: A naturalistic study of the abortion decision. In Selman R, Yando R (eds): *New Directions in Child Development: Clinical-Developmental Psychology.* San Francisco, Jossey-Bass, 1982, pp 69–90.
46. Haan N: *Coping and Defending: Processes of Self-Environment Organization.* New York, Academic Press, 1977.
47. Haan N: Two moralities in action contents: relationship to thought, ego regulation, and development. *J Pers Soc Psychol* 36:286–305, 1978.
48. Haan N: An interactional morality of everyday life. In Haan N, Bellah R, Rabinow P, Sullivan W (eds): *Social Science as Moral Inquiry.* New York, Columbia University Press, 1983.
49. Haan N, Aerts E, Cooper B: *On Moral Grounds.* New York, New York University Press, 1985.
50. Hall E: *Moral development levels of athletes in sport specific and general social situations.* Unpublished doctoral dissertation, Texas Woman's University, 1981.
51. Harter S: The perceived competence scale for children. *Child Dev* 53:87–97, 1982.
52. Hartup WW: The social worlds of childhood. *Am Psychol* 34:944–950, 1979.
53. Henkel SA, Earls NF: The moral judgment of physical education teachers. *J Teach Physical Educ* 4:178–189, 1985.
54. Higgins A, Power C, Kohlberg L: The relationship of moral atmosphere to judgments of responsibility. In Kurtines W, Gerwitz J (eds): *Morality, Moral Behavior, and Moral Development.* New York, John Wiley & Sons, 1984, pp 74–106.
55. Hoffman ML: Moral internalization, parental power, and the nature of parent-child interaction. *Dev Psychol* 5:45–57, 1967.
56. Hoffman ML: Moral internalization. In Berkowitz L (ed): *Advances in Experimental Social Psychology.* New York, Academic Press, 1977, pp 86–135.
57. Hoffman ML: Empathy, its development and prosocial implication. In Keasey CB (ed): *Nebraska Symposium on Motivation* (Vol. 25). Lincoln, University of Nebraska Press, 1977, pp 169–217.
58. Horn TS: Coaches' feedback and changes in children's perceptions of their physical competence. *J Educ Psychol* 77:174–186, 1985.

59. Horn TS, Hasbrook CA: Informational components influencing children's perceptions of their physical competence. In Weiss M, Gould D (eds): *Sport for Children and Youth.* Champaign, IL: Human Kinetics, 1986, pp 81–88.

60. Horn TS, Hasbrook CA: Psychological characteristics and the criteria children use for self-evaluation. *J Sport Psychol* 9:208–221, 1987.

61. Horn TS, Weiss MR: A developmental analysis of children's self-ability judgements in the physical domain. *Dev Psychol* (submitted for publication).

62. Hyde JS: How large are gender differences in aggression? A developmental meta-analysis. *Dev Psychol* 20:722–736, 1984.

63. Jantz RM: Moral thinking in male elementary pupils as reflected by perception of basketball rules. *Res Q* 46:414–421, 1975.

64. Kagan J: Introduction. In Kagan J, Lamb S (eds): *The Emergence of Morality in Young Children.* Chicago, IL, University of Chicago Press, 1987, pp ix–xx.

65. Kleiber DA, Roberts GC: The effects of sports experience in the development of social character: an exploratory investigation. *J Sport Psychol* 3:114–122, 1981.

66. Knoppers A, Zuidema M, Meyer BB: Playing to win or playing to play? *Sociol Sport J* 6:70–76, 1989.

67. Kohlberg L: Stage and sequence: The cognitive-developmental approach to socialization. In Goslin D (ed): *Handbook of Socialization Theory and Research.* Chicago, Rand-McNally, 1969.

68. Kohlberg L: Moral stages and moralization: The cognitive-developmental approach. In Lickona T (ed): *Moral Development and Behavior.* New York, Holt, Rinehart & Winston, 1976, pp 31–53.

69. Kohlberg L: *Essays on Moral Development, Vol. 1: The Philosophy of Moral Development.* New York, Harper and Row, 1981.

70. Kohlberg L: *Essays on Moral Development, Vol. 2: The Psychology of Moral Development.* New York, Harper and Row, 1984.

71. Kohlberg L, Candee D: The relationship of moral judgment to moral action. In Kurtinez W, Gerwitz J (eds): *Morality, Moral Behavior, and Moral Development.* New York, John Wiley & Sons, 1984, pp 52–73.

72. Lewko JH, Greendorfer SL: Family influences in sport socialization of children and adolescents. In Smoll F, Magill R, Ash M (eds): *Children in Sport.* ed. 3. Champaign, IL, Human Kinetics, 1988, pp 287–300.

73. Lickona T: Critical issues in the study of moral development and behavior. In Lickona T (ed): *Moral Development and Behavior: Theory, Research and Social Issues.* New York, Holt, Rinehart & Winston, 1976, pp 3–27.

74. Liebert RM: Observational learning: Some social applications. In Elich PJ (ed): *The Fourth Western Symposium on Learning: Social Learning.* Bellingham, WA, Washington State College, 1973.

75. Lyons N: *Two orientations to morality; Rights and care: A coding manual.* Unpublished doctoral dissertation. Harvard University, 1982.

76. Marantz M: Fostering prosocial behavior in the early childhood classroom: Review of the research. *J Moral Educ* 17:27–39, 1988.

77. Martens R: *Joy and Sadness in Children's Sport.* Champaign, IL, Human Kinetics, 1978.

78. Martens R: Youth sport in the USA. In Weiss MR, Gould D (eds): *Sport for Children and Youths.* Champaign, IL, Human Kinetics, 1986.

79. Martens R, Seefeldt V: *Bill of Rights for Young Athletes.* Washington D.C., AAHPERD, 1976.

80. McCloy C: Character building through physical education. *Res Q* 1:41–59, 1930.

81. Miller PH: *Theories of Developmental Psychology.* ed 2. New York, WH Freeman, 1989.

82. Mischel W, Moore B: Effects of attention to symbolically presented rewards upon self-control. *J Pers Soc Psychol* 3:390–396, 1966.

83. Mugno D, Feltz D: *The social learning of aggression in youth football.* Paper presented at the 1984 International Olympic Scientific Congress, Eugene, OR, July 1984.

84. Murphy JJ, Gilligan C: Moral development in late adolescence and adulthood: a critique and reconstruction of Kohlberg's theory. *Hum Dev* 23:77–104, 1980.
85. Nicholls JG: The development of the concepts of effort and ability, perception of academic attainment, and the understanding that difficult tasks require more ability. *Child Dev* 49:800–814, 1978.
86. Noddings N: *Caring: A Feminine Approach to Ethics and Moral Education.* Berkeley, University of California Press, 1984.
87. Nunner-Winkler G: Two moralities? A critical discussion of an ethic of care and responsibility versus an ethic of rights and justice. In Kurtines W, Gerwitz J (eds): *Morality, Moral Behavior, and Moral Development.* New York, John Wiley & Sons, 1984.
88. Orlick T: Positive socialization via cooperative games. *Dev Psychol* 17:126–129, 1981.
89. Park R: Three major issues: The Academy takes a stand. *JOPERD* 54:52–53, 1983.
90. Parsons TW: Gamesmanship and sport ethics. *Coaching Rev* 71:28–30, 1984.
91. Peck RF, Havighurst RJ: *The Psychology of Character Development.* New York, John Wiley & Sons, 1960.
92. Piaget J: *The Moral Judgment of the Child.* Glencoe, IL, Free Press, 1965.
93. Rest JR: *Development in Judging Moral Issues.* Minneapolis, University of Minnesota Press, 1979.
94. Rest JR: The Major Components of Morality. In Kurtinez W, Gerwitz J (eds): *Morality, Moral Behavior, and Moral Development.* New York, John Wiley & Sons, 1984.
95. Romance TJ: A program to promote moral development through elementary school physical education. Doctoral dissertation, University of Oregon, Eugene, OR, 1984.
96. Romance TJ, Weiss MR, Bockoven J: A program to promote moral development through elementary physical education. *J Teach Physical Educ* 5:126–136, 1986.
97. Sage G: Orientations toward sport and male and female intercollegiate athletes. *J Sport Psychol* 2:355–362, 1980.
98. Scanlan TK: Social evaluation and the competition process: a developmental perspective. In Smoll F, Magill R, Ash M (eds): *Children in Sport.* ed 3. Champaign, IL, Human Kinetics, 1988, pp 135–148.
99. Seefeldt V: *The Code of Ethics for Youth Sport Coaches.* East Lansing, MI, Institute for the Study of Youth Sports, 1982.
100. Selman RL: The relation of role-taking to the development of moral judgment in children. *Child Dev* 42:79–92, 1971.
101. Selman RL: Social-cognitive understanding: A guide to educational and clinical practice. In Lickona T (ed): *Moral Development and Behavior: Theory, Research and Social Issues.* New York, Holt, Rinehart & Winston, 1976, pp 299–316.
102. Shields D: *Growing Beyond Prejudices.* Mystic, CT, Twenty-third Publications, 1986.
103. Shields D, Bredemeier B: Sport and moral growth: A structural developmental Perspective. In Straub W, Williams J (eds): *Cognitive Sport Psychology.* New York, Sport Science Associates, 1984, pp 89–101.
104. Shields D, Bredemeier B: Moral reasoning, judgment, and action in sport. In Goldstein J (ed): *Sports, Games and Play: Social and Psychological Viewpoints.* ed 2. Hillsdale, NJ, Erlbaum Associates, 1989, pp 59–81.
105. Smith MD: Significant others' influence on the assaultive behavior of young hockey players. *Int Rev Sport Sociol* 3:45–56, 1974.
106. Smith MD: Social learning of violence in minor hockey. In Smoll FL, Smith RE (eds): *Psychological Perspectives in Youth Sport.* Washington D.C., Hemisphere, 1978.
107. Smith MD: Interpersonal sources of violence in hockey: The influence of parents, coaches, and teammates. In Smoll F, Magill R, Ash M (eds): *Children in Sport.* ed 3. Champaign, IL, Human Kinetics, 1988, pp 301–314.
108. Smith RE, Smoll FL, Curtis B: Coach effectiveness training: a cognitive-behavioral approach to enhancing relationship skills in youth sport coaches. *J Sport Psychol* 1:59–75, 1979.

109. Stipek D, MacIver D: Developmental change in children's assessment of intellectual competence. *Child Dev* 60:521–538, 1989,
110. Telander R, Noden M: The death of an athlete. *Sports Illustrated* 70:68–78, 1989.
111. Turiel E: *The Development of Social Knowledge:. Morality and Convention.* New York, Cambridge University Press, 1987.
112. Tutko T, Ogilvie B: Sport: If you want to build character, try something else. *Psychology Today* 5:60–63, 1971.
113. Webb H: Professionalization of attitudes toward play among adolescents. In Kenyon GS (ed): *Aspects of Contemporary Sport Sociology.* Chicago, The Athletic Institute, 1969.
114. Weiss MR, Friedrichs WD: The influence of leader behaviors, coach attributes, and institutional variables on performance on satisfaction of collegiate basketball teams. *J Sport Psychol* 8:332–346, 1986.
115. Westre KR, Weiss MR: The relationship between leadership behaviors and group cohesion in high school football teams. *Res Q Exerc Sport* (submitted for publication).
116. Wiggins DK: A history of organized play and highly competitive sport for American children. In Gould D, Weiss M (eds): *Advances in Pediatric Sport Sciences, Vol. 2: Behavioral Issues.* Champaign, IL, Human Kinetics, 1987, pp 1–24.

13
Effect of Exercise on Depression

T. CHRISTIAN NORTH, Ph.D.
PENNY McCULLAGH, Ph.D
ZUNG VU TRAN, Ph.D.

"Mens sana in corpore sano," "a sound mind in a sound body," was initially espoused by Homer in ancient Greece. The recent development of psychosomatic medicine attests to our modern day belief in Homer's philosophy, and there is currently substantial interest in psychosomatic medicine in using exercise for treating depression [56].

Depression is one of the most common complaints of adults who seek psychotherapy [10], and mood disorders are the most prevalent disorder in western society [79]. In fact, the American Psychiatric Association (see Ref. 4, p. 229) reports that 4.5–9.3% of females and 2.3–3.2% of males in the United States currently have a major depressive disorder. One potential psychosomatic treatment for reducing depression is exercise. However, some recent studies indicate that exercise may be an antidepressant [17, 26, 38, 41, 42] and others have shown no significant effect of exercise on depression [62, 63, 66]. From a clinical perspective, Greist [38], a psychiatrist, suggests that many patients would do better if they used running rather than psychoanalysis to decrease their depression. Greist qualifies this statement by suggesting that running does not resolve an individual's existential problems, but may offer temporary relief (similar to aspirin for a headache).

Previous reviews of the effect of exercise on depression have used the traditional approach, from which only subjective conclusions could be drawn. Therefore, relationships between such variables as exercise mode, length of exercise program, initial depression level, and the effect of exercise on depression are not yet clear. Thus, an objective statistical integration of studies investigating the effects of exercise on depression would help clarify this area of research. The purpose of this chapter is to provide a comprehensive review of the literature on the effect of exercise on depression using both meta-analysis and traditional review methodologies. This chapter presents the meta-analysis data first, followed by a review of proposed mechanisms for the antidepressant effect of exercise.

379

REVIEW OF RELATED LITERATURE

At the time of writing this chapter (June 1989), four published reviews dealing specifically with the effect of exercise on depression had been located [5, 54, 73, 85]. In addition, other reviews were found that were partially devoted to this topic [15, 23, 31, 48, 50, 57, 59, 68, 69, 78]. The following four reviews dealt exclusively with the effect of exercise on depression.

Antonelli [5] in an address to the Italian Federation of Sport Medicine advocated noncompetitive jogging as an antidepressant. In his noncritical selective review he cited mostly anecdotal, but some scientific, evidence to support his claim that running could be used in addition to other therapeutic instruments for treating depression.

A more traditional review on the effects of running on depression was conducted by Weinstein and Meyers [85]. Four categories of depression models were described (psychoanalytic, behavioral, cognitive, and biochemical) and seven research studies were critically reviewed. The authors concluded that "there is little clear evidence to support running as a strategy for modifying depression" (p. 296), but were quick to qualify this conclusion by indicating that most of the research had been poorly designed and executed. Recommendations for future research included adequate experimental controls, improved operationalization of independent and dependent variables, and a process approach to the research.

Simons et al. [73], like Weinstein and Meyers, concluded that many of the early studies examining exercise and depression had been poorly conducted. Their criticisms of early research included lack of good experimental designs and inadequate operationalization of the exercise treatment (i.e., intensity, frequency, and duration), and inadequate assessment of outcomes. These researchers were selective in their choice of studies to review. Only published studies or papers that had been presented using experimental or quasi-experimental designs, employing multisession exercise programs with subjects diagnosed as depressed, were included. All seven studies reviewed provided evidence that exercise was an effective antidepressant. "In fact, the magnitude of changes experienced by exercise treated patients was comparable to that reported by other studies treating similarly selected patients with more standard psychotherapies" (p. 561).

Martinsen [54] was similarly selective in his review examining the role of aerobic exercise in the treatment of depression. Critical of early studies that were poorly designed, Martinsen computer searched Medline and Dialog Information from 1980 to 1986 and located nine multiple-baseline or controlled studies that used depressed subjects to study the exercise-depression relationship. Martinsen presented each study concisely, yet thoroughly described procedures, results, strengths, and weaknesses. In the discussion, Martinsen pointed out that, despite some methodological weaknesses, the results of all studies suggested that aerobic exercise was a beneficial antidepressant that may be as potent as group or individual psychotherapy in treating depression. He recommended that future research compare aerobic and anaerobic exercise, conduct longitudinal studies, and determine the mechanisms that can adequately describe the exercise-depression relationship.

A number of other published reviews were partially dedicated to the effect of exercise on depression. The earliest review by Morgan [59] included 10 articles from 1934 to 1969 but only two studies addressed the relationship between exercise and depression. Both indicated that higher levels of depression were correlated with lower levels of fitness. Morgan noted that these studies were characterized by several weaknesses and made recommendations for improved future research.

The traditional narrative review was used by Ledwidge [50] to evaluate five studies on the effectiveness of chronic exercise in the treatment of mood disorders and presented both psychological and physiological views on how aerobic exercise could act as a remedy for depression. In this review the necessity of having a fitness change to produce a psychological change was noted. Possible mediators of psychological change were discussed such as: ". . . change in daily routine, increased social interaction, weight loss, outdoor recreation, and the overcoming of what is perceived by the subjects as a difficult physical and psychological challenge" (p. 137). The three possible physiological mediators discussed were increased norepinephrine production, a decrease in depressive fatigue in depressed individuals, and an increase in slow-wave sleep. Ledwidge viewed exercise as having value for its psychodynamic properties and suggested that exercise was a valuable psychotherapeutic modality. However, he cautioned that, due to poor experimental designs, no cause and effect relationship could be drawn between exercise and the observed changes in mood. The weakness of this review was that no information was provided on inclusion criteria for the studies reviewed. The strength, on the other hand, was that all studies included had at least one subgroup of depressed subjects.

Browman [15] reviewed the effect of fitness on psychological health in both normal and clinical populations. Although methodological information was not provided, assertions such as "exercise appears to have the greatest effect on personality and mood for borderline normals" were made and referenced by studies supporting this notion. However, because of the lack of information, it is difficult to determine the validity of the statements made. Browman concluded that there was support for the premise that exercise decreases depression in some unipolar and bipolar depressives, but that not all subjects respond favorably to exercise. It was suggested that populations as well as exercise prescription guidelines need to be delineated if exercise is to become a treatment for psychopathology.

A review by Folkins and Sime [31] focused on the internal validity of studies evaluating the effect of exercise on mental health. The portion of the review specifically dedicated to depression was quite short and included one case study, two single group studies, and one experimental study. All studies utilized depressed subjects and suggested that exercise was an effective antidepressant. In their summary of clinical populations, it was suggested that the physical training studies reviewed were merely suggestive of decreases in depression, because the reported improvements could often be attributed to the Hawthorne effect or regression toward the mean.

Ransford [68] made the assumption that exercise has an antidepressant effect and reviewed 12 studies to examine potential mechanisms mediating decreases in depression. Possible mechanisms included: time out (from worrisome responsibilities), social interaction, mastery (accomplishment as the subject becomes fit), physiological changes, and the amine theory. In the conclusion, Ransford advocated a psychobiological approach that included chemical, behavioral, and cognitive factors to explain the effects of exercise on depression.

In a review by Sachs [69] the effects of running and other exercise on anxiety and depression were discussed for three studies with inconsistent results. Despite the discrepant findings, Sachs made the implicit assumption that exercise decreases depression and focused on the potential benefits of aerobic activities to support this notion. Like many other authors, Sachs, with little justification, concluded that exercise is a beneficial psychotherapeutic tool based on "the weight of the anecdotal as well as research evidence" (p. 55).

Hughes [48] provided a critical review of published studies, using experimental designs on the effect of habitual aerobic exercise on mood, personality, and cognition. Over 1100 studies were considered for inclusion in this review and 12 met the inclusion criteria. Only five of these 12 studies included data on depression, and only two conflicting studies were reviewed. One indicated positive benefits from exercise [39] and suggested that exercise may be as beneficial as psychotherapy in reducing mild to moderate levels of depression. The second study [24] reported no significant change on the depression scale of the Minnesota Multiphasic Personality Inventory after a three week exercise program using psychiatric inpatients. In summary of the five studies, Hughes suggested that the findings were discrepant, with one study having all positive outcomes, three studies all negative outcomes, and one study with both positive and negative outcomes. While this review generally provided a good critique of the methods used in studying the effect of exercise on psychological variables and discussed the need to continue to improve methodology, it is unfortunate that the review was limited to published articles since numerous dissertations with good study designs were available on this subject. Hughes concluded that, despite the widely held belief that exercise is an antidepressant, this was not substantiated in the literature.

Mellion [57] reviewed exercise as a therapeutic modality for anxiety and depression but did not provide the criteria for study selection. The three studies he reviewed indicated that exercise was beneficial in decreasing depression, at least for the groups who were initially depressed.

Taylor and colleagues [78] reviewed the positive and negative psychological effects of activity and exercise on mental health. A short review of the effects of exercise on depression was included that reviewed four studies using only depressed subjects. They concluded that there were conflicting findings on the relationship between fitness and depression.

The latest review located [23], addressed the therapeutic effect of physical fitness on a variety of personality measures. The review was restricted to published research, and depression was included as one of the subcategories of personality. Doan and Scherman classified the research into preexperimental, quasi-experimental, and experimental categories and assessed whether psychological variables (one of which was depression) improved or showed no change. Of the 24 preexperimental studies reviewed, none had depression as their focus. Four [17, 26, 49, 64] of the 24 studies reviewed in the quasi-experimental category had depression as their focus and three of the four studies demonstrated decreased depression as a result of exercise. Only one study [56] of the 14 reviewed in the experimental category had depression data, and this study reportedly indicated improvements in depression with exercise. In their concluding remarks, the authors noted a number of problems in the literature and suggested that the type of exercise programs most beneficial in decreasing depression need to be more clearly defined and that fitness gains need to be assessed and documented before the impact of fitness on psychological constructs could be assessed. They also noted the limitations of self-reported psychological concepts as dependent measures.

META-ANALYSIS OF THE EFFECT OF EXERCISE ON DEPRESSION

Understanding the current scientific data on a topic is a requisite for investigators to proceed with future research. Reviews of literature serve to differentiate which hypotheses the literature supports and which remain in question for future research. Given the discrepant findings in this area of research, it is likely that a narrative review of literature would conclude that there were no consistent findings in this body of literature. It would also be difficult for a narrative review to address the effect of independent variables like mode of exercise, subject populations, etc. on depression in these studies. Due to the proliferation of research reports on the effect of exercise on depression in recent years, a method of reviewing that is systematic, quantitative, and replicable would contribute to a more objective view of the effect of exercise on depression research.

Introduction to Meta-analysis

To overcome some of the limitations of a traditional review, Glass [33] developed a methodology for the statistical review of literature. According to Glass et al. [34], the essential characteristic of meta-analysis ". . . is the statistical analysis of the summary findings of many empirical studies" (p. 21). Meta-analysis is a quantitative approach to reviewing research that uses a variety of statistical techniques for sorting, classifying, and summarizing information from the findings of many experimental studies. It is a systematic and replicable procedure that overcomes many of the problems associated with the traditional narrative review.

The purpose of the meta-analysis methodology includes: (*a*) to increase statistical power for primary endpoints and subgroup analysis, (*b*) to resolve conflicts when studies disagree, (*c*) to improve estimates of effect size, and (*d*) to answer questions not posed by authors of individual studies [70].

Meta-analysis Procedures

PROBLEM FORMULATION. As a preface to this present meta-analysis, a pilot meta-analysis was completed, using studies evaluating the effect of exercise on depression. This pilot meta-analysis, based on a random sample of the studies that had been located for potential inclusion, helped refine the research questions and coding sheet used in the present meta-analysis. There were only two criteria for studies to be included in this meta-analysis. First, each study must have had at least one outcome measure of depression related to exercise or fitness; and second, data (published in English) must have been available prior to June 1, 1989. Cross-sectional, longitudinal, published, and unpublished studies were included.

LITERATURE SEARCH. In a meta-analysis, the literature search is analogous to the collection of data in an experimental study. Thus, the search procedures must be explicated to the extent that it could be replicated by other researchers. The literature search is the point in a meta-analysis where the greatest bias may occur. Thus, a thorough description of the search procedures used to locate studies is provided so the reader can determine the representativeness and completeness of the data base.

Initially, approximately 20 current, relevant studies, and one review of literature were read to select key words and determine important characteristics of these studies. Using these key words, an initial search was done on ERIC (Educational Resource Information Center). This search served to identify other key words and additional studies for possible inclusion. The final list of key words were then used to search title, descriptor words, and the abstract (where possible). Computer searches were conducted at the University of Colorado and included studies catalogued up to June 1, 1989. Data bases searched include: Dissertation Abstracts Online, ERIC, PsychINFO, and MESH (Medline). Computer searches, unfortunately, do not locate all pertinent studies. Tran and Weltman [82] indicated that only 35% of the studies included in their meta-analysis were identified through computer searches. Therefore, the search for studies also included the following strategies.

Books were searched through the computerized card catalog of the University of Colorado. A productive strategy was the cross-referencing of studies in the bibliographies of the literature reviews and all previously located studies on the effect of exercise on depression. Abstracts from the annual meetings of the American Psychological Association, American College of Sports Medicine, and the North American Society for the Psychology of Sport and Physical Activity were reviewed for the years 1985–1987. A bibliography of over 1400 articles on the effect of exercise on psychological parameters was obtained from Dr. Michael Sachs (personal communication) and was cross-referenced against studies already on hand. Social Science Citations and Science Citations for the years 1981 through August 1987 (the latest available volume) were hand searched. Also, seven studies that were often referenced in the studies previously obtained were used to locate updated articles in the Social Science Citations and Science Citations Indexes [31, 39–42, 49, 62].

CODING SHEET. The coding sheet included the following types of variables: publication (author, publication date, etc.), subject characteristics (age, gender, health status, etc.), design (level of internal validity, depression scale used, etc.), and exercise treatment (length of program, intensity, and duration of session, etc.).

DEFINITION OF EFFECT SIZE. Every outcome measure found in the studies included in this meta-analysis was transformed into an effect size (ES). The standardized differences between means approach to calculating ES was a logical choice for this meta-analysis because most studies had a baseline and one or more additional measures. Hedge's g [46] was chosen as the preferred ES calculation because it uses a pooled standard deviation $g = (M_1 - M_2)/s_{pooled}$. Pooling was done with the pretest values of groups being compared to increase the standard deviation reliability. Posttests were not used in pooling. On occasions where the data presented in primary research did not permit a direct calculation of ES, data transformation computations were performed using the formulas provided by Glass et al. (see Ref. 34, pp. 93–152). Exceptions were for studies that reported a correlation coefficient between fitness and depression levels. In these cases, ESs were computed using the formula by Cooper (see Ref. 21, p. 101). The initial transformation of data to an effect size is a biased estimator of ES. A correction factor $J(m)$, where $(m = N_E + N_C - 2)$ was used to correct each biased ES to an unbiased ES. This corrected ES was used in the statistical analysis [see Ref. 46, pp. 79–80).

DEFINITION OF DEPRESSION. Depression is a term used for a variety of psychophysiological states. Depression can be a primary psychological disorder, symptomatic of a primary psychological disorder, or it may be a secondary psychological disorder [4]. Classifying depression can be difficult. One method is to distinguish depression as neurotic or psychotic, thus differentiating both a difference in severity of depression, and a separateness in psychiatric illness [20]. The cause of depression is often used in its classification, distinguishing between psychogenous and endogenous types of depression. The former is primarily caused by environmental stress and the latter by biological factors. The most universally accepted classification system of mental disorders has been developed by the American Psychiatric Association [4]. Major forms of depression as the primary illness are classified as mood disorders, or organic mood syndromes. Mood disorders are divided into two major subclassifications, bipolar disorders and depressive disorders, both of which have additional subcategories (see Ref. 4, p. 214). The American Psychiatric Association [4] also lists depression as an associated feature (symptomatic of a primary disorder, or a secondary disorder) of a large variety of other psychiatric disorders including: psychosis, schizophrenia, dementia, some adjustment and anxiety disorders, and bereavement. Depression is ubiquitous as an illness, or a symptom of an illness, in both the psychological and medical literature. The aforementioned differences in definition suggest a lack of universal agreement on how to diagnose, classify, and measure depression. This meta-analysis included all reported forms of depression.

Definition of Exercise

The American College of Sports Medicine defines three types of exercise: (*a*) cardiorespiratory or aerobic endurance, (*b*) muscular strength and endurance, and (*c*) flexibility [3]. In this meta-analysis, the first two categories were considered exercise, because they both require an elevated metabolic rate. Reports of the benefits of exercise are quite encompassing both physiologically and psychologically. Among other potential benefits, there is support in the literature that cardiovascular exercise may: reduce total cholesterol and increase HDL-cholesterol [81]; reduce blood pressure [13] and percentage of body fat [12]; reduce blood sugar in some diabetics [75]; maintain or increase bone mineral density [1]; reduce anxiety [60] and depression [52]; improve the ability to handle stress [22]; and increase the restfulness of sleep [30].

Data Analysis Procedures

PROBLEMS OF INFERENTIAL TESTING. F tests with unequal Ns per cell and multiple comparison techniques are not robust with respect to violations of homogeneity of variance and normality assumptions. Therefore, tests of homogeneity of variance and normality were made. In all cases these assumptions were violated to some degree. Thus, reported p values are on the liberal side. In addition, most inferential tests assume independence of observations. In this meta-analysis, several ESs may have been calculated from a single study, each computed from the same group of subjects. Because the ES was the dependent measure in this meta-analysis, some of the ESs are correlated and therefore, not independent. Because of this correlation, reported p values may be liberal, and reported standard deviations too small.

WEIGHTING OF ES. Because large samples more frequently produce statistically significant findings and more precise estimates than do small samples, some measure of weighting should be incorporated. Precisely what weight to assign to each ES in an aggregation of data is an extremely complex question that can not be answered adequately by giving each ES equal weight regardless of sample size. Because the sampling variance of ES is approximately proportional to the inverse of sample size, the use of sample size to weigh each ES is reasonably close to optimal so this is the procedure chosen for this meta-analysis.

OVERALL RESULTS. A z test was used to determine if the overall mean ES ($\overline{\text{ES}}$) was significantly different from zero. A $\overline{\text{ES}}$ that was significantly different from zero is comparable to rejecting the null hypothesis in an experimental study. A probability level of 0.05 was used to determine statistical significance for all results.

ANALYSIS OF VARIABLES. Each variable is presented individually in a section corresponding to the research question it addresses. Descriptive, inferential, and correlational analyses are presented as appropriate. Descriptive statistics are reported for categories of the variables analyzed and include: the $\overline{\text{ES}}$, standard deviation, number of ESs (N of ESs), and number of studies those ESs came from (N of studies). Pearson correlation coefficients and point-biserial correlation coefficients are reported, where appropriate, to quantify the magnitude and direction of the relationships between independent variables and ES. Where significant correlational relationships were found, r^2 is also reported.

INFERENTIAL ANALYSIS OF CATEGORICAL VARIABLES. One-way or two-way analysis of variance (ANOVA) for categorical variables, with ES as the dependent measure, was used to determine if significant differences existed among categories in variables with two or more levels. To increase statistical power, only categories with seven or more ESs were included in the ANOVAs. The Ω^2 (omega squared) statistic was reported for each significant one-way ANOVA to provide an indication of the magnitude of the relationship between ES and the variable analyzed [45]. Categorical variables have significance of z scores reported for each variable category where appropriate. The z scores indicate whether an $\overline{ES}$ was significantly different from zero and is comparable to rejecting the null hypothesis in an experimental study. When a one-way ANOVA was significant, post hoc, pairwise multiple comparisons were computed using the Newman-Keuls multiple comparison test.

RELIABILITY OF CODING PROCEDURES. Coding of studies was done by one investigator. The reliability of this coding was checked by an independent investigator who calculated eight ESs from six randomly selected studies. The $\overline{ES}$ for the author's and independent investigator's eight ES calculations were −0.64 and −0.65, respectively. The correlation between the two sets of ESs was high ($r = 0.99$).

Research Questions

To assess both the overall effect of exercise on depression and the influence of independent variables, six research questions were proposed. (*a*) Does exercise affect depression level? (*b*) Does the source of subjects influence the outcome of the effect of exercise on depression? (*c*) Do study design, methods employed, or publication variables affect the outcome of exercise on depression studies? (*d*) What subject populations (age, gender, initial level of depression, health status, etc.) decrease depression with exercise? (*e*) What mode and duration of exercise affect depression? (*f*) What is the magnitude of the antidepressant effect of exercise compared with other treatments?

Overall Results and Discussion

Each section of the results addresses one of the research questions investigated in this meta-analysis. Data for 19 variables are reported according to the research question that each variable addresses. Most variables have missing cases due to missing or unclear information from the studies coded or too small a number of ESs in a variable category to be included in the analysis. Each variable is discussed in terms of the data presented and compared to other authors' findings where applicable. Meta-analysis methodology is still a relatively new statistical procedure, so for clarification, the following descriptions of important components of the results are provided. (*a*) A negative mean effect size ($\overline{ES}$) in this meta-analysis indicates that exercise groups decreased depression scores more than comparison groups. For example, a $\overline{ES}$ of −0.50 indicates that subjects in exercise groups decreased their depression scores an average of one-half of a standard deviation unit more than subjects in comparison groups. (*b*) The term "comparison group" is used in this meta-analysis, because all studies of the effect of exercise on depression have been included in this synthesis of studies, regardless of the type of group to which the exercise group was compared. Comparison groups included, control, leisure activity, and psychotherapy groups, among others. The influence of different comparison groups was evaluated and results presented within the variable comparison groups. (*c*) The z scores presented throughout this chapter are measures of how different an $\overline{ES}$ is from zero. An $\overline{ES}$ of zero indicates that the change in depression scores for exercise groups and comparison groups was the same. (*d*) The Ω^2 values reported with all significant one-way ANOVAs were a measure of how much variance was accounted for by the variable being analyzed (analogous to r^2 for correlations). (*e*) To increase the power of the analysis of categorical variables, only categories with seven or more ESs were analyzed. These categorical variables are presented in tables. Categories are listed in order, starting with the largest negative $\overline{ES}$ to the least negative $\overline{ES}$ except with ordinal categorical variables, and these are tabled in the order of the variable categories. (*f*) Only the overall results section includes all ESs in the analysis. In subsequent reporting of variables, all acute exercise ESs were dropped from the analysis, because they were found to be significantly different than ESs from chronic exercise and could confound the results (see overall results). Thus, all analysis presented after the overall results section includes only ESs calculated from exercise programs and follow-up measurements of exercise programs (chronic exercise).

Results and Discussion of: Does Exercise Affect Depression Level?

OVERALL RESULTS. A total of 80 studies met the criteria for inclusion in this meta-analysis and yielded 290 ESs (Table 13.1). Each study provided an average of 3.8 ESs, with a range from 1 to 36 ESs. The overall $\overline{ES}$ was -0.53, which was significantly different from zero. The range of

TABLE 13.1
Overall Effects of Exercise on Depression

	N of ESs	N of Studies	$\overline{ES} \pm SD$
Total data	290	80	-0.53 ± 0.85***
Type of measurement			
Exercise programs	226	76	-0.59 ± 0.89***
Follow-up	38	7	-0.50 ± 0.80***
Single exercise session	26	10	-0.31 ± 0.44***

Mean effect size is significantly different from zero at: *** $p < 0.001$.

ESs was -3.88 to $+2.05$. The $\overline{\text{ES}}$ indicated that in the studies coded, depression scores decreased approximately one-half of a standard deviation more in exercise groups than in comparison groups. Thus, overall, exercise groups received antidepressant benefits from exercise because they decreased depression scores more than comparison groups.

The overall results were categorized to determine if there was a difference between a single exercise session, exercise programs, and follow-up measurements, since these could be quite different. Single exercise session included all measurements of the effect of acute exercise, exercise programs measured the effect of multisession exercise programs, and follow-up measurements were measurements taken after an exercise program had been previously terminated. All three categories were significantly different from zero (Table 13.1) indicating that exercise was a beneficial antidepressant in all three situations. The one-way ANOVA type of measurement was significant ($F_{2,290} = 4.32, p < 0.02, \Omega^2 = 0.02$). Post hoc pairwise comparisons indicated that single exercise session was significantly different from exercise programs, but not different from follow-up.

In this meta-analysis, the effect of exercise on depression was different for acute exercise (single exercise session) and for exercise programs, but both were effective antidepressants. This suggests that the antidepressant effect of exercise may begin in the first session of exercise, contradicting the findings of several studies [14, 63, 83]. The group of 38 ESs in the follow-up category indicate that the effect of exercise may persist beyond the end of exercise programs. The degree that subjects continued to exercise during the follow-up periods was not reported in most of the studies coded, so it is not clear whether continued exercise is necessary for a continued antidepressant effect. However, it is encouraging to identify a method (exercise) of treating depression that apparently has both an immediate and long-term effect.

The overall results indicated that exercise was an effective antidepressant and are consistent with the findings in several previous reviews [31, 54, 59, 68, 69, 78] and contradicted other reviews [48, 85]. However, the overall results included all subject populations, modes of exercise, length of exercise programs, etc. . . , and close inspection of the data presented in this chapter offers some contradictions to several widely accepted beliefs regarding the effects of exercise on depression. Although the overall results indicated that exercise was, in general, an effective antidepressant, it is important to determine how other factors may moderate this overall effect. To accomplish this, the previously stated research questions were examined. Subsequent data reported in this chapter were determined using only ESs calculated from programs and follow-up measurements and do not include single exercise session ESs. This was done to evaluate the effect of chronic exercise on depression.

Results and Discussion of: Does the Source of Subjects Influence the Outcome of the Effect of Exercise on Depression?

SOURCE OF SUBJECTS. There were five sources of subjects analyzed for the studies coded (Table 13.2). A one-way ANOVA of source of subjects with ES indicated that the groups were heterogeneous ($F_{4,238} = 9.66, p < 0.001, \Omega^2 = 0.13$). The variance accounted for by the source of subjects was not high, but considerably greater than most other single variables analyzed in this meta-analysis.

The medical/psychological patients category included ESs from studies using subjects receiving medical and/or psychological treatment and had the largest negative $\overline{ES}$. The post hoc analysis found significant differences between the medical/psychological patient category and all other four categories, indicating that exercise decreased depression more in individuals recruited from medical or psychological facilities than individuals recruited from other locations. These findings support Folkins and Sime [31] who suggested that exercise is most effective as an antidepressant for subjects who are the most physically and psychologically unhealthy at the outset of an exercise program. In summary, the source of subjects influenced the outcome of the studies coded, and subjects receiving medical and/or psychological care demonstrated the greatest decrease in depression with exercise.

Results and Discussion of: Do Study Design, Methods Employed, or Publication Variables Affect the Outcome of Exercise on Depression Studies?

Methodological variables can influence the outcome of a meta-analysis and all meta-analyses should code for methodological weaknesses and make a posteriori rather than a priori decisions about how methodology affects study outcomes [34]. Six variables have been included in this section to address the effects of study design, methods employed, and publication information on the outcome of exercise studies on depression.

FORM OF PUBLICATION. The form of publication was important to analyze, because a previous meta-analysis by Smith [74] found that ESs

TABLE 13.2
Effect Sizes for Source of Subjects

Source of Subjects	N of ESs	N of Studies	$\overline{ES} \pm SD$
Medical/psychological patients	46	21	-0.94 ± 1.16***
High school students	12	3	-0.60 ± 0.93*
Health club members	27	2	-0.49 ± 1.31*
Community citizens	100	20	-0.49 ± 0.60***
College students/faculty	58	20	-0.16 ± 0.60*

Mean effect size is significantly different from zero at: * $p < 0.05$ and *** $p < 0.001$.

from theses and journals were not only significantly different, but also in opposite directions. There were two categories analyzed (Table 13.3). The published category included ESs from published articles and books, and the unpublished category included all unpublished doctoral dissertations and master's theses. A one-way ANOVA of form of publication was significant ($F_{1,265} = 7.30$, $p < 0.01$, $\Omega^2 = 0.02$). The published studies had a significantly larger negative $\overline{\text{ES}}$ than the unpublished studies. In other words, results of published studies showed greater decreases in depression for exercise groups than unpublished studies. These results, like Smith's [74] indicate the importance for reviewers to include unpublished studies to avoid biasing their reviews.

PURPOSE OF EXERCISE. Purpose of exercise had four categories (Table 13.3). The medical rehabilitation category included ESs from studies that used subjects receiving medical care and exercise as part of their treatment (coronary disease, pulmonary disease, kidney failure, and alcohol and drug addiction patients). The psychological rehabilitation category included ESs using exercise as a treatment for psychological problems. The general health category contained all ESs from studies that used subjects that exercised to promote and/or maintain well-being. The academic experiment category included ESs from studies where the only purpose of exercise was to participate in an academic experiment.

All groups significantly decreased depression scores (Table 13.3). A one-way ANOVA was significant ($F_{3,247} = 11.16$, $p < 0.001$, $\Omega^2 = 0.11$). Post hoc pairwise comparisons indicated that the medical rehabilitation category was significantly different from the other three categories, and no other differences were found. The decreased depression of the psychological rehabilitation group supports several previous reviews that

TABLE 13.3

Effect Sizes for Form of Publication, Purpose of Exercise, and Exercise Location

Variable	N of ESs	N of Studies	$\overline{ES}$ ± SD
Form of publication			
Published	131	42	−0.69 ± 0.99***
Unpublished	136	31	−0.37 ± 0.72***
Purpose of exercise			
Medical rehabilitation	44	13	−0.97 ± 1.24***
Academic experiment	9	5	−0.67 ± 0.44***
Psychological rehabilitation	65	15	−0.55 ± 0.76***
General Health	133	31	−0.29 ± 0.56***
Exercise location			
Home	9	3	−1.34 ± 1.63**
Medical facility	26	15	−0.68 ± 0.80***
Community center	60	8	−0.68 ± 0.68***
University/college	115	29	−0.24 ± 0.88**

Mean effect size is significantly different from zero at: ** $p < 0.01$ and *** $p < 0.001$.

have indicated that exercise is an antidepressant for subjects in need of psychotherapy to treat depression [15, 31, 50, 57, 73, 78]. Subjects in medical rehabilitation have received very little attention in most reviews and individual studies. Only one previous review has addressed the medical rehabilitation population [78] and indicated that the effect of exercise on depression in postmyocardial infarction patients was not clear. However, in this meta-analysis, the medical rehabilitation group decreased depression with exercise more than any other group. Medications were not addressed in most of the studies coded and are not accounted for in this meta-analysis, which may confound the medical rehabilitation and psychological rehabilitation results. Because depression is a common secondary symptom of individuals with physical disease, exercise may prove to be a cost-effective means to provide both physical and psychological rehabilitation for individuals with physical illness.

EXERCISE LOCATION. Exercise location was analyzed to determine if exercising in different environments influenced the outcome of the effect of exercise on depression. Exercise took place in four types of locations (Table 13.3). The one-way ANOVA with ES was significant ($F_{3,206} = 4.14$, $p < 0.01$, $\Omega^2 = 0.04$). Post hoc pairwise comparisons indicated that the home category was significantly different from the community center and university/college categories. Thus, exercising at home led to a greater decrease in depression than exercising in a university/college or community center setting. No other significant pairwise differences were found.

In this meta-analysis, exercise significantly decreased depression regardless of exercise location. The reason for the significant difference between the home and both the community center and university/college categories was not clear. The nine ESs in the home category were from only three studies, so the results need to be interpreted cautiously. Seven of the nine ESs in this category used subjects with a purpose of exercise being medical rehabilitation. The medical rehabilitation group had the largest negative $\overline{\text{ES}}$ in the variable purpose of exercise. A two-way ANOVA of exercise location and purpose of exercise with ES as the dependent measure found a significant main effect for exercise location ($F_{3,199} = 4.13$, $p < 0.001$), a significant main effect for purpose of exercise ($F_{3,199} = 7.19$, $p < 0.001$), but no significant interaction ($F_{4,199} = 0.80$, $p > 0.05$).

GROUP ASSIGNMENT. One of the criticisms of meta-analysis has been the combining of studies that have good internal validity with studies that do not [27]. Two variables (group assignment and degree of internal validity) were coded to evaluate the effect of the quality of experimental design on the outcome of the effect of exercise on depression studies. Six categories of group assignment were analyzed (Table 13.4).

All z scores were significantly different from zero, indicating that exercise groups lowered depression scores significantly more than compari-

TABLE 13.4
Effect Sizes for Group Assignment and Degree of Internal Validity

Variable	N of ESs	N of Studies	$\overline{ES} \pm SD$
Group assignment			
Random assignment	110	27	-1.30 ± 1.11***
Cross-sectional study	11	6	-0.71 ± 0.45***
Convenient groups	11	6	-0.43 ± 0.64*
Matching groups	42	5	-0.41 ± 0.51***
One group Pre-Post	9	4	-0.30 ± 0.34**
Self-selected groups	75	20	-0.27 ± 0.74***
Degree of internal validity			
High	60	11	-0.47 ± 1.14***
Medium	62	20	-0.94 ± 1.02***
Low	139	41	-0.34 ± 0.63***

Mean effect size is significantly different from zero at: * $p < 0.05$, ** $p < 0.01$, and *** $p < 0.001$.

son groups across all categories of group assignment. The one-way ANOVA was significant ($F_{5,252} = 2.63$, $p < 0.05$, $\Omega^2 = 0.03$) but no significant post hoc pairwise differences were found. Previous reviewers have been critical of the methods used for studies investigating the effect of exercise on depression [31, 48, 50, 59, 73, 85]. However, in this meta-analysis, group assignment had no differential effect on the outcome of exercise on depression level.

DEGREE OF INTERNAL VALIDITY. The variable degree of internal validity also addressed the quality of experimental design. Internal validity scores were determined according to the methods suggested by Glass et al. (see Ref. 34, p. 83) with high, medium, and low categories. All $\overline{ES}$s were significantly different from zero (Table 13.4). A one-way ANOVA of internal validity was significant ($F_{2,258} = 4.97$, $p < 0.01$, $\Omega^2 = 0.03$). Post hoc comparisons indicated that the medium category had a significantly larger negative $\overline{ES}$ than both the high and low categories. The Pearson correlation coefficient for internal validity with ES was not significant ($N = 261$, $r = -0.08$, $p > 0.05$). To determine if degree of internal validity was affected by whether a study was published or unpublished, a two-way ANOVA of the degree of internal validity with published versus unpublished, with ES as the dependent measure, was computed. There was a significant main effect for degree of internal validity ($F_{2,255} = 4.10$, $p < 0.05$), a significant main effect of published versus unpublished ($F_{1,255} = 5.11$, $p < 0.05$) but no significant interaction ($F_{2,255} = 2.13$, $p > 0.05$). The two-way ANOVA was used to determine if there was any relationship between the quality of design of studies and whether the study had been published. Because all of the unpublished studies in this meta-analysis were from dissertations or theses, it justifies the importance of including them. In this meta-analysis, exercise decreased depression regardless of the degree of internal validity of the study design. This finding may help allay the concerns pointed out by authors who have suggested that readers interpret the studies on exercise and depression cautiously because of poor study design [15, 31, 48, 73].

STATE VERSUS TRAIT MEASUREMENTS. Evaluating the effect of state and trait measurement scales on the outcome of exercise on depression studies is important. State scales reflect subjects' affect at that point in time, and trait scales reflect subjects' more enduring personality traits. Folkins and Sime [31] have suggested that exercise studies do not demonstrate global personality trait changes. A one-way ANOVA was not significant ($F_{1,251} = 2.13$, $p > 0.05$). Because trait scores are likely to change more slowly than state scores, a two-way ANOVA of state versus trait measurements and length of exercise program, with ES as the dependent measure, was computed. There was a nonsignificant main effect for state versus trait ($F_{1,216} = 0.32$, $p > 0.05$), the main effect for length of exercise program was significant ($F_{6,216} = 12.65$, $p < 0.001$), and no two-way interaction was found ($F_{3,216} = 0.11$, $p > 0.05$). The lack of interaction needs cautious interpretation because of the low number of ESs in some of the cells for analysis (Table 13.5).

Only 11% of the total number of ESs used a trait scale. Trait measurements were used primarily on middle-aged subjects (who had the largest negative $\overline{ES}$ in the variable age category) so a two-way ANOVA was performed to determine if there was an interaction between state versus trait measurements and age category, using ES as the dependent measure. The main effect for state versus trait measurements was not significant ($F_{1,214} = 1.37$, $p > 0.05$), the main effect of age category was significant ($F_{2,214} = 4.00$, $p < 0.05$), and there was no significant interaction ($F_{1,214} = 0.16$, $p > 0.05$). In this meta-analysis, ESs using trait scales had as large a negative mean value as ESs using state scales. The two-way ANOVAs performed were not able to explain this finding. The data suggest that in the studies coded, exercise changed depression as a personality trait, as well as a temporary mood state, contradicting two previous reviews [15, 31]. No interactions were found between state and trait measures and length of exercise program, or age category. Future studies with serial comparisons using both state and trait depression scales simultaneously may be able to provide insight into any interaction that may exist between state and trait depression changes and length of exercise programs.

TABLE 13.5
Effect Sizes for State versus Trait Measurements

State vs. Trait	N of ESs	N of Studies	$\overline{ES} \pm SD$
Trait	27	16	-0.91 ± 0.83***
State	226	59	-0.45 ± 0.90***

Mean effect size is significantly different from zero at: *** $p < 0.001$.

Results and Discussion of: What Subject Populations Decrease Depression with Exercise?

Determining who (what subject populations) can decrease depression with exercise was addressed by analyzing the seven variables discussed in this section.

MEAN AGE AND AGE CATEGORY. The age of subjects from the ESs analyzed ranged from 11 to 55 years. The mean age for all ESs was 31.8 ± 12.4 years. A significant, negative correlational relationship was found between mean age and ES ($N = 170$, $r = -0.16$, $p < 0.05$). A negative relationship suggests that the older the subjects, the greater the decrease in depression with exercise. Age category was coded, because many studies did not provide a mean age, but did provide enough information to determine the age category of study subjects (Table 13.6). The z scores indicate that exercise significantly decreased depression across all age categories. The one-way ANOVA was significant ($F_{2,230} = 3.83$, $p < 0.003$, $\Omega^2 = 0.02$); however, no significant post hoc differences were found. In this meta-analysis, exercise significantly decreased depression in all age groups analyzed; unfortunately, there were not enough data on the elderly population to include in the analysis.

GENDER. Gender included the ESs from studies that used either 100% male, or 100% female subjects (Table 13.6). The $\overline{ES}$s for males and females were not significantly different ($F_{1,133} = 0.20$, $p > 0.05$). These data suggest that exercise was an equally effective antidepressant for both genders.

HEALTH STATUS. Health status was analyzed to help determine which subject populations benefit from exercise as an antidepressant (Table 13.7).

Mean ESs ranged from -2.31 for the hemodialysis category, to -0.29 for the apparently healthy category (Table 13.7). Mean ESs of all categories of health status were significantly different from zero, indicating that exercise was an effective antidepressant for all groups analyzed. A one-way ANOVA was significant ($F_{6,245} = 9.75$, $p < 0.001$, $\Omega^2 = 0.17$). Post hoc pairwise comparisons of means indicated that the hemodialysis

TABLE 13.6
Effect Sizes for Age Category and Gender

Variable	N of ESs	N of Studies	$\overline{ES} \pm SD$
Age category			
Middle aged (25–64 years)	161	41	-0.74 ± 0.95***
College (18–24 years)	55	17	-0.23 ± 0.62**
Young (<18 years)	17	5	-0.49 ± 0.78*
Gender			
Males	53	20	-0.82 ± 1.09***
Females	82	16	-0.45 ± 0.86***

Mean effect size is significantly different from zero at: * $p < 0.05$, ** $p < 0.01$, and *** $p < 0.001$.

TABLE 13.7
Effect Sizes for Health Status and Healthy and Unhealthy Subjects

Variable	N of ESs	N of Studies	$\overline{ES} \pm SD$
Health status			
Hemodialysis patient	7	3	-2.31 ± 1.02***
Schizophrenic	7	1	-1.43 ± 1.07***[a]
Postmyocardial infarction	19	7	-0.95 ± 1.28***[a]
Depressed	100	21	-0.55 ± 0.90***[a,b]
Athlete	7	6	-0.42 ± 0.33***[a,b]
Feeling down	18	1	-0.36 ± 0.43***[a,b]
Apparently healthy	94	33	-0.29 ± 0.62***[a,b]
Healthy and unhealthy subjects			
Under medical treatment	26	9	-0.97 ± 1.32***
Requiring psychological treatment	132	27	-0.60 ± 0.87***
Apparently healthy	105	40	-0.31 ± 0.60***

Mean effect size is significantly different from zero at: *** $p < 0.001$.
[a] Significantly different from hemodialysis patient ($p < 0.05$).
[b] Significantly different from postmyocardial infarction ($p < 0.05$).

category was significantly different from all other groups; schizophrenic was significantly different from depressed, athlete, feeling down, and apparently healthy groups; and the postmyocardial infarction group was significantly different from the feeling down and the apparently healthy groups.

The subjects in the postmyocardial infarction category showed a large decrease in depression with exercise, contradicting several individual studies [55, 64, 76, 77] and a review [78] that suggested that the antidepressant effect of exercise is not clearly documented in postmyocardial infarction patients. However, these data are in agreement with Kavanaugh et al. [49] who found a significant reduction in depression in postmyocardial infarction patients who participated in a 4-year running program.

The data in this meta-analysis suggest that exercise substantially reduced depression in all the health status categories analyzed. Health status had one of the largest Ω^2 values in this meta-analysis, indicating that the health of the population being studied accounted for more of the variance than most of the other variables coded. This meta-analysis of studies suggests that apparently healthy subjects significantly decreased depression scores with exercise, contrary to some previous research [31, 62, 73], but in agreement with the findings of Folkins et al. [30]. The effect of the initial level of subjects' health is analyzed further in the next two variables.

HEALTHY AND UNHEALTHY SUBJECTS. The variable healthy and unhealthy subjects had three categories, apparently healthy subjects, subjects under medical treatment, and subjects requiring psychological treatment (Table 13.7). This variable was analyzed to determine if there was a difference in the response to exercise in these three subject populations. The subjects under medical treatment group consisted of ESs from studies that used medical rehabilitation patients as subjects (post-myocardial infarction, high cardiovascular risk, pulmonary, and hemo-dialysis patients). The category of subjects requiring psychological treatment was ES from studies using subjects who had been identified in need of psychotherapy or were requesting help for mood problems. The apparently healthy group included all ESs from studies that used subjects who were generally healthy and not in need of either medical rehabilitation or psychotherapy (like subjects exercising for general health, athletes, etc.).

All three $\overline{ES}$s were significantly different from zero. The one-way ANOVA was significant ($F_{2,260} = 17.15$, $p < 0.001$, $\Omega^2 = 0.11$). Post hoc pairwise comparisons indicated that the medical group was significantly different from both the healthy and psychological groups, but there was no significant difference between the psychological and healthy groups. Some studies and reviews have stated that exercise may only help decrease depression in subjects that are already depressed [31, 62, 73]. These results indicate that all three groups decreased depression with exercise and the apparently healthy population decreased depression with exercise to a similar extent as subjects seeking psychotherapy, but less than subjects receiving medical treatment.

INITIAL DEPRESSION LEVEL. Initial depression level is a dichotomous variable that was analyzed to evaluate the antidepressant effect of exercise on subjects who were initially depressed and nondepressed (Table 13.8). Browman [15] has stated that there is a relationship between the initial level of anxiety or depression, and the amount of change in depression with exercise. In a similar vein, Simons et al. [73] have suggested that clinically depressed populations can decrease depression with exercise, but evidence in nonclinical populations needs clarification.

Both the depressed and nondepressed categories were significantly different from zero and no significant difference was found between

TABLE 13.8
Effect Sizes for Initial Depression Level and Depression Category

Variable	N of ESs	N of Studies	$\overline{ES} \pm SD$
Initial depression level			
Nondepressed	143	53	-0.59 ± 0.91***
Depressed	120	22	-0.53 ± 0.84***
Depression category			
Reactive	3	2	-0.67 ± 0.65*
Situational	2	2	-0.75 ± 0.03***
Major	1	1	-0.61
Unipolar	14	2	-0.60 ± 0.83**
Dysphoric	1	1	-0.10

Mean effect size is significantly different from zero at: * $p < 0.05$, ** $p < 0.01$, and *** $p < 0.001$.

these categories ($F_{1,261} = 1.22$, $p > 0.05$). In this meta-analysis, ES was not related to the initial depression level, and both subjects who were initially depressed and nondepressed decreased depression with exercise, contradicting statements of several authors who have indicated that exercise may be useful only in decreasing depression in subjects who are initially depressed [31, 62, 73].

DEPRESSION CATEGORY. Depression category was included on the coding sheet in an attempt to determine how subjects with different depression diagnoses were affected by exercise. Exercise has been stated to be beneficial to individuals who are mildly or moderately depressed [15, 50, 57]. Depression categories were determined by the classification provided by the author(s) of each coded study. A total of 21 ESs from eight studies had depression category coded (Table 13.8). The three categories that had more than one ES were significantly different from zero. Thus, in the studies coded, exercise was an effective antidepressant for subjects diagnosed with unipolar, reactive, and situational depression. Because there are so few studies using subjects with diagnosed depression, additional studies are needed to clarify how exercise effects depression in each diagnostic group.

Results and Discussion of: What Mode and Duration of Exercise Affect Depression?

To evaluate the effect of mode and duration of exercise programs on depression, three variables were analyzed and their results are presented.

PRIMARY MODE OF EXERCISE. Five categories of primary mode of exercise were coded (Table 13.9). The various aerobic categories included ESs from studies where subjects used a variety of forms of aerobic activity like jogging and swimming rather than just one aerobic activity.

Walk and/or jog and jogging were the most frequent forms of exercise treatments in the studies coded. The z scores indicate that all modes of exercise analyzed were effective antidepressants. The one-way ANOVA of primary mode of exercise was significant ($F_{4,224} = 3.59$, $p < 0.01$, $\Omega^2 = $

TABLE 13.9
Effect Sizes for Primary Mode of Exercise

Primary Exercise	*N of ESs*	*N of Studies*	$\overline{ES} \pm SD$
Weight training	7	2	-1.78 ± 0.82***
Various aerobic	54	18	-0.67 ± 1.22***
Walk and/or jog	89	24	-0.55 ± 0.92***
Aerobic class	13	7	-0.56 ± 0.74**
Jogging	66	15	-0.48 ± 0.38***

Mean effect size is significantly different from zero at: ** $p < 0.01$ and *** $p < 0.001$.

0.04). Multiple comparisons found weight training significantly different from all the other groups. Most authors have suggested that aerobic, and not necessarily anaerobic, exercise decreases depression [5, 31, 69]. There was a sufficient number of ESs from studies using aerobic forms of exercise to suggest that aerobic exercise in general was an effective antidepressant. This finding is consistent with Sachs [69] who suggested that all exercises that are vigorous, uninterrupted for a period of time, and require less cognitive focus and decision making than daily life may be useful psychotherapeutic forms of exercise. However, the data in this meta-analysis suggest that anaerobic exercise was also an effective antidepressant. Thus, anaerobic exercise may also be psychotherapeutic. Additional research is needed before strong generalizations can be made regarding the effect of anaerobic exercise on depression.

LENGTH OF EXERCISE PROGRAM. The variable length of exercise program was divided into 4-week categories (Table 13.10). The z scores indicated that exercise was an effective antidepressant across all categories. The one-way ANOVA of length of exercise program with ES was significant ($F_{6,230} = 13.41, p < 0.001, \Omega^2 = 0.24$) and accounted for 24% of the total variance. There was a wide range of $\overline{ES}$s. The largest negative $\overline{ES}$ was at 21–24 weeks (−2.93) and the least negative ES value was at less than or equal to 4-weeks of exercise (−0.11). A post hoc pairwise comparison found 11 significant pairwise differences between means. The relationship between length of exercise program and ES is depicted in Figure 13.1.

In this integration of studies, the variable length of exercise program accounted for more of the total variance according to the Ω^2 value than any other variable analyzed. The relationship between the length of exercise program and the effect of exercise on depression level has rarely been discussed in previous reviews. Simons et al. [73] discussed the length of exercise programs in regard to the time it takes to demon-

TABLE 13.10
Effect Sizes for Length of Exercise Program

Length in Weeks	N of ESs	N of Studies	$\overline{ES} \pm SD$
>24	11	6	−2.00 ± 1.11***[b]
21–24	4	1	−2.93 ± 0.91***
17–20	6	1	−0.97 ± 0.44***[a,b]
13–16	7	6	−0.41 ± 0.39**[a,b]
9–12	94	22	−0.31 ± 0.84***[a,b]
5–8	104	22	−0.30 ± 0.71***[a,b]
≤4	11	4	−0.11 ± 1.17***[a,b]

Mean effect size is significantly different from zero at: ** $p < 0.01$ and *** $p < 0.001$.
[a] Significantly different from >24 weeks ($p < 0.05$).
[b] Significantly different from 21–24 weeks ($p < 0.05$).

FIGURE 13.1

The relationship between length of exercise program and effect size.

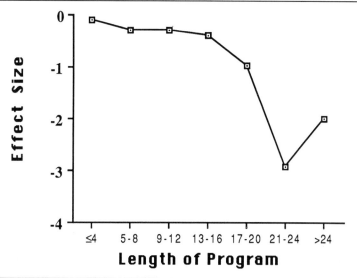

Length of Program

strate a change in cardiovascular conditioning, but not in terms of the optimal length to decrease depression. In this meta-analysis of studies, all lengths of programs significantly decreased depression, the total length of exercise programs influenced the amount of depression change, and the greatest decreases in depression were seen in programs of 17 weeks or longer.

TOTAL NUMBER OF EXERCISE SESSIONS. The variable total number of exercise sessions quantifies the total number of exercise sessions that was recommended by the research investigators that their subjects participate in during the exercise program. The mean total number of exercise sessions was 30.0 ± 34.6 with a range of 3 to 468 sessions. A significant correlational relationship was found ($N = 204$, $r = -0.27$, $p < 0.001$, $r^2 = 0.07$) between total number of exercise sessions and ES. There was one data outlier (greater than 3 standard deviations above the mean). When this outlier was dropped from the analysis, the correlation improved ($N = 203$, $r = -0.33$, $p < 0.001$, $r^2 = 0.11$). These data, like the variable length of exercise program, suggest that the longer the exercise program and greater the total number of exercise sessions, the greater the decrease in depression with exercise.

INTENSITY, FREQUENCY, AND TIME PER SESSION. Intensity of exercise was coded; however, insufficient data were found to include in the analysis. The number of times exercise was performed per week, and the length of exercise session were both found to have no influence on ES.

Results and Discussion of: What Is the Magnitude of the Antidepressant Effect of Exercise Compared with Other Treatments?

COMPARISON GROUP. The variable comparison group was analyzed to evaluate the magnitude of the antidepressant effect of exercise compared with other treatments as well as nontreatments. Eight categories were analyzed (Table 13.11) and the following is a description of these groups. The no treatment group received no treatment (the traditional control group in an experimental study); waiting list subjects were waiting to receive an antidepressant treatment; the less run/exercise comparison group participated in less exercise or running than the exercise treatment group; the relaxation group participated in relaxation therapy; the enjoyable activity ESs were from studies where subjects participated in a nonexercise activity of their choice; the psychotherapy group received psychological counseling; the anaerobic comparison group was a special situation where the two treatment groups both exercised, one aerobically and the other anaerobically (the aerobic group was coded as the exercise group and the anaerobic group was coded as the comparison group); the exercise plus psychotherapy group received both exercise and psychotherapy treatments. The z scores indicate that all comparison group categories were significantly different from zero except psychotherapy and anaerobic exercise. This suggests that exercise was as effective an antidepressant as psychotherapy and that anaerobic exercise was as effective in reducing depression as aerobic exercise. The exercise plus psychotherapy category had a significantly positive $\overline{ES}$ indicating that exercise was not as effective an antidepressant as exercise plus psychotherapy. In other words, exercise plus psychotherapy was a better antidepressant than exercise alone. The one-way ANOVA of comparison group was significant ($F_{7,168} = 8.44$, $p < 0.001$, $\Omega^2 = 0.23$). Post hoc pairwise comparisons revealed 12 pairs of significantly different $\overline{ES}$s.

TABLE 13.11
Effect Sizes for Comparison Group

Comparison Group	N of ESs	N of Studies	$\overline{ES} \pm SD$
No treatment	43	24	-0.71 ± 1.03***[a,b]
Waiting list	32	6	-0.54 ± 0.91***[a,b]
Less run/exercise	9	7	-0.29 ± 0.46***[a,b]
Relaxation	9	4	-0.50 ± 1.15[a,b]
Enjoyable activity	27	9	-0.39 ± 0.55***[a,b]
Psychotherapy	35	11	-0.19 ± 0.71[a,b]
Anaerobic exercise	14	2	$+0.20 \pm 0.67$
Exercise + psychotherapy	7	3	$+0.81 \pm 0.57$***

Mean effect size is significantly different from zero at: *** $p < 0.001$.
[a] Significantly different from anaerobic exercise.
[b] Significantly different from exercise + psychotherapy.

The first two categories, no treatment and waiting list, are control group categories. The z scores indicate that, when an exercise treatment was compared with a control group that was not receiving any treatment, exercise was an effective antidepressant. This finding is in agreement with most previous reviews [31, 54, 59, 68, 69, 78] but contradicts others [48, 85]. The less run/exercise category suggests that in the seven studies coded comparing an exercise group to an easier exercise group, the easier exercise was not as effective an antidepressant. This finding suggests that there may be an optimal level of physical activity to reduce depression. In this meta-analysis, exercise and relaxation were equally effective antidepressants. However, this finding must be viewed with caution due to the small number of ESs and studies in the relaxation category. One of the proposed mechanisms of the antidepressant effect of exercise is the time out/distraction hypothesis that states that distraction from daily worries may be the antidepressant agent, not exercise itself. The data in the enjoyable activity category indicate that exercise was a significantly better antidepressant than enjoyable activities and do not support this hypothesis.

Most studies that have evaluated the effect of exercise on depression have used aerobic activity for the exercise treatment. The 14 ESs from the two studies that used anaerobic exercise as the comparison group indicate that anaerobic exercise was at least as good of an antidepressant as aerobic exercise. Additional studies using anaerobic exercise are needed to determine the reliability of these findings.

The results comparing exercise with psychotherapy indicate that, in the studies coded, exercise was as good an antidepressant treatment as psychotherapy and is in agreement with the study by Greist et al. [41] and the review by Simons et al. [73]. However, additional data are needed to clarify this comparison.

When exercise and psychotherapy were combined as co-treatments these co-treatments decreased depression significantly more than exercise alone. These results are consistent with Simons et al. [73], who proposed that exercise may potentiate the outcome of psychotherapy in reducing depression, and Ledwidge [50], who suggested that exercise has an antidepressant effect, and would be well utilized as an adjunct to psychotherapy. The results of exercise plus psychotherapy suggest that an additive effect of treatments may exist. Due to the small number of studies available, additional data are needed to clarify how exercise and exercise plus psychotherapy, compare with psychotherapy as antidepressant treatments.

Meta-analysis Conclusions

DOES EXERCISE AFFECT DEPRESSION LEVEL? The overall results of this meta-analysis indicate that, in the studies coded, both acute and chronic exercise significantly decreased depression, and the antidepressant effect continued through follow-up measures.

DOES THE SOURCE OF SUBJECTS INFLUENCE THE OUTCOME OF EXERCISE ON DEPRESSION? All source of subject groups decreased depression with exercise, and subjects requiring medical or psychological care demonstrated the largest decreases. This variable accounted for a relatively substantial amount of the variance in this meta-analysis.

DO STUDY DESIGN, METHODS EMPLOYED, OR PUBLICATION VARIABLES AFFECT THE OUTCOME OF EXERCISE ON DEPRESSION STUDIES? Six variables were analyzed to address the above question: form of publication, purpose of exercise, exercise location, group assignment, degree of internal validity, and state versus trait measurements. Published studies reported a significantly larger decrease in depression than unpublished studies. Medical rehabilitation subjects demonstrated a greater decrease in depression than did other groups in the purpose of exercise category. The degree of internal validity affected the outcome of the studies included. Both state and trait depression scores decreased with exercise.

WHAT SUBJECT POPULATIONS DECREASE DEPRESSION WITH EXERCISE? Subjects from most of the populations coded demonstrated decreased depression with exercise including: all age groups, both males and females, subjects in all categories of health status, apparently healthy subjects, subjects involved in medical or psychological rehabilitation, subjects who were initially depressed, and those who were not depressed.

WHAT MODE AND DURATION OF EXERCISE AFFECT DEPRESSION? In this meta-analysis, all modes of exercise were effective antidepressants including anaerobic exercise. The longer the exercise program and the greater the total number of exercise sessions, the larger the decrease in depression.

WHAT IS THE MAGNITUDE OF THE ANTIDEPRESSANT EFFECT OF EXERCISE COMPARED WITH OTHER TREATMENTS? Exercise was a better antidepressant than relaxation and enjoyable activities. Exercise was as effective in decreasing depression as was psychotherapy. Anaerobic exercise was as potent an antidepressant as aerobic exercise. Exercise plus psychotherapy was better than exercise alone in reducing depression.

REVIEW OF PROPOSED MECHANISMS OF THE ANTIDEPRESSANT EFFECT OF EXERCISE

Because the meta-analysis data presented in this chapter indicate that both acute and chronic exercise is associated with an antidepressant effect, it is important to evaluate what the antidepressant mechanism(s) associated with exercise may be. The antidepressant effect of exercise is most likely mediated by psychological and/or physiological/biochemical mechanisms. This section of the chapter reviews previously proposed psychological and physiological/biochemical mechanisms that could explain all, or a portion, of the antidepressant effect of exercise using traditional review methodologies.

Proposed Psychological Mechanisms of the Antidepressant Effect of Exercise

COGNITIVE-BEHAVIORAL HYPOTHESIS. One of the most frequently proposed mechanisms for the antidepressant effect of exercise is the positive cognitive-behavioral change subjects often experience with exercise [42, 48, 68, 86]. The proposed cognitive-behavioral mechanism of the antidepressant effect of exercise is consistent with the negative-cognitive set model of depression originally proposed by Beck [9]. Beck's model [9] has three main theoretical components: (*a*) the presence of automatic negative thoughts, (*b*) the presence of systematic logical errors, and (*c*) the presence of depressogenic schemata. Simons et al. [73] have proposed that exercise releases positive thoughts and feelings. If this is true, then these feelings could break the downward thought-affect spiral that characterizes Beck's model of depression. Weinstein and Meyers [85] suggested that exercise may account for decreases in depression level due to an interaction between changes in overt behavior and changes in cognitive process. They suggest that running in particular may catalyze a transformation, or interruption, in a maladaptive cognitive set. A change in maladaptive cognitive set would break Beck's downward thought-affect spiral that causes depression.

There are a variety of related components that may mediate the cognitive-behavioral mechanism, including mastery of a difficult skill [7, 41, 42, 48, 85], increased self-efficacy [26], feeling successful [41, 72], and increased internal locus of control [26, 72]. One of the most prominent theories of behavior change is Bandura's self-efficacy theory [7]. Bandura's work has suggested that individuals who master something that they perceive as difficult, experience a positive change in their psychological state that leads to increased self-confidence, self efficacy, and ability to cope with personal problems. Because exercise is usually perceived as a difficult task for individuals who have not been regular exercisers, becoming a regular exerciser would likely lead to an enhanced positive affect. All of the proposed components of the cognitive-behavioral hypothesis would help break the downward thought-affect spiral Beck has associated with causing depression and this is a viable hypothesis, especially for chronic exercise.

SOCIAL INTERACTION HYPOTHESIS. Social group interaction, pleasure, or the personal attention subjects receive while exercising could account for the antidepressant effect of exercise [26, 68]. The meta-analysis data presented in this chapter, however, do not support the social interaction hypothesis as the only mediator of the antidepressant effect of exercise, a result that is in agreement with the findings of Brown et al. [17]. The data in this meta-analysis indicate that exercise was a significantly better antidepressant than enjoyable activities, and these activities were primarily group activities. Additionally, the meta-analysis data indicate that subjects who exercised alone at home demonstrated larger decreases in depression than subjects exercising at other treatment locations (usually in groups). This finding is contradictory to the finding of Heinzelman and Bagley [47] who reported that 90% of a sample of 195 exercisers stated that they either preferred, or would have preferred, exercising with others. However, the meta-analysis data do not adequately address the issue of exercise location. It may be that social interaction is more important at the beginning of an exercise program (because it is an external motivator), and the social interaction effect may diminish as the rewards of exercise become internalized. Additional research is needed to determine the role social interaction plays in the antidepressant effect of exercise and if an interaction exists between the length of exercise program and social interaction with depression level.

TIME OUT/DISTRACTION HYPOTHESIS. Sachs [69] proposed that distraction from daily worries could account for the antidepressant effect of exercise. Similarly, Bahrke and Morgan [6] hypothesized that the psychological benefits associated with exercise may be the result of subjects being distracted from their psychological stress. Greist et al. [41] have stated that the physical stress induced by running may temporarily interrupt ruminating over one's worries and problems and have also stated that subjects who run perceive an alteration of consciousness.

The results of the meta-analysis in this chapter generally do not support the time out/distraction hypothesis. In this meta-analysis, exercise decreased depression more than relaxation (time out) or enjoyable activities (distraction). Thus, chronic exercise may be a more effective long-term antidepressant than habitual relaxation. The time out/distraction hypothesis is generally not supported by the findings in the meta-analysis for chronic exercise, but could account for at least a portion of the antidepressant effect of acute exercise.

Proposed Physiological/Biochemical Mechanisms of the Antidepressant Effect of Exercise

CARDIOVASCULAR FITNESS HYPOTHESIS. The antidepressant effect of exercise could be mediated by cardiovascular (aerobic) fitness level. This hypothesis has been proposed ever since a negative correlational relationship was found between aerobic fitness level and depression [58]. However, several studies have noted that the antidepressant effect of exercise takes place within the first few weeks of treatment, prior to subjects experiencing a substantial change in cardiovascular fitness level

[25, 32, 56]. This meta-analysis found significant decreases in depression as the result of a single exercise session, and after only 4 and 6 weeks of exercise. The American College of Sports Medicine [3] recommends a minimum of 15–20 weeks of aerobic conditioning to demonstrate a significant change in cardiovascular fitness. Thus, significant depression level changes probably occur prior to significant changes in cardiovascular fitness. Additionally, in this meta-analysis, anaerobic forms of exercise decreased depression the same or more than aerobic forms of exercise, even though anaerobic forms of exercise are not normally recommended for increasing cardiovascular fitness [3].

The data in this meta-analysis do not indicate that aerobic fitness level is the sole mediator (mechanism) of depression level change with exercise, because depression change occurred more quickly than aerobic fitness improvement could occur. However, both the length of the exercise program and the total number of exercise sessions had significant correlational relationships with ES, indicating that the longer the subjects were involved in exercise programs the greater the decrease in depression. This relationship indicates that cardiovascular fitness level may mediate a portion of the antidepressant effect of exercise, but some other physiological/biochemical or psychological factor must also account for the short-term antidepressant effect.

AMINE HYPOTHESIS. Three monoamine neurotransmitters, serotonin [8], dopamine [51], and norepinephrine [18, 71], have been suggested to possibly have roles in the antidepressant effect of exercise. Evidence indicates that depressed individuals have decreased secretion of amine metabolites [29]. Current, effective, somatic treatments for depression include tricyclic antidepressants, monoamine oxidase inhibitors and electroconvulsive therapy, all of which increase aminergic transmission [35–37]. It has also been found that chronically exercised rats have improved emotionality [80, 84] and levels of brain norepinephrine [16]. Two previous reviews by Ransford [68] and Morgan [61] have indicated that the amine hypothesis is a tenable explanation of the antidepressant effect of exercise; however, additional research is needed to substantiate this hypothesis.

ENDORPHIN HYPOTHESIS. A current popular hypothesis to explain the antidepressant effect of exercise is the endorphin hypothesis [61, 65, 68]. Endorphins are produced in the pituitary gland, brain, and other tissues in the body and have "morphine-like" qualities in reducing pain and producing a euphoric state [61]. Pert and Bowie [67], in an exercise study with rats, found that exercise, per se, was associated with an increase in opiate (endorphin) receptor occupancy in the brain, and rats must feel euphoric due to the associated increase in opiate receptor occupancy. Central nervous system (CNS) endorphin level changes versus changes outside of the CNS would most directly affect mood. Endorphin research in humans has been done by examining changes in blood serum endorphin levels [19, 28], or by blocking endorphin receptors with naloxone [43]. These techniques do not measure CNS endorphin changes, only peripheral endorphin changes, and Morgan [61] stated that the relationship between brain and plasma levels of endorphins is relatively small. However, this does not rule out the potential influence on mood of endorphins found in blood plasma. Additional research is needed to fully comprehend the role of endorphins as antidepressant agents. The specific endorphin(s) that act as antidepressants need to be identified, and the relationship between these endorphins and exercise needs to be clarified.

Summary of Proposed Antidepressant Mechanisms

These authors are in agreement with previous reviewers Ransford [68] and Morgan [61] who have suggested that a psychobiological model will most likely explain the antidepressant effect of exercise better than any singular partisan model. Any proposed model of the antidepressant effect of exercise needs to address possible differences in the antidepressant effect of acute (single session), short-term, and habitual exercise. It seems likely that both physiological/biochemical and psychological adaptations to exercise are related to the total amount of exercise and length of exercise program.

RECOMMENDATIONS

The following recommendations are offered for future research and to future reviewers: Additional studies are needed using the following subject populations: subjects exercising in their home, young, elderly, patients with diagnosed mood disorders, and patients with diagnosed medical illnesses (drugs need to be controlled in these studies). Studies using serial measurements of both state and trait depression scales are needed to help clarify the onset and magnitude of the antidepressant effect of exercise. Cardiovascular, and muscular strength measurements need to be evaluated in regard to changes in depression level with exercise. Different forms of exercise, particularly strength training and other anaerobic exercises, need additional evaluation for their potential antidepressant effects. Intensity of exercise needs to be quantified to determine if there is a differential effect. Follow-up studies are needed to determine if the antidepressant effect is maintained as exercise is continued or discontinued. Methodology needs to be addressed to continue to improve the validity of the studies in this area. Additional studies are needed to determine the effectiveness of exercise as a cotreatment with psychotherapy in treating depression. A theoretical model of the antidepressant effect of exercise that includes the effects of acute, short-term, and habitual exercise needs to be developed.

ACKNOWLEDGMENTS

The authors gratefully acknowledge T.P. and Norma North for their superb editorial assistance and encouragement, Chris Schuster for her laborious hours to obtain pertinent studies, Karen Matzkanin for editorial assistance, and Michael Sachs and Brad Hatfield for their constructive reviews of the manuscript.

LISTING OF CODED STUDIES

Beal RK: The effect of a dance/movement activity program on the successful adjustment to aging in the active/independent older adult (Dissertation). Cincinnati, OH, University of Cincinnati, 46:3127A, 1986.

Bennett J, Carmack MA, Gardner VJ: The effects of a program of physical exercise on depression in older adults. *The Physical Educ Phi Epsilon Kappa* 39:21–24, 1982.

Berger BG, Owen DR: Mood alterations with swimming—swimmers really do "feel better." *Psychosom Med* 45:425–433, 1983.

Boutcher SH: The effects of running and nicotine on mood states (Dissertation). Tempe, AZ, Arizona State University, 47:2499A, 1987.

Boyll JR: The effects of active exercise and passive electrical muscle stimulation on self-concept, anxiety, and depression (Dissertation). Flagstaff, AZ, Northern Arizona University, 47:2219B, 1986.

Brown JD, Lawton M: Stress and well-being in adolescence: the moderating role of physical exercise. *J Human Stress* 12:125–131, 1986.

Brown RS, Ramirez DE, Taub JM: The prescription of exercise for depression. *Physician Sports Med* 6:34–45, 1978.

Burrus MJ: The effects of running treatment program on depressed adolescents (Dissertation). Miami, FL, University of Miami, 45:2446A, 1985.

Byron JM: The effects of cardiovascular fitness program on depression, anxiety, self-concept, and perceived physical fitness in college women (Dissertation). Fresno, CA, California School of Professional Psychology, 45:1907B, 1984.

Carney RM, Harter HR, Templeton BA, Schechtman KB, Goldberg AP: Exercise improves depression and psychosocial functioning in hemodialysis patients. *Clin Res* 31:294A, 1983.

Carney RM, McKevitt PM, Goldberg AP, Hagberg J, Delmez JA, Harter HR: Psychological effects of exercise training in hemodialysis patients. *Nephron* 33:179–181, 1983.

Carney RM, Templeton B, Hong BA, Harter HR, Hagberg JM, Schechtman KB, Goldberg AP: Exercise training reduces depression and increases the performance of pleasant activities in hemodialysis patients. *Nephron* 47:194–198, 1987.

Carney RM, Wetzel RD, Hagberg J, Goldberg AP: The relationship between depression and aerobic capacity in hemodialysis patients. *Psychosom Med* 48:143–147, 1986.

Cunningham J: The effects of exercise and relaxation training upon psychological variables in coronary heart patients (Dissertation). Kansas City, MO, University of Missouri, 41:2313–2314B, 1980.

Dalton RB: Effects of exercise and vitamin B_{12} supplementation on the depression scale scores of a wheelchair-confined population (Dissertation). Columbia: MO, University of Missouri, 41:4063B, 1980.

Doyne EJ: Aerobic exercise as a treatment for depression in women (Dissertation). Athens, GA: University of Georgia, 42:2050–2051B, 1981.

Doyne EJ, Ossip-Klein DJ, Bowman ED, Osborn KM, McDougall-Wilson IB, Weimeyer RA: Running versus weight lifting in the treatment of depression. *J Consult Clin Psychol* 55:748–754, 1987.

Dyer JB III, Crouch JG: Effects of running on moods: a time series study. *Percept Mot Skills* 64:783–789, 1987.

Eby JM: An investigation into the effects of aerobic exercise on anxiety and depression (Dissertation). Toronto, Canada, University of Toronto, 46:1734B, 1984.

Einhaus LB: A comparison of the effects of two exercise programs on children's self-concept, locus of control, and mood (Dissertation). Richmond, VA, Virginia Commonwealth University, 46:299, 1985.

Epstein, D: Aerobic activity versus group cognitive therapy: an evaluative study of contrasting interventions for the alleviation of clinical depression (Dissertation) Reno NV, University of Nevada, 47:3952B, 1987.

Fetsch RJ: A comparison of psychological effects of running and transactional analysis stroking for the relief of reactive depression in adults (Dissertation). Laramie, WY, University of Wyoming, 40:4999B, 1979.

Fetsch RJ, Sprinkle RL: Effects of running on depressed adults. *Am Ment Health Counselor's Ass J* 5:75, 1983.

Folkins CH: Effects of physical training on mood. *J Clin Psychol* 32:385–388, 1976.

Folkins CH, Lynch S, Gardner MM: Psychological fitness as a function of physical fitness. *Arch Phys Med Rehabil* 53:503–508, 1972.

Francis KT, Carter R: Psychological characteristics of joggers. *J Sports Med* 22:386–390, 1982.

Fremont J, Craighead LW: Aerobic exercise and cognitive therapy in the treatment of dysphoric moods. *Cognit Ther Res* 11:241–251, 1987.

Gondola JC, Tuckman BW: Extent of training and mood enhancement in women runners. *Percept Mot Skills* 57:333–334, 1983.

Gondola JC, Tuckman BW: Psychological mood state in "average" marathon runners. *Percept Mot Skills* 55:1295–1300, 1982.

Hannaford CP: The psychophysiological effects of a running program on depression, self-esteem and anxiety (Dissertation). Denton, TX, North Texas State University, 44:3527B, 1984.

Hatfield BD, Goldfarb AH, Sforzo GA, Flynn MG: Serum beta-endorphin and affective responses to graded exercise in young and elderly men. *J Gerontol* 42:429–431, 1987.

Hayden RM: Relationship between aerobic exercise, anxiety and depression: convergent validation by knowledgeable informants. *J Sports Med Phys Fitness* 24:69–74, 1982.

Hess-Homeier MJ: A comparison of Beck's cognitive therapy and jogging as treatments for depression (Dissertation). Missoula, MT, University of Montana, 42:1175B, 1981.

Hill DL: The effects of a walk-jog program on depression and state-trait anxiety in depressed psychiatric patients (Masters Thesis). Winston-Salem, NC, Wake Forest University, 1978.

Hughes JR, Casal DC, Leon AS: Psychological effects of exercise—a randomized cross-over trial. *J Psychosom Res* 30:355–360, 1986.

Janda AR: The relationship of depression and physical fitness in a group of ambulatory schizophrenics (Dissertation). San Diego, CA, United States International University, 42:772B, 1981.

Jasnoski ML, Holmes DS: Influence of initial aerobic fitness, aerobic training and changes in aerobic fitness on personality functioning. *J Psychosom Res* 25:553–556, 1981.

Joesting J: Running and depression. *Percept Mot Skills* 52:442, 1981.

Kavanaugh T, Shephard RJ, Tuck RJ, Tuck JA, Qureshi S: Depression following myocardial infarction: the effects of distance running. *Ann NY Acad Sci* 301:1029–1038, 1977.

Klein MH, Greist JH, Gurman AS, Neimeyer RA, Lesser DR, Bushness NJ, Smith RE: A comparative outcome study of group psychotherapy versus exercise treatment for depression. *Int J Mental Health* 13:148–176, 1985.

Levin SL: The effects of a ten-week jogging program as an adjunctive treatment for patients in a social rehabilitation clinic (Dissertation). Garden City, NY, Aldelphi University School of Social Work, 44:1925A, 1983.

Lichtman S, Proser EG: The effects of exercise on mood and cognitive functioning. *J Psychosom Res* 27:43–52, 1983.

Lobstein DD, Mosbacher BJ, Ismail AH: Depression as a powerful discriminator between physically active and sedentary middle-aged men. *J Psychosom Res* 27:69–76, 1983.

MacMannis DR: Factors influencing the psychological impact of running (Dissertation). San Diego, CA, California School of Professional Psychology, 40:3949–3950B, 1980.

Marblestone RA: Psychological effects of fitness running normal women (Dissertation). Garden City, NY, Adelphi University, 41:1514B, 1980.

Markoff RA, Ryan P, Young T: Endorphins and mood changes in long-distance running. *Med Sci Sports Exerc* 14:11–15, 1982.

Marshall MP: The relationship of aerobic exercise training and workouts to lower levels of anxiety and depression (Dissertation). Kansas City, MO, University of Missouri, 44:3716–3717B, 1984.

Martinsen EW, Medhus A, Sandvik L: Effects of aerobic exercise on depression: a controlled study. *Br Med J* 291:109, 1985.

McCann IL, Holmes DS: Influence of aerobic exercise on depression. *J Pers Soc Psychol* 46:1142–1147, 1984.

Moreau ME: The effectiveness of jogging as a treatment for depression (Dissertation). Burnaby, Canada: Simon Fraser University, 42:4202B, 1982.

Moran DJ: Comparative effects of participation in a physical fitness training program versus a physical education class on mood and self-image in adolescents (Dissertation). Knoxville, TN: University of Tennessee, 46:309B, 1985.

Morgan WP: A pilot investigation of physical working capacity in depressed and non-depressed psychiatric males. *Res Q* 40:859–861, 1969.

Morgan WP, Pollock ML: Physical activity and cardiovascular health: psychological aspects. In Landry F, Orban W (eds): *Physical Activity and Human Well-Being: A Collection of Formal Papers Presented at the International Congress of Physical Activity Sciences, Quebec City, July 11–16, 1976.* Miami, Symposia Specialties, 1:163–181, 1978.

Morgan WP, Roberts JA, Brand FR, Feinerman AD: Psychological effect of chronic physical activity. *Med Sci Sports* 2:213–217, 1970.

Morgan WP, Roberts JA, Feinerman AD: Psychological effect of acute physical activity. *Arch Phys Med Rehabil* 52:422–425, 1971.

Murphy JB, Bennett RN, Hagen JM, Russell MW: Some suggestive data regarding the relationship of physical fitness to emotional difficulties. *News Res Psychol* 14:15–17, 1972.

Nowlis D, Greenberg N: Empirical description of effects of exercise on mood. *Percept Mot Skills* 49:1001–1002, 1979.

Orth DK: Clinical treatments of depression (Dissertation). Morgantown, WV, West Virginia University, 40:6154A, 1980.

Penny GF, Rust JO: Effect of a walking-jogging program on personality characteristics of middle-aged females. *J Sports Med Phys Fitness* 20:221–226, 1980.

Perri S, Templer DI: The effects of an aerobic exercise program on psychological variables in older adults. *Int J Aging Hum Dev* 20:167–172, 1984–85.

Pistacchio TM: The development of a psychobiologic profile of individuals who experience and those who do not experience exercise-related mood-enhancement (Dissertation). Denton, TX, North Texas State University, 46:3286A, 1986.

Prosser G, Carson P, Phillips R, Gelson A, Buch N, Tucker H, Neophytou M, Lloyd M, Simpson T: Morale in coronary patients following an exercise programme. *J Psychosom Res* 25:587–593, 1981.

Rape RN: Running and depression. *Percept Mot Skills* 64:1303–1310, 1987.

Setaro JL: Aerobic exercise and group counseling in the treatment of anxiety and depression (Dissertation). College Park, MD, University of Maryland, 47:2633B, 1986.

Simons CW Birkimer JC: An exploration of factors predicting the effects of aerobic conditioning on mood state. *J Psychosom Res* 32:63–75, 1988.

Sothman MS, Ismail AH: Relationships between urinary catecholamine metabolites, particularly MHPG, and selected personality and physical fitness characteristics in normal subjects. *Psychosom Med* 46:523–533, 1984.

Stern MJ, Cleary PC: National exercise and heart disease project psychosocial changes observed during a low-level exercise program. *Arch Intern Med* 141:1463–1467, 1981.

Taylor CB, Houston-Miller N, Ahn DK, Haskell W, DeBusk RF: The effects of exercise training programs on psychosocial improvement in uncomplicated post myocardial infarction patients. *J Psychosom Res* 30:581–587, 1986.

Tern MJ, Cleary PC: The national exercise and heart disease project long-term psychosocial outcome. *Arch Intern Med* 142:1093–1098, 1982.

Toomman ME: The effect of running and its deprivation on muscle tension, mood and anxiety (Masters Thesis). University Park, PA, The Pennsylvania State University, 1982.

Valliant PM, Asa ME: Exercise and its effects on cognition and physiology in older adults. *Percept Mot Skills* 61:1031–1038, 1985.

VanderHoek DD: Long slow distance running as a treatment for moderate depression of outpatients (Masters Thesis). Kalamazoo, MI, Western Michigan University, 22:185, 1983.

Weaver DC: A study to determine the effect of exercise on depression in middle-aged women (Dissertation). Murfreesboro, TN, Middle Tennessee State University, 45:2033A, 1985.

Weinstein JB: The influence of physical fitness on mood and self-esteem in a young adult population: a learned efficacy model (Dissertation). Albany, NY, State University of New York, 47:2637–2638B, 1986.

Weiman JB: Running as treatment for depression: a theoretical basis (Dissertation). Fresno, CA, California School of Professional Psychology, 41:1935–1936B, 1980.

Wilfley D, Junce J: Differential physical and psychological effects of exercise. *J Counsel Psychol* 33:337–342, 1986.

Williams GH: The effects of aerobic training and a mood control workshop on depression in male college students (Dissertation). Atlanta, GA, Georgia State University, 40:2861B, 1979.

Williams JM, Getty D: Effect of levels of exercise on psychological mood states, physical fitness and plasma beta-endorphin. *Percept Mot Skills* 63:1099–1105, 1986.

Wilson LP: The effects of an exercise conditioning program on reducing the stress response in nurses (Dissertation). Detroit, MI, Wayne State University, 47:577B, 1986.

Wilson VE, Morley NC, Bird EI: Mood profiles of marathon runners, joggers and non-exercisers. *Percept Mot Skills* 50:117–118, 1980.

REFERENCES

1. Aloia JF, Cohen SH, Ostune JA, Cane R, Ellis K: Prevention of involutional bone loss by exercise. *Ann Intern Med* 89:356–358, 1978.

2. American College of Sports Medicine: Position statement on the recommended quantity and quality of exercise for developing and maintaining fitness in healthy adults. *Med Sci Sports Exerc* 10:3, 1978.

3. American College of Sports Medicine: *Guidelines for Exercise Testing and Prescription.* ed 3. Philadelphia, Lea & Febiger, 1986.

4. American Psychiatric Association: *Diagnostic and Statistical Manual of Mental Disorders.* 3rd rev ed. Washington D.C., American Psychiatric Association, 1987.

5. Antonelli F: Sport and depression therapy. *Int J Sport Psychol* 13:187–193, 1982.

6. Bahrke MS, Morgan WP: Anxiety reduction following exercise and meditation. *Cognit Ther Res* 2:323–333, 1978.

7. Bandura A: Self-efficacy: toward a unifying theory of behavioral change. *Psychol Rev* 2:191–215, 1977.

8. Barchas JD, Freedman DX: Brain amines: response to physiological stress. *Biochem Pharmacol* 12:1232–1235, 1963.
9. Beck AT: *Depression: Causes and Treatment.* Philadelphia, University of Pennsylvania Press, 1967.
10. Beck AT: *The Diagnosis and Management of Depression.* Philadelphia, University of Pennsylvania Press, 1973.
11. Beck AT: *Cognitive Therapy and the Emotional Disorders.* New York, International Universities Press, 1976.
12. Blackburn H: Physical activity and cardiovascular health: The epidemiological evidence. In Landry F, Orban W (eds): *Physical Activity and Human Well Being.* Miami, Symposia Specialists, 1978.
13. Boyer JL, Kasch FW: Exercise therapy in hypertensive men. *JAMA* 211:1668–1671, 1970.
14. Browman CP, Tepas DI: The effects of presleep activity on all-night sleep. *Psychophysiology* 13:536–540, 1976.
15. Browman CP: Physical activity as a therapy for psychopathology: a reappraisal. *J Sports Med Phys Fitness* 21:192–197, 1981.
16. Brown BS, Van Huss WD: Exercise and rat brain catecholamines. *J Appl Physiol* 34:664–669, 1973.
17. Brown RS, Ramirez DE, Taub JM: The prescription of exercise for depression. *Physician Sportmed* 6:34–37; 40–41; 44–45, 1978.
18. Bunney WE Jr, Davis JM: Norepinephrine in depressive reactions. *Arch Gen Psychiatry* 13:483–494, 1965.
19. Carr DB, Bullen BA, Skirnar GS, Arnold MA, Rosenblatt M, Beitins IZ, Martin JB, McArthur JW: Physical conditioning facilitates the exercise-induced secretion of beta-endorphine and beta-lipoprotein in women. *N Engl J Med* 305:560–562, 1981.
20. Claridge G: *Origins of Mental Illness.* New York, Basil Blackwell, 1985.
21. Cooper HM: *The Integrative Research Review: A Systematic Approach.* Applied Social Research Methods Series. Beverly Hills, CA, Sage Publications, 1984.
22. Crews DJ, Landers DM: A meta-analytic review of aerobic fitness and reactivity to psychosocial stressors. *Med Sci Sports Exerc* 19:114–120, 1987.
23. Doan RE, Scherman A: The therapeutic effect of physical fitness on measures of personality: A literature review. *J Counsel Dev* 66:28–36, 1987.
24. Dodson LC, Mullens WR: Some effects of jogging on psychiatric hospital patients. *Res Q* 39:1037–1043, 1969.
25. Doyne EJ, Bowman ED, Ossip-klein DJ, Osborn KM, McDougal-Wilson I, Neimer RA: A comparison of aerobic and nonaerobic exercise in the treatment of depression. Paper presented at the Meeting for the Association for the Advancement of Behavior Therapy. Washington D.C., 1983.
26. Doyne EJ, Chambless DL, Beutler LE: Aerobic exercise as a treatment for depression in women. *Behav Ther* 14:434–440, 1983.
27. Eysenck JH: An exercise in mega-illness. *Am Psychol* 33:517b, 1978.
28. Farrell PA, Gates WK, Maksud MG, Morgan WP: Increases in plasma beta-endorphin/beta-lipotropin immunoreactivity after treadmill running in humans. *J Appl Physiol* 52:1245–1249, 1982.
29. Fawcett J, Mass JW, Dekirmenjiar H: Depression and MHPG excretion. *Arch Gen Psychiatry* 26:246–251, 1972.
30. Folkins CH, Lynch S, Gardner MM: Psychological fitness as a function of physical fitness. *Arch Phys Med Rehabil* 53:503–508, 1972.
31. Folkins CH, Sime WE: Physical fitness training and mental health. *Am Psychol* 36:373–389, 1981.
32. Fremont J, Craighead LW: Aerobic exercise and cognitive therapy for mild/moderate depression. Paper presented at the Association for Advancement of Behavior Therapy. Philadelphia, PA, 1984.

33. Glass GV: Primary, secondary and meta-analysis of research. *Educ Res* 5:3–8, 1976.
34. Glass GV, McGaw B, Smith ML: *Meta-Analysis in Social Research.* Beverly Hills, CA, Sage Publications, 1981.
35. Glowinski J, Axelrod J: Inhibition of uptake of titrated noradrenaline in the intact rat brain by imipramine and structurally related compounds. *Nature* 204:1318–1319, 1964.
36. Glowinski J, Baldessarini RJ: Metabolism of norepinephrine in the central nervous system. *Pharmacol Rev* 18:1201–1238, 1966.
37. Grahame-Smith DG, Green AR, Costain DW: Mechanism of the antidepressant action of electro-convulsive therapy. *Lancet* 1:254–256, 1978.
38. Greist JH: *Run to Reality.* Milwaukee, Bulfin, 1977.
39. Greist JH, Eischens RR, Klein MH, Faris JW: Antidepressant Running. *Psychiat Ann* 9:23–33, 1979.
40. Greist JH, Klein MH, Eischens RR, Faris J: Running as a treatment for non-psychotic depression. *Behav Med* 5:19–24, 1978.
41. Greist JH, Klein MH, Eischens RR, Faris J, Gurman AS, Morgan WP: Running through your mind. *J Psychosom Res* 22:259–294, 1978.
42. Greist JH, Klein MH, Eischens RR, Faris J, Gurman AS, Morgan WP: Running as a treatment for depression. *Compr Psychiatry* 20:41–54, 1979.
43. Haier RJ, Quaid K, Mills JSC: Naloxone alters pain perception after jogging. *Psychiatry Res* 5:231–232, 1981.
44. Hanson DL: Influence of the Hawthorne effect upon physical education research. *Res Q* 38:723–724, 1967.
45. Hays WL: *Statistics for the Social Sciences.* New York, Holt, Rinehart & Winston, 1973.
46. Hedges LV, Olkin I: *Statistical Methods for Meta-Analysis.* New York, Academic Press, 1985.
47. Heinzelman F, Bagley RW: Response to physical activity programs and their effects on health behavior. *Public Health Rep* 85:905–911, 1970.
48. Hughes JR: Psychological effects of habitual aerobic exercise: a critical review. *Prev Med* 13:66–84, 1984.
49. Kavanaugh T, Shephard RJ, Tuck JA, Qureshi S: Depression following myocardial infarction: the effects of distance running. *Ann NY Acad Sci* 301:1029–1038, 1977.
50. Ledwidge B: Run for your mind: aerobic exercise as a means of alleviating anxiety and depression. *Can J Behav Sci* 12:127–140, 1980.
51. Lipton MA: Neuropsychopharmacology of monoamines and their regulatory enzymes. In Usdin E (ed): *Advances in Biochemical Psychopharmacology.* New York, Raven Press, 1974, p. 451.
52. Lobstein DD, Mosbacher BJ, Ismail AH: Depression as a powerful discriminator between physically active and sedentary middle-aged men. *J Psychosom Res* 27:69–76, 1983.
53. Markoff RA, Ryan P, Young T: Endorphins and mood changes in long distance running. *Med Sci Sports Exerc* 14:11–15, 1982.
54. Martinsen EW: The role of aerobic exercise in the treatment of depression. *Stress Med* 3:93–100, 1987.
55. Mayou A: A controlled trial of early rehabilitation after myocardial infarction. *J Cardiac Rehabil* 6:387–402, 1983.
56. McCann IL, Holmes DS: Influence of aerobic exercise on depression. *J Pers Soc Psychol* 46:1143–1147, 1984.
57. Mellion MB: Exercise therapy for anxiety and depression. *Postgrad Med* 77:59–66, 1985.
58. Morgan WP: A pilot investigation of physical working capacity in depressed and non-depressed males. *Res Q* 40:859–861, 1969.
59. Morgan WP: Physical fitness and emotional health: a review. *Am Correct Ther J* 23:124–127, 1969.

60. Morgan WP: Anxiety reduction following acute physical activity. *Psychiatr Ann* 9:36–45, 1979.
61. Morgan WP: Affective beneficence of vigorous physical activity. *Med Sci Sports Exerc* 17:94–100, 1985.
62. Morgan WP, Roberts JA, Brand FR, Feinerman AD: Psychological effect of chronic physical activity. *Med Sci Sports* 2:213–217, 1970.
63. Morgan WP, Roberts JA, Feinerman AD: Psychological effect of physical activity. *Arch Phys Med Rehabil* 52:422–425, 1971.
64. Naughton J, Bruhn JG, Lategola MT: Effects of physical training on physiological and behavioral characteristics of cardiac patients. *Arch Phys Med Rehabil* 49:131–137, 1968.
65. Pargman D, Baker MC: Running high: enkephalin indicted. *J Drug Issues* 10:341–349, 1980.
66. Perri S, Templer DI: The effects of an aerobic exercise program on psychological variables in older adults. *Int J Aging Hum Dev* 20:167–172, 1985.
67. Pert CB, Bowie DL: Behavioral manipulation of rats causes alterations in opiate receptor occupancy. In Usdin E, Bunney WE, Kline NS (eds): *Endorphins in Mental Health.* New York, Oxford University Press, 1979, pp 93–104.
68. Ransford CP: A role for amines in the antidepressant effect of exercise: a review. *Med Sci Sports Exerc* 14:1–10, 1982.
69. Sachs ML: Exercise and running: effects on anxiety, depression, and psychology. *Humanistic Educ Dev* 21:51–57, 1982.
70. Sacks HS, Berrier K, Reitman D, Ancona-Bark VA, Chalmer TC: Meta-analysis of randomized controlled trials. *N Engl J Med* 316:450–455, 1987.
71. Schildkraut JJ: The catecholamine hypothesis of affective disorders: a review of supporting evidence. *Am J Psychiatry* 122:509–522, 1965.
72. Seligman MEP: Learned helplessness. *Annu Rev Med* 23:407–412, 1972.
73. Simons AD, Epstein LH, McGowan CR, Kupfer DJ, Robertson RJ: Exercise as a treatment for depression: an update. *Clin Psychol Rev* 5:553–568, 1985.
74. Smith ML: Sex bias in counseling and psychotherapy. *Psychol Bull* 87:392–407, 1980.
75. Soman VR, Koivisto VA, Deibert D, Felig P, Defronzon RA: Increased insulin sensitivity and insulin binding to monocytes after physical training. *N Engl J Med* 301:1200–1204, 1979.
76. Stern MJ, Cleary PC: The national exercise and heart disease project long-term psychosocial outcome. *Arch Intern Med* 142:1093–1098, 1982.
77. Stern MJ, Gorman PA, Kaslow KL: The group counseling versus exercise therapy study. A controlled intervention with subjects following myocardial infarction. *Arch Intern Med* 143:719–725, 1983.
78. Taylor CB, Sallis JF, Needle R: The relation of physical activity and exercise to mental health. *Public Health Rep* 100:195–202, 1985.
79. Taylor MA, Abrams R: Prediction of treatment response in mania. *Arch Gen Psychiatry* 38:800–802, 1981.
80. Tharp GD, Carson WH: Emotionality changes in rats following chronic exercise. *Med Sci Sports Exerc* 7:123–126, 1975.
81. Tran ZV: The effects of exercise on blood lipids and lipoproteins: A meta-analysis of studies (Dissertation). Boulder, CO, University of Colorado 43:1081A, 1982.
82. Tran ZV, Weltman A: Differential effects of exercise on serum lipid and lipoprotein levels seen with changes in body weight: a meta-analysis. *JAMA* 254:919–923, 1985.
83. Walker JM, Floyd TC, Fein G, Cavness C, Lualhati R, Feinberg I: Effects of exercise on sleep. *J App Physiol* 44:945–951, 1978.
84. Weber JC, Lee RA: Effects of differing prepuberty exercise programs on the emotionality of male albino rats. *Res Q* 39:748–751, 1968.
85. Weinstein WS, Meyers AW: Running as a treatment for depression: Is it worth it? *J Sports Psychol* 5:288–301, 1983.

14
Application of Epidemiological Methodology to Sports and Exercise Science Research

STEPHEN D. WALTER, Ph.D.
LAWRENCE E. HART, M.B., B.Ch., M.Sc., F.R.C.P.(C)

INTRODUCTION

This review paper has two main objectives. First, it will introduce the reader to the general principles of epidemiology and indicate how epidemiologic designs can be applied to various areas of sports and exercise science research. The methodologic strengths and weaknesses of different research designs will be discussed. Second, we will present a systematic review of the current research literature in sports and exercise science, in which research papers are classified according to the design they have employed. This empirical evaluation of the literature will indicate the current trends in the choice of research design and suggest relatively deficient areas where further work may be needed.

We have organized our presentation as follows. First, we give an overview of sports and exercise science research and its interface with epidemiology. We then describe the concept of epidemiology rather generally, including its foundations in etiology and its more recent applications in the clinical setting. Next is a review of the various epidemiological designs, beginning with an extended discussion of the popular case series method. Some of the interpretational difficulties of this approach are indicated. There then follows discussion on other observational designs, including the prospective cohort method, the retrospective case-control method, and the cross-sectional survey method, followed by a summary of the types of data and the relative strengths of these designs. An outline of the preferred methodology for randomized controlled trials is given. We then indicate some common statistical issues encountered in all types of epidemiological studies. Finally, we present the results of a systematic survey of the sports and exercise science research literature, classifying all the articles appearing in a selection of relevant journals according to their various design features.

SCOPE OF PAPER

Because a study design reflects only the *process* of research rather than the underlying scientific question that is being addressed, it is helpful to

417

list the important research areas that are commonly identified by sports and exercise science investigators and which lend themselves to the application of epidemiologic techniques. These are as follows:

1. *Estimation of the burden of morbidity and/or mortality in populations of athletes.* For example, we may wish to evaluate the type and frequency of musculoskeletal injuries in members of a college track team.
2. *Identification of risk factors and high risk participants.* For example, we may wish to study the relationship of weekly running mileage or other aspects of training and equipment to the injury rate. Also, endogenous factors such as age, gender, and body build may be predictive of injury risk.
3. *Development of preventive interventions.* Having identified significant risk factors, it is logical to consider modifications of training or equipment to reduce the risk of morbidity or mortality.
4. *Evaluation of diagnosis and therapy.* When, despite our best efforts at prevention, injuries and illness do occur, we need to optimally diagnose and manage them.
5. *Physiological and biomechanical studies of exercise and sports.* These basic sciences are used to study the mechanisms of injury or illness. In addition, there is often interest in the underlying physiologic response to exercise or the biomechanical aspects of sports performance without direct concern for adverse health outcomes.

In addition, there are several other areas of investigation that occur less frequently in the sports science literature, such as the psychology of sports performance, medical knowledge of coaches and trainers, provision of sports medicine facilities and services, sports science education for health and other professionals, and sociopolitical issues. Epidemiologic methods are appropriate and used in some of these.

Indeed "sports and exercise science" is such a broad and multidisciplinary area of research that it is clearly not feasible to discuss all of its facets in detail in a single article. In order to limit the scope, we have chosen to emphasize areas where there is direct concern with human health in relation to exercise and sports, and where the epidemiologic approach may be correctly applied. However, the basic sciences have not been excluded, because many studies of this type have important (if indirect) implications for human health. In fact, in the second part of this paper describing our survey of current sports and exercise science literature, we were guided by the empirical definition that "sports and exercise science research" is what sports and exercise science researchers "do"; therefore *all* articles in the selected journals were included and classified.

EPIDEMIOLOGY

Classical Epidemiology

Epidemiology has been defined as "the study of the distribution of a disease or a physiological condition in human populations and of factors that influence this distribution" [27]. As such, epidemiology has been traditionally concerned with etiologic questions. Thus, in *descriptive* epidemiology, one addresses issues of the distribution of a health event, such as disease or illness. The event may be described using incidence rates, prevalence rates, or the duration of the disease or illness in question. Time trends are also of interest. In routine descriptive reports, such as annual vital statistics dealing with national mortality data, it is usual to adjust for possible changes in the age structure of the population by a technique known as age standardization; this technique avoids potentially misleading comparisons between unadjusted crude rates [6]. Less commonly, adjustment for other covariates is made; two examples are the adjustment of cancer incidence rates for differences between urban and rural areas [1], and subgroup reporting of vital statistics to allow for racial differences in vital rates [40]. The ability to allow for covariates in this way is usually limited by the availability of routinely collected data.

In contrast, *analytic epidemiology* is concerned with the determinants of morbidity and mortality. Analytic studies are usually based on data collected specially for a given project, rather than relying on routinely available official data. Information may be gathered directly from study subjects, using interviews or physical examinations, or from medical records in hospitals, clinics or physician files. Data of this type are almost always observational (as opposed to experimental) in nature; therefore, in attempting to demonstrate an association between a postulated risk factor and a disease outcome, one must be alert to the possibility of confounding of the association by some third variable. Much of the statistical methodology used in analytic epidemiology is directed at recognizing and correcting confounding effects; therefore, it tends to be more complex than methods used for descriptive studies. Furthermore, there are many sources of bias and imprecision that affect observational epidemiologic data. The likelihood of these adverse effects occurring depends partly on the choice of study design, as is discussed in more detail later.

Clinical Epidemiology

In recent years there has been growing interest in applying epidemiologic methods to problems with greater clinical content. It has been suggested that "it should be possible to take a set of epidemiologic and biostatistical strategies to study the distribution and determinants of disease in groups and populations, recast them in a clinical perspective, and use them to improve our clinical performance" [43]. This translation of "classical" epidemiologic techniques to the clinical arena leads to a more systematic evaluation of diagnostic strategies and therapeutic choices and also permits effective critical appraisal of the medical literature.

Prominent among these developments has been the evolution of the randomized controlled trial (RCT) as the preferred method for assessing new methods of therapy. Randomization greatly reduces the chance of confounding and thereby provides a real advantage over otherwise comparable unrandomized designs, thus alleviating some of the problems of statistical analysis. However, many of the methodologic challenges in executing a trial of therapy relate to the practical implementation of the study. For instance, it is necessary to carefully specify and account for all the patients for whom the therapy is intended, even if not all patients adhere to the therapy to which they are randomized. Issues of this kind are discussed more fully in our later section dealing with trials.

Whether one is investigating a question of description, etiology, diagnosis, or therapy, the epidemiologic method is uniquely characterized by its study of *groups* of individuals. Many scientific researchers, who have been primarily concerned with decision making in individual patients, find it difficult to evaluate statistical patterns in groups of patients. Some of the method's detractors might argue that one is effectively replacing the "art of medicine" with an irrelevant science. However, thorough integration of the epidemiologic method (with its underlying basic science and clinical applications) can be used "to explain and to teach, not replace, the art of medicine" [43]. As is demonstrated later in this paper, epidemiologic methods have already been successfully used in several areas of sports science.

CHOICE OF EPIDEMIOLOGICAL STUDY DESIGN IN SPORTS AND EXERCISE SCIENCE RESEARCH

The most important epidemiological study designs that appear relevant to questions of sports and exercise science include case series and case reports, comparative observational studies, and randomized controlled trials. For each design, we will give a brief outline of the method, some of its methodologic advantages and disadvantages, and some typical examples from the literature.

Case Series

The case series method is usually employed by clinicians to describe various characteristics of some number of their recent patients. In epidemiological terms, this is a *numerator-based* design, because information is only available from "cases," i.e., persons who are injured or ill. There are usually no corresponding data on people in the population "at risk," that yielded the cases under study.

One of the main uses of the case series design is to establish the relative frequencies of different types of injury. For instance, one may wish to estimate the annual numbers of injuries treated at a clinic among athletes from different sports; DeHaven and Lintner [8] undertook a study of this sort using 4551 athletes from among professional, intercollegiate, high school, intramural, and unorganized sports groups. Similarly, it may be of interest to determine the relative "importance" (as indicated by frequency) of various types of injury among a single type of athlete, such as the numbers of different musculoskeletal injuries seen in runners.

Interpretational Difficulties of Case Series Data

Even simple results like the relative frequency of injury are subject to idiosyncrasies, such as local differences in the clinical referral pattern of injured athletes. Operational definitions of injury groups, and even the type of injuries to be included, may vary between studies, leading to differences in the apparent relative importance of the various categories of injury.

As an example, Table 14.1 gives the percentages and ranked frequencies of various running injuries by body site, according to the investigators in four case series studies [4, 25, 36, 37]. First, we note that the set of injuries included and how they have been categorized is not uniform; several sites were not included in one study [25]. Second, there is variation in the relative importance of various injuries; for example, foot injuries show almost a 3-fold variation as a percentage of all injuries, and the knee a 2-fold variation. These inconsistencies likely reflect differences in the study populations, and in referral preferences of athletes to clinicians. Thus, for instance, studies with podiatrists involved as investigators are likely to find foot injuries as a more frequent problem.

Another possible explanation of the differences in the rankings is in the study methodology. For instance, studies based on clinic patient records may produce different results from those using self-reporting of injuries by the runners themselves. The extent and accuracy of the data may well depend on the way they are collected, thus affecting the final study results. In other areas of medicine, it has been shown that the agreement of the patient with medical records concerning details of potentially serious illness is only moderately good, at best [52]. Unpublished data from a cohort study of ours on running injuries suggests that, compared to the findings on blinded clinical examination, runners are able to accurately report the body site of a musculoskeletal injury,

TABLE 14.1
Relative Frequency of Various Types of Injury in Runners,
in Four Case Series

Body Site		Study (Reference No.)			
		(37)	(4)	(36)	(25)
Back	No[a]	39	58	15	
	%	1.5	4	1.4	
	Rank	8	8	8	
Hip	No	44	90	28	
	%	1.7	5	2.6	7
	Rank	7	5	6	6
Groin	No	3	6	6	
	%	0.01	0.3	0.6	
	Rank	9	9	9	
Thigh	No	65	70	18	
	%	2.4	4	2	6
	Rank	6	6	7	7
Knee	No	671	761	220	
	%	25.7	42	21	25
	Rank	2	1	2	1
Leg	No	345	291	114	
	%	13.2	16	11	22
	Rank	3	3	3	3
Ankle	No	107	53	97	
	%	4.1	3	9	11
	Rank	5	7	4	5
Achilles tendon	No	147	113	61	
	%	5.6	7	6	18
	Rank	4	4	5	4
Foot	No	1187	227	335	
	%	45.5	16	31	24
	Rank	1	2	1	2

[a] Each cell shows the number of injuries, the percentage of all injuries found at body site, and the site ranking within each study.

but are inaccurate in describing the involved tissue; definitive diagnosis almost certainly requires clinical examination.

For the above reasons, we must conclude that there may be difficulties in interpreting case series data, even at a simple level. However, when we wish to examine possible risk factors for injury, the case series design is even more problematic. Consider the following hypothetical example.

Suppose one wishes to test the hypothesis that habitual training on hills is a significant risk factor for injury among recreational runners. To investigate this question, we decide to study all runners presenting with injuries at a sports medicine clinic over a 12-month period. The injured athletes are asked to give details of their training practices with particular emphasis on their use of hill running. After a year, there have been 375 injured runners who provided data; 250 of these indicated that they did habitually use hill training methods, while 125 said they did not.

Because the majority of injured runners reported that they used hill training, it is perhaps tempting to conclude that running on hills is indeed a risk factor for injury. However, this is potentially a completely incorrect inference. Suppose that in fact the 375 injured runners came from a population "at risk" of 1000 runners, as shown in Table 14.2. In the entire population, 750 runners would be classified as habitual hill runners, while 250 would not have included this practice in their training routines. (This additional information on the general population is, of course, not available through the case series mechanism of data collection.)

Now, expressing the risk of injury as a percentage of the number of runners in each group, we see that hill runners have an estimated annual injury rate of 250/750 or 33%, whereas nonhill runners have a rate of 125/250 or 50%. Thus, the risk in hill runners is actually *lower* than for the other group. Although not important to the general methodological point, and bearing in mind that this is only an (unlikely) scenario that has been used to demonstrate a statistical misconception, we may take this example through to its conclusion by inferring that appropriate use of hill training may actually promote extensibility of the leg musculature and thereby reduce the risk of subsequent lower limb injury. The main lesson from this example is that, without the additional information on the prevalence of the risk factor exposure in the general population at risk, inferences from the case data alone really amount to little more than intuition.

Case series data may also be distorted by a referral process bias, which skews the distribution of injury severity. For instance, while severe injuries are very likely to be treated, there may be a certain number of moderate or mild injuries that are not seen by a health professional. The resulting distribution of severity among cases seen at a health care facility will then have a disproportionate representation of severe cases. This tendency will be accentuated in the case series of tertiary referral centers.

These are not hypothetical situations. Even those injured runners who

TABLE 14.2
Example of Incorrect Inference on a Risk Factor for Injury from Case Series Data

	Using Hill Training		
	Yes	*No*	*Total*
Number of injured runners (reported in case series)	250	125	375
Number of uninjured runners (not studied in case series)	500	125	625
Total	750	250	1000
Injury rate (%)	33%	50%	37%

do present to health care facilities may delay before doing so: in one study, about one-half of injured recreational runners who sought medical care delayed their first visit for at least a week following the injury, and one-third delayed for 2 weeks or more [53]. More than half of the injured runners who sought care did so only when the injury had progressed to the point of actually limiting their running activity. Other investigators have shown that runners often continue to run while injured [18]. Furthermore, many injuries are never assessed by health care professionals: for about one-quarter of injuries, no help is sought, and a significant amount of advice is obtained from other sources such as fellow runners, books, or magazines [18, 53]. Although times from injury to seeking treatment and the numbers of untreated injuries will vary in different populations, the main methodological message is clear, i.e., that clinically based case series are unlikely to represent the spectrum of injuries in the general population. The only exception to this might be in the context of close medical monitoring of elite athletes or teams.

Examples of Interpretational Difficulty in Sports Medicine Case Series

For all of the above reasons, we must treat case series with considerable caution. However, the case series approach is commonly used in both general medical research and in addressing pertinent questions in the sports sciences. Many of these studies include inferences on risk factors and other aspects of etiology that are not necessarily justified. Without wishing to cast doubt on specific studies (because their inferences may, in fact, be correct), the following quotes are offered as examples of *potentially* misleading conclusions from case series data in the sports medicine literature.

First, in a clinic-based series of overuse running injuries [4], it was noted that "women under age 30 had the greatest risk." This is a classic example of the missing denominator problem alluded to earlier. In order to support the conclusion that the *rate* of injuries was highest among young women, one would need to know the relative numbers of runners in each age-sex group "at risk" of injury (and being seen at the clinic) among the population in which the injuries occurred. Otherwise, the larger *numbers* of injuries in the younger women might simply reflect a relatively large number of runners in this group generally and/or a greater tendency for injured runners in this group to be referred to the specific investigators undertaking this study.

Second, in a case series study of roller-skating injuries, it was noted that "inexperienced skaters were involved in 77% of all accidents," with the implicit inference that "inexperience" was a risk factor for injury [11]. Again, however, to support this conclusion the available data from the injured participants would need to be supplemented with information on the general level of "experience" in all skaters. Assuming that no other factors are involved, the inference would be false if there were more than 77% of inexperienced skaters in the population; in this situation one would conclude that *experienced* skaters were the ones at higher risk of injury, perhaps because they skated at a higher speed.

As a final example, in a case series of stress fractures [32], data were gathered from the injured runners on factors such as the use of "improper" footwear and training "errors" such as rapid changes in running intensity. Having ascertained that these factors occurred quite frequently among their cases, the authors concluded that they were probable causes of the injuries. As usual, of course, the corresponding information would be required from the general population, in order to compare the *relative* frequency of these attributes in injured and noninjured runners.

These are not isolated examples. Indeed almost all case series reports in the literature are accompanied by statements about postulated risk factors or mechanisms of injury. The astute and critical consumer of the medical literature will recognize the potential pitfalls of these claims, that are perhaps best regarded as hypothesis generating rather than hypothesis testing.

Summary of Strengths and Weaknesses of the Case Series Method

The major strengths of the case series method include: (*a*) it is a relatively simple design that can easily be implemented into routine clinical practice; (*b*) it can validly be used to estimate the total morbidity load on a health facility; and (*c*) it can be used to estimate the relative frequency of different types of injuries treated in any given practice.

The major disadvantages are: (*a*) the cases are usually not representative of the morbidity in the general population; (*b*) one cannot calculate absolute risks of injury for athletes in the general population; and (*c*) it is not possible to assess relative risks of injury for athletes in subgroups of interest. Therefore, one cannot identify high risk athletes or detect factors that increase the risk of injury.

Despite the difficulties inherent in their interpretation, the case series approach has been widely used in a great range of sports. A previous review [54] found examples of the case series method in sports as diverse as baseball, freestyle skiing, trampoline, darts, skateboarding, and parachuting. For some of these (e.g., baseball and parachuting), population denominator data is relatively easy to acquire, whereas for others (e.g., darts and skateboarding), participation may be on an intermittent or casual basis, thus making it more difficult to identify and study, with the intention of deriving population denominators, a well-specified group of athletes.

The sample sizes for case series studies vary enormously. There are many "series" that actually report clinical details of diagnosis and/or management for only one or two especially interesting or unusual cases

[26, 28, 39]. We designate these as "case reports" in our review of current literature. At the opposite extreme, the largest series we found was in a centralized register of 24,000 injuries in martial arts [2].

Further details of the recent use of the case series method are given later, in our literature review. We now move on to discuss the various types of comparative observational epidemiologic designs that may eliminate some of the deficiencies of case series.

Comparative Observational Studies

In epidemiologic designs, the specification of a population denominator is often as important as the choice of the case numerator. Various denominators can be adopted, depending on the research question posed and on the availability of data. Some typical examples of denominators are:

> the number of entrants in a road race;
> the number of children in a school (e.g., for a study of school athletic injuries);
> the number of climbers registered at a park (in a study of climbing injuries);
> the number of parachute jumps; and
> the number of player-games played by a team.

These denominators typically lead to the estimation of a rate of injury *per athlete*. Sometimes, however, the number of times a particular individual participates cannot easily be linked in the data base, so the rate may instead be expressed *per occasion;* an example of this would be the estimation of the risk of injury per parachute jump. In other situations, there may be changing membership of the participant group. For instance, when team membership varies over the playing season, it may be more convenient to express the risk in *person-time units* (e.g., in player-games or athlete-hours), without direct linkage of the denominator contributions of each specific athlete.

Another important component in the choice of epidemiologic design is the treatment of the time dimension, in its relation to the development of injuries or the therapies under study. There are three major types of design: prospective, retrospective, and cross-sectional. These differ fundamentally in the way their comparison groups are defined and sampled over time. This in turn affects the type and quality of data they provide and the reliability of their findings.

Prospective Design

This design is perhaps the most natural to conceptualize, because it is oriented *forward* in time, from initial risk states to subsequent outcomes.

As a simple example in the context of identifying risk factors for injury, one might assemble a group of athletes at baseline and measure all the variables that are thought to be prognostic of injury. The group is then followed prospectively for a period of time, during which the occurrence of all injuries is monitored and documented. After the follow-up is complete, one may calculate an absolute rate of injury for the entire group or for specific subgroups of interest. If the subgroups are defined at baseline (e.g., by age, sex, training mileage, etc.), then comparisons among them will help to identify significant risk factors for injury. The prospective design is also referred to as the *cohort* design, with the study group of athletes constituting the cohort.

In our Ontario running study [53] we used the cohort design. Approximately 1700 runners were enrolled at baseline, using the entrants to community road races as the sampling frame. Our baseline assessments included a listing of the characteristics of the runners (such as training habits, experience in running and racing, history of previous injury, participation in other sports and exercise, and anthropometric traits). The cohort was followed for 1 year, with several contacts by phone or mail to ascertain all injuries experienced. It was therefore possible to compute an annual risk of injury for various subgroups of the sample. A typical analysis compared the risk of injury for males and females (49 versus 46%), yielding a statistically nonsignificant difference. It was possible to examine in similar fashion a wide variety of risk factors (either singly or in combination), to obtain absolute estimates of the risk of injury.

For purposes of this study, an injury had to be "severe enough to reduce the number of miles run, take medicine, or see a health professional." Injuries were ascertained by self-report from the athlete, with new injuries being distinguished from recurrences. Note also that this definition allows for the inclusion of untreated injuries.

The Ontario study gave absolute risks of injury per year. In other circumstances, it may be of interest to compute the risk in other ways: e.g., in a study of the risk of sudden cardiac death [48], we might want to express the risk of death per exercise session or to estimate the lifetime risk of cardiac death among habitual exercisers versus sedentary individuals [51]. These and other absolute estimates of risk are all achievable with an appropriate prospective design.

It is possible to cite a number of interesting examples from prospective studies where the choice of denominator for the risk of injury is crucial to the interpretation of the entire study. Our first example is taken from North American football where it has been suggested that it is very important to take account of the actual time that individual players participate in the game. For instance, the number of players available and the amount of time on the field varies considerably between quarterbacks, defensive linebackers, and so on [45]. Individual data of this type

may be hard to acquire, so an alternative way of expressing player exposures is by classifying them into groups such as regular starters, special
teams, and tryouts [17].

A second example is from a cohort study of teams in a soccer league
[10], where exposure time was divided into practice hours and game
hours. It was found that the incidence of injury *per player-hour* was approximately twice as high in games as in practice. Finally, a similar analysis was made in a study of women's gymnastic injuries, showing an even
higher relative risk during competition compared to practice [16].

As mentioned earlier, we must always consider the appropriateness of
the individual subjects chosen for the study denominator. For studies
that use athletic events for their sampling frame, we must, for instance,
consider the likelihood of selection bias. By this, we mean the possibility
that injured athletes are less likely to enter the event than the surviving
athletes who remain injury-free. An example of this phenomenon is
given in a study by Nicholl and Williams [33, 34], who showed that
proportionately more male than female runners had failed to enter a
marathon because of injuries experienced in prerace training.

Similarly, there may be another form of selection bias present if there
are some casual athletes in the population who never enter organized
events. Such individuals cannot, by definition, be included in the study
cohort, thus reducing the generalizability of the study results. Even
when athletes are enrolled in this type of study, we should be concerned
about bias arising from differential drop-out rates during the follow-up
period. For instance, people without injuries might be more likely to
drop out of the study, because they have less motivation to continue,
having less health events to report.

Selection bias is often difficult to study, because of the limited amount
of information typically available for nonparticipants in any particular
study. In the Ontario runner's study, we were able to compare age and
sex distributions for runners who did or did not participate and also
compare the injury rates in groups of runners defined by the degree of
difficulty in enrolling them initially [53]. After making these comparisons, we felt that selection bias was unimportant in our study.

In addition to observational studies of etiology, the cohort design is
also used frequently in the clinical context to describe the outcome experience of a series of patients given a particular therapy or for evaluating
all patients seen at a given health facility. Patient subgroups of interest
can be examined in the same way as for injury studies. For instance,
patients on different forms of therapy can be compared. Also, several
outcomes (e.g., a variety of physiologic variables) can be examined in the
same study.

Caution is required if there has been no randomization of patients to
therapeutic groups, because of possible conscious or subconscious selection of patients by their clinicians. For example, there may be a tendency

for only the more severe cases of injury to be referred to invasive surgery, so that a comparison of surgically treated patients with others would be difficult to interpret. Randomized controlled trials (to be discussed later) avoid this type of problem more successfully.

Observational clinical cohorts are sometimes assembled using previous medical records, and hence the studies are often referred to as "retrospective" (because they go back in time to obtain the data). However, the essential nature of the analysis of such data is prospective, working forward in time from the point of therapy initiation to subsequent clinical and functional outcomes. To avoid confusion with truly retrospective (case-control) studies, cohort studies using previously collected data are sometimes referred to as "nonconcurrent" cohort studies [27].

The prospective design for studies of injury is generally more difficult to execute than the case series method, because of the necessity to establish the cohort and then follow its members for a period of time (often quite lengthy) to record their injury experience. These tasks may be simple to execute in the context of team management, where athletes are already under regular scrutiny, even before they become injured. However, for sports where there is no routine clinical monitoring of participants (which is the situation for the majority of sports), the cohort design is not feasible in the context of normal clinical activities. Special research resources must then be obtained to use this method, and a mechanism to identify and follow the cohort outside the clinical setting needs to be carefully considered.

Despite problems of selection and other forms of bias, and possible difficulties in generalizability of the results, the cohort design is generally regarded as the strongest of the comparative designs, from the methodologic point of view. Its greatest strength lies in the fact that the risk profile for each study subject is established *before* the outcome is observed. In contrast, when the risk profile must be established after the injury has occurred (as in case-control studies), many more problems of bias may arise.

Retrospective Design

An alternative to the cohort method that may require considerably less resource is the retrospective design. With a retrospective design, one samples injured athletes and uninjured controls; the risk profile for each group is then established retrospectively, by obtaining information about postulated antecedent risk factors. The retrospective design, also referred to as the case-control design, is so-called because of the nature of its data collection. It is *rearward* looking in time, examining risk exposures that took place *before* the injuries occurred.

The statistical analysis is based on the calculation of *relative* exposure rates to the various risk factors among the injured and uninjured athletes. To avoid prevalence-incidence bias (discussed in the next section), it is usual to require that the cases be newly diagnosed (i.e., investigators need to examine an *incident* series of cases, rather than using previously diagnosed *prevalent* cases). An example of a case-control study was reported by Johnson et al. [20] who identified a large series of injured skiers over a 7-year period at a Vermont resort. A sample of uninjured skiers was obtained from the same location. Both groups were interviewed about their skiing habits, physique, ability, and the equipment they used. Differences in the distributions of these variables between the two groups indirectly suggested potential risk factors for injury, with the risk being measured in terms of *relative* risk.

In this example, as in many case-control studies, the information on risk was derived through an interview requiring memory recall on the part of the respondents. Depending on the particular variables and the time period of recall under study, this may be a difficult task. Thus, the reliability and validity of data obtained in this way may be inferior. In some extreme situations, the risk information must be gathered indirectly through a proxy respondent, e.g., a coach or spouse. This approach was necessary in a study of cases of sudden death in squash players [35]. With proxy respondents the quality of data is presumably suspect, but for reasons of comparability one might wish to use such respondents even for the living controls.

A related concern is the problem of case-control bias, which can arise in several ways. Cases, by virtue of their injury, may feel more motivated to provide an accurate exposure history, whereas uninjured controls may have little motivation to do so. When using interviewers or self-reported questionnaires, care must be taken to deliver questions in exactly the same way for both the case and control groups, avoiding unnecessary probing of cases in relation to the controls. Ideally, interviewers should be blinded, so that they are unaware of which group each respondent comes from.

Finally, both controls and cases must be sampled from the same population. Because the source population for the cases is sometimes hard to define, one may end up sampling controls from a slightly different population. For instance, if one samples randomly identified athletes in the community as controls for cases seen at a sports injury clinic, there is the possibility that the controls will tend to be less "elite" than the cases, who have a greater chance of using a specialized sports medicine facility. Hence "eliteness" or "ability" would confound any differences observed between cases and controls.

While retrospective designs are generally more efficient than prospective ones, bias is a much greater concern among the former. For injury studies, a prospective investigation often requires a large sample size and a lengthy follow-up period to obtain a sufficient number of outcome events to support a meaningful statistical analysis. For instance, if one wished to study stress fractures in runners, it would likely be necessary to enroll hundreds of athletes and study them over several years in order to derive more than a trivial number of cases. Although the majority of study participants would not experience stress fractures, they would nevertheless consume a large portion of the study resources.

In contrast, a case-control study is more efficient in its ability to more closely balance the relative numbers of injured and noninjured study subjects. Equal sized case and control groups are often used, although this is not strictly necessary [49, 50, 55]. Balanced sample sizes improve the power of the study, providing a greater likelihood of identifying important risk factors, for the same total sample size. Furthermore, less resource per subject is consumed in the retrospective design, because it is not necessary to track subjects over time, as is usually required in the prospective approach.

The case-control method seems somewhat less appropriate for evaluations of therapy. Prospective cohort studies of therapy can usually be mounted more easily than those designed to study injury, because the outcome events in therapeutic evaluations (cure, return to normal function, etc.) are not rare. Also, one can often exploit data that are routinely collected as part of the normal patient management system, so that relatively little expense is required to organize the data for analysis.

Cross-sectional Design

The essence of this design is that the information on injury (or other outcome) status and risk factors is collected simultaneously, usually in the form of *current* information, or *prevalence* rates. In practice, such studies may also involve collecting retrospective information on the same variables for a short period before the cross-sectional survey itself, for instance, concerning all injuries in the past 6 months.

One example of a cross-sectional survey concerned injuries and risk factors among tennis players [19]. Information was gathered by questionnaire on all injuries in the past 2 months and postulated risk factors such as ability and hand grip size. Another example of this design is the readership survey of *Runner's World* [41], in which there were questions about a wide range of risk factors. We should note that this survey had a rather low response rate, which raises concern about the representativeness of its respondents. Also, the sampling frame of subscribers may have included nonrunners, which complicates the interpretation of the resulting estimates of injury rates.

Under its strict definition, a cross-sectional study will only record injuries actually present at the time of the survey. Unfortunately, because of the problem known as prevalence-incidence bias [42], these prevalent cases of injury are clearly not a representative sample of all injuries in the population. Because of the prevalence-incidence bias, prevalent cases are proportionately more likely to be those of long duration, for instance those with a pattern of slow, chronic onset and resolution. More acute and rapidly resolved injuries have a much lower probability of being included at the time of a cross-sectional survey. This nonrepresentativeness fundamentally limits the interpretation of cross-sectional data.

Even with the use of a more liberal definition, which might include some injuries from the recent past, the same difficulty applies, but now to the estimate of prevalence of disease during a period of time. Also, as in retrospective studies, there are problems of memory recall for the accurate reporting of injuries and risk exposures. Finally, accurate recall of the times of past injuries may be a problem, due to memory telescoping, a tendency to recall events as more recent than is actually the case [47, 52].

Yet a further weakness of cross-sectional studies is that they only provide data for a single point in time or, at best, for a short interval of time. Thus, there is little, if any, capability to differentiate purely statistical associations from time-dependent causal relationships. For instance, two cross-sectional studies provided information on muscle tightness and musculoskeletal flexibility in soccer players [9] and gymnasts [22]. Both surveys also included nonparticipant controls, to establish normal values for these physical variables. However, even data that show differences between the athletes and controls do not necessarily support a conclusion of a causal relationship; indeed, which variable is the cause and which is the effect is open to doubt. On the one hand, one might speculate that participation in sport leads to muscle tightness, while on the other it might be conjectured that those with greater flexibility and less muscle tightness are more likely to become and continue as gymnasts. One simply cannot distinguish between these two possibilities when data from only one time point are available.

Despite these interpretational difficulties, cross-sectional designs have been used frequently in sports medicine research. Like the retrospective design, its main appeal is one of efficiency—less time is required to execute the study. A cross-sectional design is implemented (in theory) at a single point in time, when both the injury status and risk information is obtained simultaneously. Thus, there is no need to wait for cases of injury to occur on an incident basis (as in retrospective studies) or for the follow-up period to expire (as in prospective cohort studies).

Summary of Comparative Observational Designs

We have seen how the three major observational designs of epidemiologists provide risk or rate estimates of somewhat different types: the prospective cohort design yields *absolute risk* estimates of injury (or other outcome) for the study cohort or its subgroups; the retrospective case-control design gives *relative risk* estimates of exposure, comparing subgroups of interest; and the cross-sectional design gives *prevalence* rate estimates for injuries and risk factors simultaneously, with corresponding measures of association. However, all three do involve denominators, and hence have greater design strength than the case series method, which is based on numerators only.

Being observational, there is always the possibility that associations seen in these designs are not truly causal, but merely statistical. Careful attention is needed at the design stage to eliminate possible confounding by nuisance variables and to ensure the comparability of the various study subgroups.

Even if questions of internal study validity are addressed, there may still be concerns about generalizability to other populations. One should consider the possible selection mechanisms in populations being used for sports medicine research. In general, groups of subjects who can be readily accessed and studied (e.g., participants in exercise programs, athletic events, or competitive teams) may contain a relatively high proportion of "survivors" who have remained free of injury in earlier stages of their career. This survivorship form of selection bias may, in turn, affect the prediction of later outcomes for the same individuals.

Even if one has what is regarded as a completely valid conclusion concerning the risk of injury from an observational epidemiological study, caution is still needed in applying the results to clinical practice. For example, we have observed that the risk of running injuries is approximately the same for all age and sex groups [53]. What, if anything, does this say about the injury risk for persons consulting their physician for advice about starting a running program? It *may* follow that the risk of injury for new runners is also independent of age and sex (so that, for instance, there would be no need to discourage older people from taking up running), but a stricter answer to this question would require a somewhat different study design, to examine *new* runners in particular.

By their nature, many of the objectives of sports medicine research identified at the start of this paper can be addressed only by observational methods, for ethical or logistical reasons. However, there is a greater opportunity to use the experimental method (i.e., the randomized controlled trial) in the context of evaluating therapeutic interventions. The reader may note some parallels between the issues arising in observational and experimental designs, so that, to a large extent, the same methodological principles apply in both types of study.

Randomized Controlled Trials

The RCT is the design of choice for many research problems in clinical epidemiology and represents one of the main ways to apply epidemiological methods to the clinical setting. Through the randomization process, one may reduce (although not eliminate) many of the problems of bias and confounding that affect otherwise comparable nonrandomized studies. A review of 145 randomized and unrandomized trials [3] revealed that the group of unrandomized studies had a much higher percentage of studies with maldistribution of at least one prognostic covariate, compared to the randomized group; the potential for bias was correspondingly greater in the unrandomized studies.

An excellent set of criteria for critically appraising studies of therapy has been proposed by Sackett et al. [43]. These will be presented and discussed briefly in turn.

1. *Determine if the assignment of patients to treatments is really randomized.* True methods of randomization, where each patient has known assignment probabilities are acceptable. One should avoid studies with pseudorandom methods of assignment, or those in which the randomization process is not defined.
2. *Determine if all clinically relevant outcomes have been reported.* The outcome variables should be specified at the outset and constitute all the clinically relevant events.
3. *Decide if the patients in the study are similar to your own.* This is obviously a question of generalizability of the study to your own local circumstances.
4. *Decide if the clinical maneuver is feasible in your practice.* This is also a question of generalizability. The therapeutic intervention in the study should be described in sufficient detail to be reproduced elsewhere. Also, the issues of contamination (patients not receiving the therapy to which they were randomized) and cointervention (the use of additional therapies, possibly at different rates in the study comparison groups) should be addressed and solved.
5. *Assess whether both clinical and statistical significance were considered.* Studies with very large sample sizes nearly always give statistically significant results, but with absolute differences in outcome that are so small that they are clinically meaningless. In contrast, studies with very small sample sizes often show impressive differences that are not statistically significant, essentially as a chance event. Both definitions of what constitutes significance need to be specified at the design stage of a study.
6. *Ascertain if all patients entering the study were accounted for.* This is to make sure there is no bias resulting from selective reporting of only some of the patients; reporting nonrepresentative subsets of patients amounts to a type of "selection bias" at the analysis stage of a study.

Sackett et al. [43] also make the following recommendations for conducting a methodologically sound study:

a. *An inception cohort of patients should be used.* By this means, one can study the experience of a representative set of cases, rather than a biased subset enrolled some time after the initial diagnosis. This choice also avoids prevalence-incidence bias, which potentially distorts the results of studies using samples of currently available prevalent cases.

b. *The referral pattern should be described.* This allows one to relate the study results back to an underlying population.

c. *There should be complete follow-up of all patients.* This is to avoid bias, if the persons lost to follow-up have a different distribution of outcomes than those who are followed successfully.

d. *Objective outcome criteria should be developed and used.* This will tend to eliminate subjectivity, which typically adds "noise" to the system, making the study less likely to produce significant results.

e. *Blind outcome assessments should be used.* Blinding will avoid deliberate or subconscious bias. If possible, both the patient and the person assessing clinical outcomes should be blinded to the treatment assignments. Empirical evidence [3] reveals a much stronger potential for bias in unblinded studies.

f. *There should be adjustment for extraneous factors.* Adjustment for *known* extraneous factors may be warranted even in randomized studies. The advantage of randomization is that *unknown* extraneous factors are balanced, on average, between the treatment comparison groups. This is much less likely to occur in unrandomized studies.

Pocock [38] has listed some common deficiencies in published studies on therapy. These include: inadequate definition of patients, treatment, and their method of evaluation; lack of a control group (i.e., making it a noncomparative, observational study, with a very difficult interpretation); a failure to randomize to treatment groups (leading to biased comparisons); lack of objectivity in evaluating patient outcomes; and failure to use blinding, when appropriate.

SOME STATISTICAL ISSUES IN EPIDEMIOLOGICAL STUDIES

Without going into technical detail, we would like to mention several statistical issues of design and analysis that can potentially affect most types of epidemiological study, both observational and experimental.

SAMPLE SIZE. The sample size should be appropriate, with sufficient statistical power to address the study question. "Negative" studies are often reported, claiming, for instance, no statistically significant difference between two comparison groups, when in fact the study was too small to have any chance of finding a difference, even if one existed. A thorough report of a research study should give an outline of the rationale for the sample size selected; this is especially important for "negative" studies.

A survey of 71 randomized trials reported as "negative" (i.e., no difference between treatment groups) [15] revealed that virtually all of them had insufficient power to detect a real treatment effect of 25%, an effect that would often be of considerable clinical interest. Correspondingly, a majority of these studies were compatible with quite large differences in response rates, although their estimates of relative benefit were very imprecise. This implies that considerable research effort is effectively wasted through inadequate consideration of this basic design issue.

SUBGROUP ANALYSES. It is often tempting to analyze study data using a large number of variables to define subgroups of interest (e.g., by clinic, by treating physician, by age and sex of the patient, by detailed clinical characteristics of the injury, and so on). This frequently produces very small numbers in each subgroup, with inadequate power to say anything much about any of them. Subgroups should only be analyzed and reported if they were clearly specified *a priori*.

CONFOUNDING. As has been mentioned previously, it is often necessary to consider the possibility of confounding variables that might explain the effect of interest. Reduction or elimination of confounding can take place either at the design stage (by matching or stratification) or during the statistical analysis (e.g. by covariance analysis).

MULTIPLE COMPARISONS. If enough different analyses are carried out on a given set of data, some of them will produce results that are (apparently) statistically significant. This may happen, for instance, if several outcome variables are each analyzed in relation to a large number of potential predictor variables. A similar difficulty arises if a large number of subgroups are examined.

The tendency to go on so-called "fishing expeditions" for statistical significance can be preempted by clear specification of a primary scientific hypothesis that will be the object of the main analysis. Other questions or examinations of the data should be regarded as distinctly secondary, and their reported significance levels should not be taken literally. If secondary analyses are carried out, they should be regarded as hypothesis generating only.

If the investigators cannot confine themselves to a single primary hypothesis, it may be worthwhile to implement a formal statistical control for the p values of the several analyses that are regarded as primary. Techniques such as the Bonferroni method [23] ensure that the overall probability of rejecting one or more of the null hypotheses being tested, if they are all true (i.e., no differences between groups), remains at its nominal level (e.g., 5%). Having drawn attention to these issues, we should point out that the more technical statistical questions (such as the particular choice of analytic technique) are distinctly secondary to the formulation of the research question itself. Specifying and focusing the scientific question in sufficient detail is usually the most difficult and time-consuming stage of implementing an epidemiological study design.

FURTHER READING

The following are some texts that may provide useful further reading on the methodology of epidemiologic studies.

Classical texts include those by MacMahon and Pugh [29] and Mausner and Bahn [30]. More recent general introductions to epidemiology methods include texts by Lilienfeld [27] and Kelsey et al. [21]. A more technical approach to the typology of research designs is by Kleinbaum et al. [24]. Schlesselman [44] provides more details on the methods of case-control studies, while Cochran [5] and Cook and Campbell [7] discuss other aspects of observational and quasi-experimental designs.

General introductions to clinical applications of epidemiology are provided by Sackett et al. [43] and Fletcher et al. [14]. The first of these [43] is described by its authors as directed toward those who "use" (and apply) research done by others. It places strong emphasis on the development of critical appraisal skills, but also provides a broad overview of the application of methodologic principles to diagnostic and management problems in the medical sciences. This is an ideal introductory text for any aspiring clinical investigator. The second [14] is a readable and entertaining introduction to the basic principles of clinical epidemiology. This book is well organized and should appeal to those clinicians who want to learn how to utilize the fundamentals of methodology to resolve problems in the clinical setting. Fleiss [12] discusses most of the important statistical issues in clinical experimentation, whereas Colton [6] gives a more basic introduction to many of the statistical techniques required.

Two less formal texts should also be mentioned. The first, *PDQ Epidemiology* [46], is a concise text that makes epidemiology come alive. Its informal style should endear it to anyone who is looking for a solid, although easily absorbable, introduction to clinical methodology. The second is *Biomedical Bestiary* [31]. As its title infers, this irreverent little book takes a light-hearted look at the fundamentals of clinical epidemiology. By enlisting the help of 16 "beasts" (among them the Grand Confounder, the Regression Meany, and the Test Bloater, to name but a few), the *Bestiary* provides an introduction to common flaws in the design and execution of medical research. It is clinically oriented, informative, and, above all, fun to read.

REVIEW OF CURRENT LITERATURE IN SPORTS AND EXERCISE SCIENCE RESEARCH

The second major part of this paper describes our review of the current use of epidemiological techniques in sports and exercise science research. The objectives of the review were to identify the major topic areas being researched and to systematically classify the papers using epidemiological methods, according to the research design that had been adopted.

Identification of Literature Sources for Review

A preliminary task was to identify the journals that might be expected to yield a relatively high proportion of original research papers in sports and exercise science and where an epidemiological approach was likely to have been used. As discussed previously, we wanted to limit the primary focus of our literature search to papers with a direct interest in sports, exercise, and human health.

We began by examining the list of approximately 110 journals that are routinely abstracted by *Year Book of Sports Medicine*. After inspection of specimen issues of these journals, we elected to limit our systematic review to four journals: *American Journal of Sports Medicine* (AJSM), *Canadian Journal of Applied Sports Sciences* (CJASS), *Medicine and Science in Sports and Exercise* (MSSE), and *Physician and Sports Medicine* (PSM). These appeared to contain a reasonable proportion of relevant articles. For these four journals, we examined *all* the papers published in issues dated in 1988. News items, press summaries, conference reports, and abstracts were not included.

In addition, we reviewed all entries in the 1988 *Year Book of Sports Medicine* (YB), in order to include some of the important articles found outside the four selected journals. *YB* reproduces the original abstract for each article and sometimes shows some tables or figures from the original paper. There is also a short editorial comment on each of the papers cited.

By scrutinizing *YB*, we were able to identify a substantial number of articles from a diverse set of journals where the proportional yield of relevant work would have been small. These are included in our review. For instance, *YB* reports sports and exercise science articles published in general clinical journals such as *British Medical Journal, Clinical Science,* and *Lancet,* and specialized journals such as *Journal of Urology, Thorax,* and *Journal of Gerontology*. It was clearly impractical for us to scan these journals in their entirety, but the use of *YB* abstractions did permit a more comprehensive coverage of the entire sports and exercise science literature.

The entries in *YB* are divided into the following categories: exercise physiology and medicine, fitness, biomechanics, sports injuries, pediatric sports medicine, women in sports, and athletic training. Because, on inspection, we were able to find examples of epidemiological studies within each of these categories, we elected to review all entries from *YB*, even though this greatly increased the total number of articles that needed to be assessed and even though a relatively high proportion of entries in some categories were nonepidemiological in nature.

The vast majority of entries in the 1988 *YB* are papers published in 1987. Thus, because the four journals previously selected for systematic review are all abstracted by *YB*, we actually achieved coverage of these four journals for 2 calendar years. However, for the sake of simplicity, the results from *YB* will be presented in aggregate, with no distinction made for the journals of origin.

Classification of Selected Articles

First, each paper was initially classified into one of the following types: case reports; original studies (except case reports); and reviews or editorials. Second, each article was categorized according to its content and methods area(s). The areas were: biomechanics, diagnosis, epidemiology, physiology, psychology, therapy, and other. Multiple entries were allowed, so that a given paper could be counted in more than one content area. For example, there were many papers that dealt with both diagnosis and therapy.

Papers were counted in the epidemiology category either if they addressed a "pure" epidemiologic question of etiology using descriptive or analytic methods (e.g., determination of risk factors for injury in a cohort of soccer players), or if they used epidemiological methods to address a topic in another content area (e.g., use of a cohort design to study the outcomes of patients on a particular therapy).

The "diagnosis" category also included studies dealing with the natural history of disease. The "therapy" section included studies of prognosis, management, and prophylaxis. Papers in physiology were not counted as epidemiological if they were restricted to the study of normal physiological values or to short-term physiologic responses to experimental stimuli. However, physiology papers were categorized as epidemiological if they concerned ill or diseased patients or if they studied long-term effects outside a laboratory situation. For instance, the effects of exercise on bone mass or enzyme levels in general populations would meet our criteria in this category. The "other" category contained papers mostly on nonresearch issues, such as the history of sport, training for sport health professionals, didactic papers on clinical topics, sociopolitical subjects, and the organization of sports health care services. These types of publications did not appear in large numbers.

Any article that was uniquely or jointly classified into the epidemiology group was further characterized according to its research design. As described previously, these were the case series design, the prospective (cohort) design, the retrospective (case-control) design, the cross-sectional survey design, and the randomized controlled trial. For the epidemiology group, we also recorded the primary content area, with categories: diagnosis and therapy, injuries and mortality, physiology and biomechanics, and other. Psychology was included in other because of the relatively small number of papers in this area. The study sample sizes were recorded for all papers in the epidemiology group.

A minor difficulty arose in distinguishing "case report" papers from "case series" in the epidemiology group. This was because a case series might be regarded as a set of case reports and hence might be viewed as methodologically similar. We adopted a convention whereby a paper would be classified as a case report if it gave clinical details of each of the patients being described; conversely, it was classified as a case series if only aggregated statistics on patients were provided. Although there were exceptions, this rule had the effect of classifying papers with only one or two patients into the case report group, whereas the case series group typically had larger sample sizes.

Results

Table 14.3 shows the distribution of the types of papers yielded by each of the five sources. Among the total of 756 papers examined, about 80% were original research studies. This proportion was quite similar for all of the sources, except for *PSM* which had a much higher percentage of reviews and editorials than the other journals. The total lack of case reports in *CJASS* and *MSSE* suggests that these journals are not targeting practicing clinicians. On the other hand, the more frequent reviews and editorials in *PSM* may be intended as continuing education resources for practitioners.

Table 14.4 indicates the pattern of content and methods area by source. Again, differences in the presumed readership are suggested by the lack of papers on diagnosis and therapy in *CJASS* and *MSSE* and by the higher percentages of papers on physiology in these journals. Only about 1% of all papers involved psychology. Epidemiology was involved in about 20% of all papers.

Table 14.5 shows the distribution of study design and content area for the 182 papers containing original research with an epidemiologic ap-

TABLE 14.3
Distribution of Types of Paper, by Source

Source	Case Reports	Reviews/Editorials	Original Research	Total
AJSM	20 (16%)	1 (1%)	101 (83%)	122
CJASS	0 (0%)	8 (26%)	23 (74%)	31
MSSE	0 (0%)	3 (3%)	104 (97%)	107
PSM	17 (16%)	49 (45%)	42 (39%)	108
YB	11 (3%)	41 (11%)	336 (87%)	388
Total	48 (6%)	102 (13%)	606 (80%)	756

AJSM, American Journal of Sports Medicine; CJASS, Canadian Journal of Applied Sports Sciences; MSSE, Medicine and Science in Sports and Exercise; PSM, Physician and Sports Medicine; YB, Year Book of Sports Medicine.

TABLE 14.4
Content and Methods Classification of Papers, by Source

Source	Content/Method Area						
	Biomechanics	Diagnosis	Epidemiology	Physiology	Psychology	Therapy	Other	Total
AJSM	17 (10%)	38 (22%)	52 (30%)	10 (6%)	0 (0%)	56 (32%)	1 (1%)	174
CJASS	5 (16%)	0 (0%)	8 (25%)	16 (50%)	0 (0%)	0 (0%)	3 (9%)	32
MSSE	12 (11%)	0 (0%)	11 (10%)	85 (77%)	1 (1%)	1 (1%)	0 (0%)	110
PSM	3 (2%)	33 (26%)	22 (18%)	25 (20%)	2 (2%)	30 (24%)	10 (8%)	125
YB	34 (8%)	47 (10%)	105 (23%)	160 (35%)	5 (1%)	86 (19%)	15 (3%)	452
Total	71 (8%)	118 (13%)	198 (22%)	296 (33%)	8 (1%)	173 (19%)	29 (3%)	893

Abbreviations are defined in Table 14.3.

TABLE 14.5
Content Area and Study Design of Papers Involving Original Epidemiology Research

		Content Area				
Source	Design	Diagnosis/ Therapy	Injuries/ Mortality	Physiology and Biomechanics	Other	Total
AJSM	Case series	5	1	1		7
	Cohort	23	9			32
	Case-control	1	1	2		4
	Cross-sectional	2	4	2		8
	RCT	1				1
CJASS	Case series					
	Cohort		1			1
	Case-control					
	Cross-sectional			4	2	6
	RCT			1		1
MSSE	Case series					
	Cohort		1	3		4
	Case-control		1	1		2
	Cross-sectional			2	1	3
	RCT	1				1
PSM	Case series	4	3			7
	Cohort		1	2		3
	Case-control		2			2
	Cross-sectional		4	3	3	10
	RCT					
YB	Case series	1	8			9
	Cohort	11	10	7		28
	Case-control	1	4			5
	Cross-sectional	1	13	16	7	37
	RCT	4	1	6		11
Total	Case series	10 (18%)	12 (19%)	1 (2%)	0	23 (13%)
	Cohort	34 (62%)	22 (34%)	12 (24%)	0	68 (37%)
	Case-control	2 (4%)	8 (13%)	3 (6%)	0	13 (7%)
	Cross-sectional	3 (5%)	21 (33%)	27 (55%)	13 (100%)	64 (35%)
	RCT	6 (11%)	1 (2%)	7 (14%)	0	14 (8%)
		55 (100%)	64 (100%)	50 (100%)	13 (100%)	182 (100%)

Abbreviations are defined in Table 14.3.

proach. Overall, the cohort design was the most frequent, especially in the diagnosis/therapy category. A large proportion of this group consisted of descriptive presentations of the clinical treatment and prognosis for various sets of patients, typically over periods of a few weeks or months. Many of the deficiencies noted by Pocock [38] were often evident, especially the lack of a control group and failure to use blinded assessment methods. Randomization was used in only a small proportion of studies. These were either randomized trials of therapy or basic science randomized experiments in the areas of physiology and biomechanics.

Randomization was not used (where it perhaps should have been) in approximately six of every seven studies of therapy and in two of every three studies on physiology and biomechanics. Although the practical implementation of randomization is sometimes difficult, the enormous methodologic strength it conveys makes it well worth the effort. This is clearly an area for some improvement in the future. Even if randomization is not possible, the inclusion of an observational control group adds a great deal to the interpretability of most studies.

The cross-sectional design was the next most common choice and was especially popular in the physiology/biomechanics categories. Many of these studies were on problems such as the distribution of blood chemistry and muscle strength values in various athlete groups, training patterns, use of dieting, or the relationship of smoking status to current fitness levels. This design was also used to gather historical (or retrospective) information on variables such as the lifetime history of back pain, and some investigators used the method to study teams or institutions (e.g., in determining the level of medical coverage of sports events at various schools).

The case-control method was used only infrequently. It was slightly more popular in studies of injuries and mortality, which would typically involve relatively rare outcomes and longer periods of follow-up were the cohort method to be used. For instance, there were case-control studies of factors associated with collapse during running races, development of "jumper's knee," and sports-related cases of myocardial infarction. The efficiencies of time and effort afforded by the retrospective approach are far less important for studies of therapy or basic science, where the "response" to be observed occurs relatively quickly and frequently.

Sample Sizes

Table 14.6 shows the minimum, median, and maximum sample sizes for the various designs and content areas. The median is probably the most meaningful summary statistic for these comparisons, because the generally positive skewness in the distribution of sample sizes and the presence of some extremely large studies in some groups (see below) have a substantial effect on the mean. The total number of cases and controls was counted for retrospective studies. For studies that reported the existence of nonparticipants (e.g., those who refused to respond to a questionnaire), we report only the number of compliant participants. (Obviously the response rate would be an important factor in assessing the likelihood of response bias for a particular study).

There is a tendency for studies on injuries and mortality in all design groups to have larger sample sizes, while those on physiology and biomechanics tend to contain smaller numbers. Diagnosis and therapy articles usually had samples that were intermediate in size. The size advantage of the case-control method is very noticeable in the injury category

TABLE 14.6
Minimum, Median, and Maximum Sample Sizes for Epidemiological Studies by Study Design and Content Area

							Content Area						
	Diagnosis/Therapy			Injuries/Mortality			Physiology			Other			
Design	Min	Med	Max	Min	Med	Max	Min	Med	Max	Min	Med	Max	
Case series	6	48	1,447	13	368	1,916		(11)					
Cohort	7	51	35,879	22	1,172	2,084,000	8	19	607				
Case-control		(37)		22	64	2,275		(45)					
Cross-sectional		(271)		55	278	2,762	6	53	18,073	45	110	19,110	
RCT	16	26	139		(141)		12	17	60				

Parentheses indicate median only estimated from less than five studies. Min, minimum; Med, median; Max, maximum.

where the median sample was 64, compared to a median of 1172 with the cohort method. The relatively small sample sizes in the physiology group may represent the greater effort required to record data in the context of a systematic basic science study, compared to the descriptive reporting of limited and/or existing data from medical records in studies of diagnosis, therapy, and injuries. The above remarks are obviously crude generalizations, but they did seem to apply in the majority of studies we examined.

Statistical power was not discussed in most of the articles. Indeed, sample sizes were usually reported without any comment. A rigorous determination of the appropriate sample size should include a specification of an acceptable type I error rate, a reference to the difference between comparison groups of clinical interest (e.g., the difference in rates of recovery by 6 weeks after an injury) and the statistical power required to detect this difference, if it exists. Frequently, and somewhat conventionally, the type I error rate is taken as 5% and the required power as 80%.

Unfortunately, many of the sample sizes reported in our survey would have given inadequate power to support their hypotheses. For instance, consider the median sample size of 26 reported for randomized controlled trials of therapy and assume that the 26 subjects would be divided into two equal groups of 13 each. With the usual type I error rate of 5%, such a study would have 80% power only to detect differences in recovery rates at least as large as 65 versus 5% [13]. Most clinical interventions would not be expected to produce such large effects. The power would be similarly low even if continuous outcome variables (e.g., improvement in muscle strength) were used. One must conclude that many of the reported "negative" studies have designs that are inadequate to address the scientific questions under investigation. This is similar to the situation in other areas of medicine [15].

The extremely large sample sizes reported in Table 14.6 are also worth mentioning. The largest, a cohort study of more than 2 million subjects, investigated the incidence of death during basic training of army recruits and focused, in particular, on the presence of sickle cell trait. (Only 62 such deaths were reported.) Other examples of this type included a study of injuries among almost 25,000 Boy Scouts at a 9-day jamboree and an investigation of facial and eye injuries in 171,000 hockey players. The large sample size of 18,073 for a cross-sectional study (in physiology) used the Canada Fitness Survey data base to examine the transmissibility of several fitness variables in a national population.

All of these examples are characterized by the presentation of very limited data with minimal or no interaction with most of the study subjects. For instance, the three large cohorts referred to would have been assembled essentially from paper records, with no need to examine or interview uninjured subjects. Similarly, the Canada Fitness Survey analysis was performed on existing data, although, of course, the original survey was a massive undertaking. In general, there is likely to be an inverse relationship between the number of subjects and the amount of information gathered per subject.

CONCLUSIONS

The epidemiologic method is being used frequently, either explicitly or implicitly, in the conduct of sports and exercise science research. Based on a review of the literature, we feel that the commonest methodological deficiencies encountered are: a failure to recognize the limitations of numerator-based case series and case report data; inadequate attention to power considerations in study design, especially with respect to determining appropriate sample sizes; and the lack of randomization or controls in many studies of therapy.

All of these factors potentially lead to inefficiency in the use of research resources and may induce inappropriate therapeutic strategies in clinical practice. Studies lacking appropriate population denominators or having limited statistical power or inadequate controls are more likely to yield incorrect inferences on their research question. This will, in turn, mislead future researchers in their specification of new research hypotheses and misdirect health care professionals in the application of research results in clinical practice.

We note that most of these problems can be solved without a substantial reorganization of research activity. Epidemiologic methods can and have been used already in many areas of sports and exercise science. What seems to be required is some improvement in critical appraisal of research proposals and results, by investigators, journal editors, and readers of the literature. This would have the effect of reducing unwarranted or overenthusiastic interpretations of research data based on inadequate designs, with a consequent improvement in the overall quality of research in the field.

REFERENCES

1. Bendix C, Jensen OM: *Atlas of Cancer Incidence in Denmark 1970–79*. Copenhagen, Danish Cancer Registry, Environmental Protection Agency, 1986.
2. Birrer RB, Birrer CD: Martial arts injuries. *Physician Sportsmed* 10:103–108, 1982.
3. Chalmers TC, Celano P, Sacks HS, Smith H: Bias in treatment assignment in controlled clinical trials. *N Engl J Med* 309:1358–1361, 1984.
4. Clement DB, Taunton JE, Smart GW, McNicol KL: A survey of overuse running injuries. *Physician Sportsmed* 9:47–58, 1981.
5. Cochran WG: Planning and Analysis of Observational Studies. New York, John Wiley & Sons, 1983.

6. Colton T: *Statistics in Medicine*. Boston, Little, Brown & Co., 1974.
7. Cook TD, Campbell DT: *Quasi-Experimentation Design and Analysis Issues for Field Settings*. Boston, Houghton Mifflin, 1979.
8. DeHaven KE, Lintner DM: Athletic injuries: comparison by age, sport, and gender. *Am J Sports Med* 14:218–224, 1986.
9. Ekstrand J, Gillquist J: The frequency of muscle tightness and injuries in soccer players. *Am J Sports Med* 10:75–78, 1982.
10. Ekstrand J, Gillquist J, Moller M, Oberg B, Liljedahl SO: Incidence of soccer injuries and their relation to training and team success. *Am J Sports Med* 11:63–67, 1983.
11. Ferkel RD, Mai LL, Ullis KC, Finerman GA: An analysis of roller skating injuries. *Am J Sports Med* 10:24–30, 1982.
12. Fleiss JL: *The Design and Analysis of Clinical Experiments*. New York, John Wiley & Sons, 1986.
13. Fleiss JL: *Statistical Methods for Rates and Proportions*. New York, John Wiley & Sons, 1981.
14. Fletcher RH, Fletcher SW, Wagner EH: *Clinical Epidemiology—The Essentials*. Baltimore, Williams & Wilkins, 1983, p 246.
15. Freiman JA, Chalmers C, Smith H, Kuebler RR: The importance of beta, the type II error and sample size in the design and interpretation of the randomized control trial. *N Engl J Med* 299:690–694, 1978.
16. Garrick JG, Requa RK: Epidemiology of women's gymnastics injuries. *Am J Sports Med* 8:261–264, 1980.
17. Gerberich SG: Response from Dr. Gerberich. *Am J Public Health* 74:1170, 1984.
18. Gottlieb G, White JR: Responses of recreational runners to their injuries. *Physician Sportsmed* 8:145–149, 1980.
19. Gruchow HW, Pelletier D: An epidemiologic study of tennis elbow. *Am J Sports Med* 7:234–238, 1979.
20. Johnson RJ, Ettlinger CF, Campbell RJ, Pope MH: Trends in skiing injuries. *Am J Sports Med* 8:106–112, 1980.
21. Kelsey JL, Thompson WD, Evans AS: *Methods in Observational Epidemiology*. New York, Oxford University Press, 1986.
22. Kirby RL, Simms FC, Symington VJ, Garner JB: Flexibility and musculoskeletal symptomatology in female gymnasts and age-matched controls. *Am J Sports Med* 9:160–164, 1981.
23. Kleinbaum DC, Kupper LL: *Applied Regression Analysis and Other Multivariable Methods*. North Scituate, MA, Duxbury Press, 1978.
24. Kleinbaum DG, Kupper LL, Morgenstern H: *Epidemiologic Research. Principles and Quantitative Methods*. Lifetime Learning Publications, Belmont, CA, 1982.
25. Krissoff WB, Ferris WD: Runners injuries. *Physician Sportsmed* 7:55–64, 1979.
26. Kurzweil PR, Zambett GJ, Hamilton WG: Osteochondritis disscans in the lateral patellofemoral groove. *Am J Sports Med* 6:308–310, 1988.
27. Lilienfeld AM: *Foundations of Epidemiology*. New York, Oxford University Press, 1976.
28. Loosli A, Garrick JG: The functional treatment of a third proximal phalanx fracture. *Am J Sports Med* 15:94–96, 1987.
29. MacMahon B, Pugh TF: *Epidemiology Principles and Methods*. Boston, Little Brown & Co., 1970.
30. Mausner JS, Bahn AK: *Epidemiology: An Introductory Text*. Philadelphia, WB Saunders, 1974.
31. Michael M III, Boyce WT, Wilcox AJ: *Biomedical Bestiary: An Epidemiologic Guide to Flaws and Fallacies in the Medical Literature*. Boston, Little, Brown & Co., 1984.
32. Micheli LJ, Santopietro F, Gerbino P, Crowe P: Etiologic assessment of overuse stress fractures in athletes. *Nova Scotia Med Bull* 59:43–47, 1980.
33. Nicholl JP, Williams BT: Popular marathons: forecasting casualties. *Br Med J* 285:1464–1465, 1985.

34. Nicholl JP, Williams BT: Medical problems before and after a popular marathon. *Br Med J* 285:1465–1466, 1982.
35. Northcote RJ, Evans ADB, Ballantyne D: Sudden death in squash players. *Lancet* i:148–150, 1984.
36. Pagliano JW, Jackson DW: The ultimate study of running injuries. *Runners World* November: 42–50, 1980.
37. Pagliano JW, Jackson DW: A clinical study of 3,000 long-distance runners. *Ann Sports Med* 3:88–91, 1987.
38. Pocock SJ: *Clinical Trials. A Practical Approach.* New York, John Wiley & Sons, 1983.
39. Rayan GM: Lower trunk brachial plexus compression neuropathy due to cervical rib in young athletes. *Am J Sports Med* 16:77–79, 1988.
40. Riggan WB, Creason JP, Nelson WC, Manton KG, Woodbury MA, Stallard E, Pellom AC, Beaubier J: *U.S. Cancer Mortality Rates and Trends, 1950–1979.* Washington D.C., United States Environmental Protection Agency, 1987.
41. Runners World: Who is the American runner? *Runners World* December: 36–42, 1980.
42. Sackett DL: Bias in analytic research. *J Chronic Dis* 32:51–63, 1979.
43. Sackett DL, Haynes RB, Tugwell P: *Clinical Epidemiology. A Basic Science for Clinical Medicine.* Boston, Little, Brown & Co., 1985.
44. Schlesselman JJ: *Case-Control Studies.* New York, Oxford University Press, 1982.
45. Schor SS: Relation of football injuries to exposure time. *Am J Public Health* 74:1169–1170, 1984.
46. Streiner DJ, Norman CR, Munroe-Blum H: *PDQ Epidemiology.* Toronto, Decker, 1989.
47. Sudman S, Bradburn NM: Effects of time and memory factors on response in surveys. *J Am Stat Assoc* 68:805–815, 1973.
48. Toronto Globe and Mail: Guru of jogging promoted value of physical fitness. Toronto, July 23, 1984.
49. Walter SD: Determination of significant relative risks and optimal sampling procedures in prospective and retrospective studies of various sizes. *Am J Epidemiol* 105:387–397, 1977.
50. Walter SD: The author replies. *Am J Epidemiol* 106:437–438, 1977.
51. Walter SD: The risks of exercising: sudden cardiac death and injuries. In Bouchard C, Shephard RJ, Stephens T, Sutton JR, McPherson BD (eds): *Exercise, Fitness and Health: A Consensus of Current Knowledge.* Champaign, IL, Human Kinetics, 1990, pp 715–720.
52. Walter SD, Clarke EA, Hatcher J, Stitt LW: A comparison of physician and patient reports of Pap smear histories. *J Clin Epidemiol* 41:401–410, 1988.
53. Walter SD, Hart LE, Sutton JR, McIntosh JM, Gauld M: Training habits and injury experience in distance runners: age and sex related factors. *Physician Sportsmed* 16:101–113, 1988.
54. Walter SD, Sutton JR, McIntosh JM, Connolly C: The aetiology of sport injuries. A review of methodologies. *Sports Med* 2:47–58, 1985.
55. Yanagawa T, Blot WJ: Optimal sampling ratios for proportion studies. *Am J Epidemiol* 106:436–437, 1977.

Index

Page numbers in *italics* denote figures; those followed by *t* denote tables.

449